DEATH BY CALCIUM

DEATH BY CALCIUM

by Thomas E. Levy, MD, JD

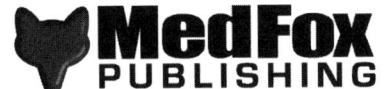

Copyright © 2013 by Thomas E. Levy, MD, JD

First Edition: 2013

Library of Congress Control Number: 2013951742

ISBN: Soft cover 978-0-615-88960-3

All rights reserved. No part of this book may be reproduced or transmitted in any form or by any means, electronic or mechanical, including photocopying, recording, or by any information storage and retrieval system, without permission in writing from the copyright owner.

This book was printed in the United States of America.

To order additional copies of this book, contact:
MedFox Publishing, LLC
1-866-359-5589
www.MedFoxPub.com
Orders@MedFoxPub.com
2654 W. Horizon Ridge Pkwy - Suite B5 #233
Henderson, NV 89052

To my good friend and mentor,
Hal A. Huggins, DDS, MS,
who gave me the guidance that I so
desperately needed.

Acknowledgments

To Les and Cindy Nachman, whose friendships and professional support have been invaluable to me. Without their help and guidance, most of the medical information that I have wanted to tell the world would have never reached the many doctors and individuals who are now living healthier lives because of it. A book unread is no better than a paperweight.

To Dave Nicol, who has been invaluable in helping me get the thoughts out of my head and onto paper. His editing, organization, and oftentimes rewriting of my words have allowed me to better express important concepts than I thought possible. His help has also made many of my previous books much better than they were before his input.

To Ron Hunninghake, friend and colleague, who has been invaluable in helping me move forward with my thoughts and research, both in this book and in other collaborations.

To my wife, Lis, and my daughter, Daniela, who keep me grounded and aware of what life is really all about on a daily basis.

To my precious Mother, Catherine, and my sister, Cathy, whose love and support have always been unqualified.

And to Hal Huggins, for unlocking my mind and setting me free.

Foreword

by Ron Hunninghake, MD

The Personal Dimension of My Concern

"Dr. Ron, we've got to figure out this family osteoporosis curse!"

My cousin's pleading words stopped me in my tracks outside the church where we had just attended her mother's funeral service. Aunt Lucile was the fifth of nine beautiful sisters to die a horrible death of intractable pain and prolonged disability from a series of severe spinal compression fractures.

As a family physician, I was perplexed. My deceased aunts had grown up on the farm in a close-knit family. Except for one sister, they had not smoked. They ate well and were active. Except for hypertension and one instance of coronary artery disease, they were all relatively healthy. Despite this, they had each died with profound osteoporosis.

My mother attended Lucile's funeral. She was second to the youngest of the nine and still alive in her early eighties. She too had lost several inches of height and complained of back pain. She was taking her bisphosphonate medication, her calcium supplement, and walking fairly regularly. Her DEXA scans were nevertheless dismal. I kept asking myself: what was missing?

Then it struck me: *were they getting too much of something?*

Since people in the United States consume more supplemental calcium than anywhere else on the planet, why does the U.S. have a higher incidence of osteoporosis than any other country?

Could the entire modern paradigm of osteoporosis prevention and care be based upon a false assumption? Were my aunts victims of a calcium mythology born of the aggressive marketing of dairy and the overly simplistic viewpoint that weak bones are just a calcium deficiency?

Originally, the government's Recommended Daily Allowances (RDAs) were advanced in wartime to assure the bare minimums of human nutrition. Over time, the RDAs came to ignore circumstances surrounding their original formulation in the admittedly complex issues that surround nutritional science. RDA committees often "sold out" to the marketing interests of the U.S.D.A. over the actual nutritional needs of the American consumer. This collusion evolved into a complex web of nutritional mythology and marketplace salesmanship that has left the United States ranked 33rd in overall life expectancy, and #1 in cost of health care.

Broadening My View of Clinical Nutrition

In 1989 my medical career took a surprising turn. I became the medical director of the esteemed Riordan Clinic in Wichita, Kansas. Its founder, the late Dr. Hugh Riordan, was a medical maverick who believed that the complex importance of human

Foreword

nutrition could not be reduced to such Madison Avenue platitudes as "Got milk?" or "Eat bananas for potassium!"

Under Dr. Riordan's mentorship I learned to question this mass marketing of nutritional assumptions. Instead, I sent thousands of seriously ill and frustrated patients for testing at one of the first truly nutritional labs, the Bio-Center Laboratory, an arm of the Riordan Clinic. I wanted to objectively assess their nutrient reserves, hormonal imbalances, digestive disorders, food intolerances, undiagnosed infections, and environmental toxicities in a medically disciplined way. My goal was to discern correctable underlying causes of their sustained illness. Dr. Riordan's dream was for a new medical paradigm of solid clinical nutrition.

Dr. Roger Williams, a famous nutritional pioneer, taught that quality nutrition is not simply *more* or *less*. Quality in this context means the *right* amount of the correct nutrients and whole foods geared appropriately to the individual's needs.

What is right and correct for the individual has to be informed by standards of scientific evidence gathered from both large population studies and measurements of each individual's unique genetic and epigenetic requirements and tempered with a lot of common sense.

Even as billions upon billions are spent on medical research and treatments, millions of victims go on suffering and dying from cancer, heart disease, extreme osteoporosis, chronic fatigue syndrome, diabetes, obesity, mental illness, and autoimmune disorders. When questions arise as to *why*, the answer is all too often, "We just don't know why these diseases occur."

This is not a complaint against the many dedicated and often selfless health professionals that spend their lives fighting disease. As one of my former partners so aptly lamented, his whole medical career had been largely consumed by the diagnosis and careful documentation of the prolonged demise of his patients. He was a fantastic primary care doc. Then he himself died of renal cancer.

Applied Clinical Nutrition Comes of Age

Isolated nutrients were never meant to work by themselves. They work cooperatively and synergistically as team members. Calcium is no different. We need calcium. We need it for healthy bones, teeth, and many other functions. In this amazing book, Dr. Levy eloquently shows us that we don't need **too much** calcium! We need the right amount of calcium as part of a balanced team of nutrients.

Orthomolecular medicine is a term that was first coined by the great two-time Nobel prizewinner, Dr. Linus Pauling. "Ortho" means "right" or "correct." Not too much or too little. Nowhere is "ortho" more important than in the field of nutrition.

Rather than a simple rant against excess calcium, Dr. Tom Levy paints a comprehensive portrait of a new nutritional medicine — an "ortho" molecular medicine — where we as a culture once again recognize our organic roots in nature. Our bodies depend on the correct balance of the right nutrients ideally coming from natural whole foods in the context of a well-lived, balanced lifestyle. That's where *health* comes from!

Modern medications are important tools, but they cannot substitute for comprehensive nutritional and lifestyle care. More and better synthetic molecules are not going to save us from the ongoing harm we are ignorantly doing to ourselves.

The Path to Health Requires a Radical Shift in Thinking

My cousins, my mother, my patients, and my community have been looking to me for help. *They are afraid.* All around they see average people getting hit with devastating illnesses for which the treatment options are either exorbitantly expensive or fraught with serious side effects... or they are simply not working. This is especially true for many of the new osteoporosis medications.

Victory against any and all diseases will not be won until we begin to think correctly about health. Dr. Levy is a master at gathering pertinent data from the medical literature and distilling that data into comprehensive protocols that address the real sources of sickness and disease. Rather than promoting a magic bullet, he offers the truth along with a sound and practical way of using it to achieve real and lasting health.

Death by Calcium provides a powerful reorientation that I believe will help the reader find his or her way back to healthier bones, cleaner arteries, less inflamed joints, better immunity, higher energy levels, and a lowered risk of diabetes and cancer.

Although written with the layman in mind, the information, science, and substantiation that Dr. Levy has interwoven throughout the book are hefty enough to convince the critical medical professional who is willing to lay aside prejudice long enough to evaluate the evidence.

If the general direction of medicine in America is going to ever move away from a business-model to a nutrition-based healing paradigm, it is going to take people like Dr. Levy and books like this one to keep clearing the path.

And it can be done. I have seen it work in over 10,000 "co-learners" who have showed me IT CAN WORK for the past 24 years of my medical practice at the Riordan Clinic. This book scientifically validates what I and these patients have worked so hard to create: *a rational approach to better nutrition, less infection and toxicity, resulting in a more hardy constitution in those who are willing to do the hard detective work of learning how to take better care of themselves.*

Ron Hunninghake, MD
Chief Medical Officer
Riordan Clinic
Wichita, Kansas

Preface

Twenty years ago, at the age of 43, I was still practicing the "traditional" form of cardiology, diagnosing angina pectoris, performing angiograms and angioplasties, and sometimes referring patients for coronary artery bypass surgery. I believed then, and I still believe, that my practice of mainstream cardiology helped many individuals to live longer and less symptomatic lives. However, the true meaning of the word "prevention" was not part of my mindset, any more than it was for any other physician practicing pharmaceutical-driven medicine. And in general, as long as you are performing your job in the same manner as all of your peers, you are led to believe that you are doing the right thing.

However, I now know that so much more can be done to prevent the chest pain, the balloon angioplasty, and the often-inevitable coronary bypass surgery, from ever having to occur. Cardiologists and most allopathic doctors still believe that by telling patients to avoid butter, eggs, and fat (three things that are actually part of a healthy diet), their preventive medicine obligations have been fulfilled. This is not only ridiculous, but what is not being told to so many patients is truly a deadly omission.

While I generally felt I was helping my patients, I could not help but feel there was more that could be done. It was a deep "something-just-isn't right" disturbance that I could not put into words. Then I met Dr. Hal Huggins, a dentist who ended up teaching me more medicine than any physician I have ever known.

For roughly half a century now, Dr. Huggins has been leading the movement against toxic dentistry. He has worked tirelessly to educate dentists and physicians on the enormous negative impact on health by root canal-treated teeth, chronically infected gums, residual toxin-filled cavitations in the jawbones, mercury-containing amalgam fillings, other toxic dental metals and materials, and even dental implants. Countless individuals have been spared an enormous amount of disease, suffering, and shortened lifespans, because of his work. However, when one considers the innumerable millions who still have not been exposed to the truth that Dr. Huggins uncovered, it's obvious that there is so much more work that remains. I greatly hope that I can be an effective tool in further disseminating the truth about the toxic roots of all medical diseases, along with the highly effective ways in which they can be managed and treated.

When I first began working as a medical consultant for Dr. Huggins, helping as best I could with the initial evaluations and then long-term follow-up of the patients from around the world who were seeking his help, I repeatedly encountered abnormal laboratory tests that I could not explain. For that matter, there were many results to be interpreted from tests with which I had never worked, and that I did not really understand. Patiently, Dr. Huggins explained them all to me, a physician board-certified in both internal medicine and cardiovascular disease!

One thing that especially intrigued me was the results of the hair analysis examinations done on all of the patients who visited Dr. Huggins' clinic. Just about everybody, myself included, had mild to massively elevated levels of calcium that had accumulated in the hair samples sent for testing. I really had no idea what to make of this. I even thought it could well be a common and persistent misleading artifact.

However, I learned from Dr. Huggins that the American diet subjected almost everyone to enormous amounts of calcium, and by the time people were older adults they had routinely accumulated too much calcium in their bodies. He also told me that this excess calcium — with its dire health consequences — could gradually, over several years, be remedied. However, it would require removal of dental toxicity, a consistent regimen of quality supplementation, and an avoidance of calcium in both the diet and supplementation.

I had my root canal removed, followed his recommendations, and after several years my hair calcium levels normalized just as he said they would.

So in a way, this book began with my work with Dr. Huggins 20 years ago. At that time, however, I had neither the medical experience nor the knowledge of basic physiology and biochemistry to produce a scientifically sound argument that most adults are needlessly suffering from years of calcium accumulation throughout their bodies. For years circumstantial evidence of the damage that excess calcium has wreaked upon our society has been visible. However, in the last few years — from 2010 to 2013 to be precise — overwhelmingly compelling indictments of the enormous toxicity of calcium supplementation and excess dairy consumption have been published in the medical literature. Until this writing, very little of this vital research has seen the light of day. Volumes of important medical information are buried in seldom read journals. Sadly these discoveries never influence routine medical practice or benefit the sick and dying. The objective of this book is to herald the dangers of excess calcium and to highlight the path of escape. Whether the research displayed herein gets the exposure and the dissemination it deserves remains to be seen.

When the world stops supplementing calcium and having their mouths filled with a mind-numbing variety of infections and toxins, Dr. Huggins will have had his day. I only pray that he does. A Nobel Prize would not be recognition enough.

Thomas E. Levy, MD, JD

Table of Contents

Foreword - 9
Preface - 15
Introduction - 27

SECTION ONE: The Huge Problem with Calcium

Chapter 1 - 33
Is Calcium Really a Killer?
Impartial Science Delivers a "Guilty" Verdict

Excess Calcium Promotes Heart Disease 35
Excess Calcium Promotes Cancer. 38
Excess Calcium & Toxins Promote Increased
   Cellular Dysfunction and Death. 41
Excess Calcium Increases Death Rate from All Diseases . . . 43
The Toxicity of Calcium Supplementation 45

Chapter 2 - 47
Limiting Calcium Promotes Health
More Proof That Excess Calcium Promotes Death

How Cells Limit Calcium Levels. 48
The Benefits of Limiting Calcium Influx into Cells 48
Calcium Channel Blockers Effectively Treat
   Many Degenerative Diseases. 49
The Calcium Channel Blocker Shocker 50
Summary. 51

Chapter 3 - 53
Calcium's Deadly Myths
Untangling Fact from Fiction

Myth #1: "Calcium supplementation and increased dietary
   calcium are good for you.". 55
Myth #2: "You cannot get enough calcium in your diet
   without dairy products.". 57
Myth #3: "Everyone with osteoporosis has a
   calcium deficiency.". 59

Myth #4: "Calcium supplementation prevents fractures." . 60
Myth #5: "Increased bone density always means
   stronger bones." 63
Myth #6: "The biggest danger faced by someone with
   osteoporosis is disability or death
   following a fracture." 65
Myth #7: "Vitamin D just serves to increase
   calcium absorption.". 68
Myth #8: "You get all the vitamin D you need
   from the sun." 70

Chapter 4 - 71
The Truth About Osteoporosis
The Real Reason Bones Become Brittle and Calcium Deficient
The Root Cause of Osteoporosis 73
Vitamin C, Bones, and Osteoporosis 74
Vitamin C Prevents Bone Loss and Fractures 77
Vitamin C Deficiency, Osteoporosis, and Coronary
   Heart Disease. 79

SECTION TWO: Agents for Reversing Osteoporosis

Chapter 5 - 85
Building a Fracture-Resistant Frame
Vitamin C: The Foundation and Cornerstone of Strong Bones
Vitamin C: Essential in Bone Physiology —
   From Start to Finish 86
Vitamin C: Frontline Defender Against Oxidative Stress . . 89
Vitamin C Supplementation Increases Bone Density 90
Vitamin C Supplementation Lowers Fracture Risk 91
Vitamin C Supplementation Accelerates and Improves
   Quality of Bone Healing 92
Vitamin C Supplementation Protects Against
   Dangerous Calcifications. 93
Vitamin C Supplementation Protects Against
   Calcium-Laden Kidney Stones 94
Vitamin C Supplementation Lowers All-Cause Mortality . . 97
Safety of vitamin C Supplementation 98
Supplementing with Vitamin C 99
Summary 101

Table of Contents

Chapter 6 — 103

Nature's Calcium Channel Blocker
Magnesium: Its Importance and Life-Saving Power

The Calcium-Magnesium "Tug-o-War" 104
The Calcium-Related Importance of
 Magnesium Supplementation. 105
The Biological Importance of Magnesium Supplementation 105
Magnesium Supplementation Lowers All-Cause Mortality . 106
Safety of Magnesium Supplementation 109
Important Magnesium Supplementation Considerations . . 110
Summary 111

Chapter 7 — 113

Ignored Yet Essential Weapon Against Osteoporosis
Vitamin K: Dissolves Unwanted Calcium Deposits, Reduces Fracture Risk

Multiple Members of the Vitamin K Family 114
Vitamin K Supplementation and Blood Coagulation 115
Vitamin K Supplementation Inhibits and
 Reverses Abnormal Calcification 115
Vitamin K Supplementation Lowers All-Cause Mortality . . 117
Vitamin K Supplementation and Cancer Prevention 118
Vitamin K Supplementation and Bone Health 119
The Synergistic Effect of Vitamin K and
 Other Anti-Osteoporotic Agents 124
Safety of Vitamin K Supplementation 126
Vitamin K Supplementation Considerations 127
Summary 127

Chapter 8 — 129

Needed: Immediate Divorce
Vitamin D: Works Wonders Apart from Calcium Supplementation

Why Calcium and Vitamin D Should Not Be
 Consumed Together 130
Vitamin D and Bone Health 130
The Biological Importance of Vitamin D Supplementation . 131
Vitamin D Lowers All-Cause Mortality 133
The Importance of Maintaining Vitamin D Levels
 in the Normal Range 134
Safety of Vitamin D Supplementation 136

Important Vitamin D Supplementation Considerations. . . 136
Summary. 137

Chapter 9 — 139
Stronger Bones and More Calcium Channel Blocking
Omega-3 Fatty Acids
Combat Calcium Toxicity

What Are Essential Fatty Acids? 139
Omega-3 Fatty Acids and Bone Health 141
Omega-3 Fatty Acid Supplementation
   Lowers All-Cause Mortality. 144
Safety of Omega-3 Fatty Acid Supplementation 146
Omega-3 Fatty Acid Dosing Considerations 147
Summary. 148

Chapter 10 — 149
Bone Health: The Hormonal Component
Estrogen, Testosterone, and Thyroid

Estrogen
Estrogen Therapy Inhibits Abnormal Calcification 150
Estrogen and Bone Health 151
Estrogen Therapy Side Effects and Impact on
   Mortality Risk 152
Estrogen Therapy Considerations 156
  1. Estrogen Dosing. 157
  2. Estrogen Types 157
  3. Estrogen Formulations 158
  4. Other Hormone Administration 158
  5. Routes of Estrogen Administration 158
     • Oral Estrogen 158
     • Non-Oral Estrogens 158
     • Transdermal Estrogen 159
  6. Duration of Administration 160
  7. Timing of Initial Administration 161
  8. Concurrent Antioxidant Administration 161
  9. Serial Clinical Correlation 161
 10. Serial Laboratory Testing 162
Estrogen Summary and
   General Recommendations. 163

Testosterone
Testosterone and Bone Health 165

Testosterone, Cardiovascular Health, and
   All-Cause Mortality 166
Testosterone Therapy Side Effects 168
Testosterone Therapy Dosing Considerations 170
Testosterone Summary and General Recommendations . . 173

Thyroid

Thyroid and Bone Health 174
Thyroid, Cardiovascular Health, and All-Cause Mortality . . 177
Thyroid Therapy Side Effects and Dosing Considerations . 178
Hormone Replacement Summary. 179

SECTION THREE: What's Right with Calcium

Chapter 11 - 183

More Than Teeth and Bones
The Vital Roles of Calcium

General Information About Calcium 184
Calcium's Roles in Healthy Non-Bone Metabolism 185
Calcium Homeostasis: Hormones that Help Keep
   Calcium Levels in Balance 185
Summary. 192

Chapter 12 - 193

Getting Calcium in Balance
Where You Get It, How Much You Really Need

Calcium: What the Government Says You Need 193
Calcium: What You Actually Need 195
Dietary Sources of Calcium 198

SECTION FOUR: Osteoporosis and Toxins

Chapter 13 - 207

Toxin Exposure and Degenerative Disease
Eliminating Hidden Causes of Osteoporosis

1) Digestive Sources of Disease-Causing
   Oxidative Stress. 210
2) Dental Sources of Disease-Causing
   Oxidative Stress. 212

Chapter 14 — 213
Cleansing the Foul Mouth
The Overlooked Source of Infections and Toxins

Root Canal-Treated Teeth: A Death Sentence
Physiology of a Root Canal. 215
All Root Canal-Treated Teeth Are Dangerously Toxic . . 216
How Root Canal-Treated Teeth Poison and Kill 217
Why Lasers Do Not and Cannot Eliminate
Root Canal Infection. 219
Root Canal-Treated Teeth: Efficient Toxin Pumps . . . 220
Dental Research Recognizes the Danger of
Root Canal-Treated Teeth 220
Root-Canal Treated Teeth: A Final Appeal. 222

Dental Cavitations: Perpetually Toxic Wells
Physiology of a Cavitation 223
The Toxic Consequences of Cavitations. 224
Repair of Cavitations and Removal of
Root Canal-Treated Teeth 226
The Problems with Dental Implants 227

Most Dental Materials: Highly Toxic
Amalgam Dental Fillings Are Astonishingly Toxic. . . . 229
Toxic Reconstruction Materials Used in
Implants, Bridges, and Crowns. 230
Biocompatibility Testing Provides Helpful Guidance . . 231
Periodontal (Gum) Disease Is Hazardous to Health, Too 231
Conclusion 232

SECTION FIVE: Now What?

Chapter 15 — 235
Getting Good Care in a Sea of Bad Medicine
Work with a Physician Who Will Work with You

Chapter 16 — 239
Reversing Bone Damage
Suggested Osteoporosis Protection/Reversal Protocol
1) Minimize New Toxin Exposure 239
2) Eradicate Old Infections. 243
3) Eliminate Old Toxins 244
4) Correct Critical Hormone Deficiencies 245

Table of Contents

    5) Optimize Antioxidant Levels 245
    6) Appropriate Prescription Medication Use 246

Chapter 17 - 251
  Decalcifying Coronary Arteries
    Suggested Heart Disease Protection/Reversal Protocol
    1) Minimize New Toxin Exposure 252
    2) Eradicate Old Infections. 254
    3) Eliminate Old Toxins 255
    4) Correct Critical Hormone Deficiencies 256
    5) Optimize Antioxidant Levels 258
    6) Appropriate Prescription Medication Use 260

Chapter 18 - 263
  Neutralizing the Mutagenic Effects of Calcium
    Suggested Cancer Protection/Reversal Protocol
    1) Minimize New Toxin Exposure 264
    2) Eradicate Old Infections. 266
    3) Eliminate Old Toxins 266
    4) Correct Critical Hormone Deficiencies 267
    5) Optimize Antioxidant Levels 268
    6) Appropriate Prescription Medication Use 272

Chapter 19 - 275
  Tracking the Progress of a Treatment Protocol
    How Do You Know If It's Working?
    Specific Tests for Tracking Progress of
      Atherosclerosis Protocols 276
    Specific Tests for Tracking Progress of Cancer Protocols 277
    General Chronic Degenerative Disease
      Protocol and Testing. 278
    Recap 280

Chapter 20 - 281
  "But I really like milk!"
    How to Have Some Dairy and Good Health, Too
    Calcium Intake 282
    Calcium Excretion 283
    Recap 285

Appendix A - 287
  More About Calcium Channel Blockers

Appendix B 293
A Guide to Effective Administration of Vitamin C

Important Factors in the Effective Administration of Vitamin C

1) Dose: The Most Critical Factor for Effective Results . . 294
2) Route: What's the Best Avenue for Vitamin C Administration? 298
3) Rate: How Fast Should Vitamin C Be Administered?. . . 298
4) Frequency: What's the Optimal Interval Between Vitamin C Administrations? 302
5) Duration: How Long Should Vitamin C Administrations Be Continued?. 303
6) Type: What's the Best Chemical Form of Vitamin C to Use?. 303
7) Adjunct Therapies: Will Vitamin C Administration Compete with Other Treatments? . . . 309
8) Safety: How Safe is Vitamin C? 310
9) Overall Protocol of Administration 312

Multi-C Protocol

1) Liposome-Encapsulated Vitamin C 313
2) Sodium Ascorbate Powder. 315
3) Ascorbyl Palmitate 317
4) Intravenous Vitamin C (IVC). 317
Practical IVC Considerations 319
Mop-Up IVC. 224
Recap 327

Appendix C 329
The Cause of All Disease: A Unified Theory

Overview. 329
Toxins, Vitamin C, and Electrons 332
Infections and Toxins 336
Reduction-Oxidation [Redox] Chemistry 337
Reactive Oxygen Species (ROS) 339
Toxin Properties and Variables 340
Levels of Intracellular Oxidative Stress 345
Summary. 348

References 349

Resources 415

Index 417

Introduction

We now know that accepted geographical wisdom during the time of Christopher Columbus was built upon shaky ground. In the fifteenth century, "truth" of a flat earth seemed self-evident and was not to be questioned.

Our global perspectives have morphed much since then. Today, it's almost impossible to imagine how anyone could concoct such a simplistic, two-dimensional concept of our planet.

Before we get too smug, however, we need to realize that humans are still very much in the business of fabricating flawed models of reality. Far too frequently theories are formed with little supporting evidence and touted as truth, while boatloads of evidence to the contrary are ignored and even altered. Oftentimes, fairytale realities are embraced as true because we want or need them to be true. It is all too common for scientists and lay people alike to risk their professional and personal reputations clinging to their foregone conclusions with a white-knuckled grip — even after their irrefutable "facts" are shown to be false.

Such is the case with calcium.

It is dogmatically taught as self-evident medical wisdom that the best prevention and treatment for osteoporosis requires an increased intake of calcium. Certainly it is true that bones have a large calcium content. It is also true that osteoporosis involves a significant calcium loss from the bones. On the basis of these two isolated facts and nothing more, it is concluded that upping calcium consumption will prevent and possibly reverse this condition. Unfortunately nothing could be further from reality.

Calcium is essential for bodily function. That is not what is being called into question. The research and conclusions presented in *Death by Calcium* are not intended to incite a crusade against this essential nutrient. The goal is to expose the real and grave danger of pumping excessive amounts of calcium into our bodies. Just like iron and copper, calcium is absolutely essential for good health. However, excess levels of these three nutrient elements are very toxic. Deficiencies of these nutrients are certainly not desirable, but they are only rarely encountered in the United States. An irrational fear of such rare and easily treated deficiencies should not be allowed to fuel the chronic intake of enormously toxic excesses.

Most of us are careening toward a host of health problems because of bad food and lifestyle choices. Influenced by what is widely accepted as healthy dietary practice, the typical American menu is laden with calcium-saturated foods. To make matters worse, we are frequently admonished that everyone, especially post-menopausal women, should fortify their daily calcium intake with calcium supplementation. When heeded this counsel greatly increases the odds of heart attack, kidney failure, stroke, and other undesirable outcomes. A legitimate body-wide deficiency of calcium is virtually non-existent, but too much calcium is very common and highly toxic, and it reliably leads to great suffering and premature death. Also reversing a long-standing excess of calcium in the body is a difficult and involved process.

Actually, the amount of calcium needed for healthy cellular function is infinitesimally small relative to the amount of calcium found in bones. Most of the adult population has no need for significant calcium intake and the amount needed rapidly decreases with age, as older individuals are already significantly accumulating calcium.

Introduction

Like iron and copper, calcium quickly becomes toxic as concentrations barely inch over required levels. Almost without exception, osteoporotic individuals have toxic excesses of calcium outside the bounds of bone tissue. This fact alone highlights the fallacy of calcium supplementation for the treatment of osteoporosis. It is this excess of ingested calcium along with calcium chronically released from osteoporotic bone that poses the most dangerous threat to health and life as it moves in and around all of the cells in the body, promoting disease wherever it accumulates. This notably includes heart disease, high blood pressure, strokes, and cancer. However, truth be known, it fuels and accelerates all chronic degenerative diseases.

Once calcium deposition in non-bone structures begins, the body's compensatory responses pull even more calcium from the bones as the deposited calcium is taken out of circulation. Predictably this prompts prescriptions for additional calcium intake, which further promotes health-damaging deposits throughout the body.

When a body-wide state of excess calcium already exists, any added calcium is too much as it promotes abnormal cellular, glandular, and bodily function. That is why supplemental calcium needs to be stopped, excess dietary calcium needs to be curtailed, and all calcium-rich, vitamin D-fortified foods need to be avoided.

In the following pages you will see the truly astounding evidence documenting the toxicity of the excess calcium already present in most older adults today. You'll find out why supplemental calcium does not help osteoporosis, while it truly worsens all known chronic degenerative diseases. You will also learn methods that you and your doctor can use to achieve and maintain optimal nutrient levels for managing osteoporosis as well as many other diseases. Properly treated, osteoporosis and most other diseases currently considered to be largely irreversible can be improved dramatically.

It is my hope that as the truths in *Death by Calcium*

are applied, you and countless others will be spared the painful consequences of the easily avoidable toxicity of excess calcium.

May the truth propel us to longer and healthier lives.

SECTION ONE:

The Huge Problem with Calcium

CHAPTER 1

Is Calcium Really a Killer?

Impartial Science Delivers a "Guilty" Verdict

Blowing the whistle on the toxic effects of excess calcium will undoubtedly provoke a firestorm of deafening propaganda. The dairy industry, the medical establishment, and supplement companies have invested untold time, money, and talent in promoting the necessity of increased calcium consumption along with calcium supplementation in the prevention and treatment of osteoporosis. To implicate calcium — a universally-accepted nutritional "good guy" — as a cause of disease and death will incite retaliation from challenged egos and threatened bank accounts. However, once the evidence gets widespread exposure the fear of class action lawsuits will muster spin-doctors and lawyers to fast and furious action in an effort to limit damage and protect many self-serving interests.

Déjà vu here we come again... During the 50's most of America watched the tobacco industry battle efforts to debunk their claim that smoking was actually a healthy habit. Once they lost that skirmish the fight moved to years of vehement "not true" and "you can't prove it" claims against any attempt to link tobacco and cancer.

Defeated once again, they finally tried to convince the state attorneys general and the public that they were completely ignorant of ties between smoking and lung cancer. At massive cost to their reputation and capital they finally lost! Today no one doubts the veracity of the initial indictments against tobacco. Yet how many unfortunate smokers suffered enormously and had their lives shortened because of an industry's greed?

The real problem is not a lack of calcium in the diet, but rather a "relocation" of calcium from the bones to other areas of the body.

In like fashion recent scientific data provides an overwhelming case against calcium. What follows is based on research studies published in peer-reviewed medical journals. When considered as a whole the evidence delivers a resounding "guilty" verdict on the common existence and enormous toxicity of calcium excess in the adult population today.

At the time of this writing little consideration is given to the possibility that anyone, especially the elderly, may be suffering from a toxic calcium excess, even as they continue to dose, and overdose on it. Deeply etched and often-parroted warnings from doctors, the popular press, the dairy industry, and supplement suppliers assert that calcium deficiency is a common and nearly universal problem in postmenopausal women and aging men.

The evidence provided in this chapter shows that the opposite is true. Osteoporosis, by definition, is a degenerative condition of the bone associated with a significant calcium deficiency in the bony structural matrix. Somehow the observation of a calcium-deficient state in osteoporotic bone is promoted as proof of a general, body-wide, calcium deficiency.

Is Calcium Really a Killer?

The scientific evidence, however, paints a much different picture: the degree of calcium deficiency in osteoporotic bone is actually an indicator of the amount of excess calcium that has taken up residence in non-bone tissues. The real problem is not a lack of calcium in the diet, but rather a "relocation" of calcium from the bones to other areas of the body. [1,2,3]

The body-wide distribution of excess calcium is of far greater concern to the longevity and well-being of an older person than any of the problems associated with osteoporosis. Not only does increasing calcium intake fail to improve bone strength, it fuels calcium excess everywhere in the body.

You are 30% more likely to have a heart attack and up to 20% more likely to have a stroke if you take an extra 500 mg of calcium per day.

This excess calcium in non-bone tissues been shown to increase mortality from all causes. Not only that, it has specifically been linked to a substantially greater risk of death from America's two deadliest diseases: coronary heart disease and cancer. Consider this sobering evidence...

Excess Calcium Promotes Heart Disease

You are 30% more likely to have a heart attack and up to 20% more likely to have a stroke if you take an extra 500 mg of calcium or more per day — that's the consensus derived from a comprehensive review of 15 independent clinical investigations. The reviewing researchers reported that subjects taking calcium supplements (500 mg or more per day) had a 27 to 31% higher risk of heart attack and a 12 to 20% greater risk of stroke. [4-6]

Dump more calcium into the caldron and the brew becomes even more deadly. A study of over 61,000 participants viewed over a 19-year period concludes that those with calcium intakes over 1,400 mg/day had an alarming 40% increased risk of death from cardiovascular disease in general and a 114% increase in risk of death from a reduced flow of blood to the heart muscle (ischemic heart disease).[7]

Over one-third of Americans over the age of 45 have evidence of arterial calcification.

Another recent clinical trial compared individuals who regularly supplemented with calcium with individuals who took no supplements at all. These researchers also concluded that those who take supplements had a significantly increased risk of heart attack.[8] The same study further found that calcium supplementation significantly increased total cholesterol levels in postmenopausal women. Total cholesterol is a factor generally considered to be an important measure of coronary artery disease risk.

Healthy postmenopausal women taking calcium supplements were the subjects of a large, 5-year population study. Investigators reported a substantial increase in vascular event rates, such as heart attacks and strokes. Higher calcium intake was further implicated because these vascular events were even more pronounced in women who claimed to be highly compliant in taking their supplements, which would suggest a larger total ingestion of calcium.[9,10]

Perhaps even more conclusive evidence is found through the use of computed tomography (CT Scans). This powerful diagnostic tool uses computer technology and x-rays to produce cross-sectional "slices" or images of bodily structures. CT Scans reveal that over one-third of Americans over the age of 45 have evidence of arterial calcification.[11] This percentage rises drastically with greater age, literally skyrocketing in postmenopausal women as well as in testosterone-deficient males. The calcification of arteries is so intrinsically related to coronary disease that the measurement of calcification in these vessels is used to assess the development and progress of the disease.[12,13] A 1990 study demonstrated that calcium content in arterial plaque increases as the plaque develops. The earliest clearly visible evidence of atherosclerosis appears as fatty streaks in the arterial walls. Investigators reported that these fatty streaks had 13 times more calcium than healthy arterial tissues. Moderately evolved plaques had 25 times more calcium than normal, and fully developed plaques had 80 times more calcium. Roughly 50% of the dry weight of the advanced plaques was comprised of calcium salts. Early stages of atherosclerosis appeared cholesterol-laden, while the advanced plaques were very calcium-rich.[14]

> Roughly 50% of the dry weight of the advanced plaques was comprised of calcium salts.

Other investigators also report that older patients had increased calcium content in their atherosclerotic plaques when compared to younger patients.[15] This is clearly consistent with the increasing degrees of excess calcium ingestion observed in older patients.

There is also evidence that calcium is playing an important role in the early development of atherosclerosis, even when the coronary artery calcium score is zero. Plaques are not only present in individuals with zero scores,[16] the distribution of the plaques is similar to that seen in patients with calcified plaques.[17,18]

This strongly suggests that a younger person with plaque should still have the same concerns of calcium excess since calcium likely plays just as important a role in the early evolution of plaque, before it finally becomes detectable by a CT Scan. Plaque does not just appear one day with an easily detectable calcium load without an earlier stage of development when it was not detectable. A coronary calcium score of zero would be spectacular in an 80-year old, but in a 40-year old it needs to be correlated with other laboratory data and clinical observations. In the case of the younger person with a minimal calcium load and a coronary artery calcium score of zero it should never be assumed that lifestyle does not need modifications because the stage for detectable calcium accumulation might already be set. Lifestyle and risk factor modification is best begun when calcium has not yet accumulated to a detectable level.

Calcifications in the thyroid gland were found to increase the incidence of malignancy.

Excess Calcium Promotes Cancer

Calcium and cancer are frequent bedfellows. That fact has been evident for decades. However, medical researchers not wanting to implicate this near-sacred nutrient in the initiation and development of cancer have been reluctant to connect the dots.

Both microscopic and easily visible calcifications are frequently seen in malignant tissues. Such deposits tend to occur at points of inflammation and antioxidant deficiency. However, if the calcium/phosphorus metabolism is sufficiently out of balance, deposition can occur without inflammation. Once calcium begins to accumulate — with or without an initiating point of inflammation — the presence of calcification often initiates or increases inflammation that facilitates further deposition.

These tissue calcifications are commonly seen in cancer patients, and evidence suggests that there is a significant causal link between the two. For example, calcifications in the thyroid gland were found to increase the incidence of malignancy.[19]

Several studies clearly demonstrate the friendly relationship between excess calcium and cancer. In one such study, investigators used advanced magnetic resonance imaging (MRI) techniques to detect calcification in 22 of 23 (95%) malignant prostate glands.[20]

> *Advanced MRI techniques detected calcification in 95% of malignant prostate glands.*

Granted, just because calcium and cancer often occupy the same space doesn't prove calcium's causative role. But we have a smoking gun: a mechanism scientists call "oxidative stress." The following two facts establish an indisputable link between excess calcium and cancer:

1) Oxidative stress is a well-known causal factor of all degenerative diseases, especially cancer.

2) Increased intracellular calcium always increases oxidative stress, even in the absence of detectable calcification.

It also appears that the aggressiveness of some cancers is directly related to the concentration of calcium in the cells. In small cell lung carcinoma — a highly malignant cancer — the cancer cells actually multiply through a chemical process that increases the calcium concentration inside the cells. Several researchers have demonstrated that as the concentration of intracellular calcium increases, the invasive nature of cancer also increases, resulting in a metastatic spread. [21-24]

Other research shows a strong correlation between bone mass and risk of malignancy. Women with the highest bone mass were found to have an increased risk of developing breast cancer. [25-28] Interestingly none of these authors could satisfactorily explain how higher bone mass could ever be undesirable, and furthermore how it could have anything to do with the development of breast cancer. An understandable and probable mechanism emerges as three other relationships are considered.

1) High bone mass readings do not necessarily mean healthier bone but rather suggest that women with the highest bone mass are those who ingest and supplement the most calcium and therefore are prone to the highest levels of excess calcium.

2) Continued exposure to excess calcium results in calcium deposition in non-bone tissues including the breasts. Women with breast cancer frequently have macro- and microcalcifications on mammography. [29,30] In fact many breast biopsies are performed because of the presence of such calcifications. [31]

3) And finally, calcium deposits in breast tissue allow and promote calcium migration into individual breast cells (increased intracellular calcium) increasing cancer-promoting oxidative stress.

In addition, studies show that breast cancer patients with calcifications are less likely to survive their battle with the disease. [32]

There is however, a cancer/calcium partnership that provides even more solid proof of calcium having a cancer-promoting activity. Cancer cells seem to need, or at least want to acquire, increased intracellular calcium. Many cancer cells actually develop an increased number of calcium channels. These channels facilitate and promote the flow of calcium into cells, helping to cause a state of increased intracellular calcium.[33] This influx increases oxidative stress and promotes the spread of cancer to other glands and organs.

This influx [of calcium] increases oxidative stress and promotes the spread of cancer.

Conversely, inhibiting calcium uptake appears to make cancers less invasive and less prone to grow new blood vessels.[34] When calcium is actually pulled out of metastasizing melanoma cells in the brain, the metastatic nature of those cancer cells is reduced. Furthermore, reduction of calcium content in such a cell resulted in a reduced degree of intracellular oxidative stress. The reduction of oxidative stress actually makes these malignant cells more resistant to chemotherapy since the chemo (toxic chemicals) attempts to kill cancerous cells by increasing intracellular oxidative stress to the point of cell death are less effective in accomplishing this goal.[35]

While excess calcium in a cell does not always result in cancer it always produces decreased cellular health through an increase in oxidative stress that can manifest itself in a number of disease states including heart disease and cancer.

Excess Calcium & Toxins Promote Increased Cellular Dysfunction and Death

Poisons are toxic primarily because they start flameless molecular fires that consume whatever they touch. In the process they generate more toxins through a chain reaction that spreads like a blaze through a forest. Scientists call these pro-oxidant "fires" oxidative stress. Antioxidants are the body's frontline defense against pro-oxidants and the oxidative stress they generate. They are able to extinguish oxidative stress and the initiating toxins — without becoming toxic themselves — as long as an unspent supply remains available.

> *If calcium levels remain too high a cascade of reactions push cells toward programmed cell death.*

The amount of calcium outside cells [extracellular calcium], depending on the type of cell, can be 1,000 to 10,000 times higher than levels inside the cell [intracellular calcium]. This difference in concentrations means that there is always calcium on the outside that wants to get inside. Through various mechanisms, calcium is able to enter the cell. Once in, if calcium levels remain too high a cascade of reactions push cells toward programmed cell death [apoptosis] or complete cell destruction [necrosis].[36]

Clear evidence shows that several known toxins greatly facilitate calcium's passage through cell membranes. Formaldehyde, for example, induces escalated intracellular calcium levels.[37] Exposure to methylmercury, an especially toxic form of mercury, also facilitates calcium's passage into cells, ultimately leading to increased cell death.[38,39] Arsenic induces an influx of calcium into cells.[40] Elevated glucose levels, as seen in diabetes, cause damage on their own, but they appear to instigate cell death by increasing intracellular levels of calcium as well.[41]

As mentioned previously, the increase in intracellular calcium in many cancer cells is fed by an increased number of calcium channels in those cells.[42] Calcium channel blockers are agents that impede calcium's entrance into cells through these channels, and in so doing they can prevent the manifestation of certain disease states. For example, calcium channel blockers prevent the appearance of neurological disorders in rats exposed to a powerful toxin [methylmercury].[43] And even in the absence of toxins high intracellular calcium levels still initiate cell injury and death in neurons.[44] Even in the absence of known toxin exposure, chronically elevated calcium levels in the cell appear to be a common denominator for most, if not all, forms of oxidant-induced cell damage and death.[45-48] It is through this very process that sustained elevations of intracellular calcium play a significant part in degenerative neurological diseases such as Lou Gehrig's disease [amyotrophic lateral sclerosis or ALS],[49] Parkinson's disease,[50] and Alzheimer's disease.[51]

A recently published study found a strong association between increased calcium levels and death from any cause.

Excess Calcium Increases Death Rate from All Diseases

As already demonstrated, coronary artery calcium scores have been shown to reliably predict cardiac events and increased risk of death from heart attack. These same scores, however, also accurately predict the risk of death from all causes (all-cause mortality).[52,53] As calcium scores rose — starting at undetectable levels of calcium — all-cause mortality also increased.[54]

Other studies have demonstrated the great significance of calcium accumulation as an independent factor that increases all-cause mortality. A recently published study conducted over a period of 8 years found a strong association between increased calcium levels and death from any cause.[55] Another study demonstrated that individuals with increasing coronary artery calcium scores — in the absence of other traditional coronary artery disease risk factors — had a substantially higher all-cause mortality rate than individuals with three or more significant risk factors but a coronary calcium score of zero.[56]

Coronary artery calcification is also associated with a greater chance of death from all causes.

Even when calcium is not being tracked in the coronary arteries its accumulation still appears to predict all-cause mortality. Calcification around the bases of the aortic and mitral valves is also associated with increased death from all causes. When compared to individuals with no calcification in either valve, calcification around one valve increased all-cause mortality risk. When both valves had calcification the risk of all-cause mortality was higher still. These valve calcifications were found to be independently associated with mortality risk,[57] indicating that the calcification process is strongly related to dying from anything, not just heart disease.

It is very important to note that coronary artery calcification is also associated with a greater chance of death from all causes. That means that even though calcium accumulation may be more easily detected in the coronary arteries than elsewhere in the body, this particular calcification demonstrates the universal role calcium has in accelerating the course of all chronic degenerative diseases. Not only is the coronary calcium score a good indicator of coronary artery disease and plaque burden,[58] it is also a good indicator of the severity of chronic degenerative diseases in general.

Additionally, other studies have found that higher serum parathyroid hormone levels were associated with increased all-cause mortality.[59-64] This is consistent with the fact that parathyroid hormone serves to increase calcium concentration in the blood by a number of mechanisms.

And finally, in the large study of over 61,000 women mentioned above, it was demonstrated that those who ingested 1,400 mg of calcium/day or more not only were much more likely to die from a vascular event, but they also had an increased mortality from all causes. Alarmingly, those with the highest calcium consumption, whether from dietary and/or supplemental sources, posted a death rate two and one-half times (257%) higher than the groups who ingested less.[65]

Identification of the milk-alkali syndrome established the toxicity of calcium supplementation long ago.

The Toxicity of Calcium Supplementation

Identification of the milk-alkali syndrome established the toxicity of calcium supplementation long ago. This condition was first identified in 1923 when peptic ulcer disease was commonly treated with milk and sodium bicarbonate.[66] Although milk and sodium bicarbonate alone were sufficient to induce the syndrome it evolved from a relatively infrequent condition to almost disappearing when proton-pump inhibitors came into widespread use by the mid-1980's for ulcers and effective treatment no longer required an intake of calcium.[67] However, when calcium carbonate, an over-the-counter antacid, largely replaced milk as the predominant source of calcium for individuals trying to self-treat their peptic ulcer diseases the incidence of the milk-alkali syndrome increased substantially.[68,69] The "current" milk-alkali syndrome, now caused by calcium carbonate and little or no milk, has become the third leading cause of hypercalcemia [excess calcium] of any degree and the second leading cause of striking hypercalcemia in patients with end stage renal disease.[70]

Of particular interest in the current version of the milk-alkali syndrome is that it has been seen with a supplemental amount of roughly 2,000 mg of calcium, along with milk ingestion and some vitamin D supplementation.[71] One woman with the syndrome deliberately supplemented only 1,000 mg of calcium carbonate daily, but was found to be taking additional calcium carbonate antacids along with 800 IU of vitamin D daily — not extraordinary amounts for many individuals.[72] This is especially important since many current recommendations for routine calcium intake/supplementation are as much as 1,500 mg daily in patients.

If the assumption is made that some calcium must be supplemented this provides little margin for error between a recommended amount of calcium and an amount that can potentially result in hypercalcemia, metabolic alkalosis, and renal insufficiency, the classical triad of the milk-alkali syndrome.[73,74] It also strongly supports the assertion that many people are ingesting far too much calcium on a regular basis. Even if they do not push themselves into a classical milk-alkali syndrome it is very clear that individuals can fuel states of calcium excess by pairing a relatively modest dose of vitamin D with "ordinary" calcium supplementation.

CHAPTER 2

Limiting Calcium Promotes Health

More Proof That Excess Calcium Promotes Death

Calcium's link to the initiation and evolution of degenerative disease is hard to ignore. Where chronic degenerative disease is found, excess calcium is also present. The demonstrated links between calcium and disease revealed in the previous chapter provide a powerfully convincing argument against bolstering calcium intake through diet or supplemental forms of this substance.

The evidence does not end there however! Substantial research provides another indictment that is as strong, if not stronger, against excess calcium. A thorough review of the scientific literature provides shocking answers to the question: what happens when calcium's access to bodily structures and cells is purposely limited? As you'll see in this chapter, health breaks out!

In grand summary then, if excessive calcium in the body leads to disease and death and limiting calcium access produces health and life, the case against calcium becomes difficult, if not impossible, to refute.

Here's the evidence, judge for yourself...

How Cells Limit Calcium Levels

To remain healthy, cells need to keep calcium levels within a specific and fairly narrow range. In the presence of large extracellular excesses of calcium the maintenance of normal levels of calcium inside the cells requires much cellular energy. First, to limit entrance, the cell must attempt to restrict access by lowering membrane permeability and by tightly controlling entrance through calcium channels that are embedded in the membrane. Once normal intracellular levels of calcium are exceeded the cell tries to limit damage through binding or buffering it [1] and/or by locking it up in intracellular compartments. [2]

Cells also attempt to manage calcium concentrations by expelling excesses through a process called extrusion. Extrusion requires the oxidation of ATP, [3] an extremely high-energy molecule, to create a "calcium pump" that is fueled by other high-energy molecules. [4,5] Because this "pump" must push the calcium out of the cell into an already high concentration of extracellular calcium, the rate and intensity of energy consumption generates a large quantity of oxidative byproducts. This is true even if intracellular calcium levels are normal or only minimally elevated.

When calcium concentrations outside the cell remain too high for too long, intracellular levels never completely return to normal and the level of oxidative stress inside the cell is perpetually elevated. This situation invites the manifestation and full-blown development of degenerative disease and highlights the need to avoid excess calcium intake.

The Benefits of Limiting Calcium Influx into Cells

Calcium channel blockers comprise a group of drugs designed to limit the influx/uptake of calcium into cells. For decades calcium channel blockers have been used effectively in the treatment of high blood pressure. They have also been used to reduce the incidence of cardiac events associated with high blood pressure, such as stroke, heart attack, angina, and heart failure. [6,7]

As previously discussed, atherosclerosis [hardening of the arteries] is a disease that can be monitored by the degree of calcification seen in the coronary arteries. Research indicates that calcium channel blockers exert an anti-atherosclerosis effect. [8]

After years and years of exhaustive research on calcium channel blockers there is no evidence for any significant mode of action other than limiting the cellular uptake of calcium. This fact certainly implicates excess calcium's roll in the development of hypertension, but there are two other interesting findings. Firstly, calcium channel blockers have been used to effectively treat a myriad of diseases that have nothing to do with hypertension. Secondly, even though these drugs have been and are widely prescribed, very rarely do they produce low blood pressure in patients who have normal blood pressures but are taking the drugs for the treatment of other diseases, strongly supporting the concept that almost all adults have a chronic state of excess calcium inside their cells.

> *Calcium channel blockers have been used to effectively treat a myriad of diseases that have nothing to do with hypertension.*

Calcium Channel Blockers Effectively Treat Many Degenerative Diseases

The widespread and effective use of calcium channel blockers in the treatment of a host of diseases provides even more clear evidence against excess calcium's role in the development of degenerative diseases.

Multiple examples of this include:
- Preterm labor [9]
- Coronary artery spasm [10]
- Angina pectoris [11]
- Pulmonary arterial hypertension [12]
- Raynaud's phenomenon [13]
- Acute head trauma [14]
- Epilepsy [15,16]
- Peripheral neuropathy induced by chemotherapy [17]
- Alzheimer's disease [18]
- Parkinson's disease [19]

Calcium channel blocker treatment of rats with removed ovaries — to simulate a menopausal state — significantly diminished the osteoporosis that normally follows such removal.[20] In another animal study, calcium channel blocker therapy was even able to rescue cells at the point of death because of pathological increases in intracellular calcium concentration.[21]

As noted above, increased intracellular calcium levels are always accompanied by increased intracellular oxidative stress and they are probably the primary cause for it. And as expected, when elevated intracellular calcium levels are significantly lowered, increased intracellular oxidative stress is reduced as well. This is the main reason that calcium channel blocker therapy produces a significant and positive impact in such a wide array of diseases.

The Calcium Channel Blocker Shocker

Long-term use of calcium channel blockers by individuals without hypertension — for conditions unrelated to high blood pressure — would be expected to display excessive drops in blood pressure if calcium levels inside the cells were in their narrow normal range. In truth however, the long-term use of these drugs in older individuals without hypertension almost never results in unwanted hypotension. Why? The logical answer is that virtually all individuals using these drugs also have chronic states of excess intracellular calcium.

Studies involving a total of over 175,000 patients and three commonly prescribed calcium channel blockers (diltiazem, verapamil, and nifedipine) revealed some shocking data, especially for a prescription drug. All three drugs significantly decreased all-cause mortality, not just cardiac-related mortality. [22-25] This evidence further confirms the conclusion that all the cells are suffering from calcium excess. It also emphasizes that limiting further calcium entry into cells promotes improved health for all diseases, not just the "big two" (heart disease and cancer).

All three [calcium channel blocker] drugs significantly decreased all-cause mortality, not just cardiac-related mortality.

Summary

- All disease is initiated and/or worsened by elevated oxidative stress.
- Elevated intracellular calcium increases oxidative stress inside the cells.
- Calcium channel blockers decrease intracellular calcium.
- One would expect calcium channel blockers to produce a significant reduction in the symptoms and the mortality resulting from all diseases.
- Significant long-term research confirms that calcium channel blockers do lower all-cause mortality. (This is perhaps the

only prescription drug on the market that can make this claim. For more information about calcium channel blockers, see Appendix A.)

The evidence is clear. Once calcium in the body accumulates beyond our limited need, it becomes toxic. Make no mistake: compliance to mainstream dietary recommendations, especially in regard to calcium, will put your health and life in grave jeopardy. Even more importantly, you must reject the conventional wisdom that suggests we add calcium supplements to an already calcium-rich diet. The prevalence of bone fractures in the elderly perpetuates the commonly accepted advice that we all need to ingest more calcium. This is not science; it's unscientific hogwash!

Yes, osteoporosis is a real epidemic and it is costly. It must be addressed. But until we abandon the all-too-common myths about this degenerative disease we will only be making matters worse — much worse. In the next chapter we will use real science to dismantle those myths.

CHAPTER 3

Calcium's Deadly Myths

Untangling Fact from Fiction

Ever wonder why two scientists can look at the same data and arrive at opposing conclusions? Consider "Global Warming" for example. Regardless of how the media or politicians may spin it, there are many credible scientists on both sides of the argument. They start with the same data but come to opposite conclusions. Why? The conflict is not only in what constitutes the facts themselves, but also in the interpretation of those facts. There are always assumptions or presuppositions, opinions, prejudices, and biases that flavor interpretations. And when fame, fortune, or political power is at stake, objectivity becomes even more elusive.

This is certainly true in the nutritional and medical worlds. In particular it is hard to overestimate the role money plays in obscuring objectivity. Little do we realize how much politics, grants, and employers influence where scientists concentrate their efforts and how they evaluate the data from their research. But the corrupting enticements of fame, fortune, and power extend far beyond the laboratory. Think about it: a staggering $4,000,000,000,000 [four trillion dollars] is spent in the food and drug sector of the U.S. economy every year. Without a doubt the glare from that much gold can greatly blur the objectivity of marketers, manufacturers, government agents, medical providers, and the advertisement-driven news media.

The quest for profits can quickly transform sheer fantasy into sacred fact. Here's a simplistic example of this: Let's say a national organization of dairy farmers is concerned about the decreasing consumption of milk. To stimulate business they hire a large advertising agency and provide them with research studies that substantiate these two facts:

1) Calcium is necessary in a host of bodily functions, and

2) Cow's milk is a rich source of dietary calcium

After weeks of creative brainstorming the advertising agency makes their pitch. They suggest a multi-million-dollar nationwide marketing campaign based on the sound-byte, "Milk does a body good." Once the campaign is approved, the frenzy begins. Media outlets want their slice of the advertising pie. News desks are flooded with press releases. Misleading studies on the benefits of calcium capture headlines. Pro-calcium doctors are interviewed and appear in a flood of "osteoporosis epidemic" news features. Over time the flurry of attention and the constant repetition of the, "Milk does a body good" message — presented in genuinely entertaining commercials — ends up changing the way people think about milk. Over time it's difficult to find anyone who doesn't believe that drinking milk is healthy!

So does milk genuinely do a body good, or has fiction been presented as fact? Hopefully you can spot the faulty premise in this advertising. If not I'll give you a hint. There's an unstated assumption that increasing calcium intake is always good for the body. However, when one realizes that excessive calcium is in fact a health hazard (as was demonstrated in Chapter 1) and that most older individuals already are in a state of body-wide calcium excess, then pushing concentrations even higher will never be beneficial for the body.

Considering the high incidence of atherosclerosis — a disease in which calcification of the coronary arteries always indicates calcium excess — at least half the population over 50 is well on its way to a heart attack if some other disease does not kill them first. That means millions have embraced the milk-is-good-for-you myth and related fictions, as confirmed medical wisdom. Sadly, I contend that they have done so to the detriment of a long life and good health. Now let's address some of the more common myths that continue to be promoted as important principles leading to good health.

> *Calcification of the coronary arteries always indicates calcium excess, and at least half the population over 50 is well on its way to a heart attack.*

Myth #1: "Calcium supplementation and increased dietary calcium are good for you."

Although certainly not the only voice proclaiming this myth, the dairy industry has done an effective job in promoting it to nearly every human in America. Most of us remember: "Milk is a natural," "You never outgrow your need for milk," "Milk has something for everyone," "Milk does a body good," and lastly, "Got Milk?" Kudos to the dairy industry! With a string of very effective advertising campaigns they have helped shape the way we all think about dairy foods.

Unfortunately, the need to condense everything into a few words — or in some cases a few letters — typically results in a significant lack of truth. And who has the luxury of revisiting ideas that are already engraved in stone and held by most professionals to be self-evident? With so little time to review the dizzying influx of new information, who is going to make time for a critical review of old ideas that nobody even seems to be questioning? That's why few doctors, nutritionists, news reporters, and researchers question the nutritional wisdom of a calcium supplement and/or a calcium-rich diet.

> *Osteoporosis involves a lack of calcium in the bones. It does not mean that there is a lack of calcium in the body or the diet.*

After all, defending this myth is so simple. Aren't bones largely composed of calcium? Isn't osteoporosis a calcium deficiency of the bone? So it makes sense that drinking calcium-rich milk or downing some calcium tablets will fix the problem...right?

Using the same logic, you might decide to paint a rotten fence with a new coat of bright, white paint. There is certainly nothing wrong with making something old and decrepit look good. The important point, however, is not to make something only cosmetically appealing while continuing to let its structure deteriorate. Calcium by itself for osteoporotic bone is very much like the paint put on the rotting fence. The fence may end up looking good (or better), but it's still going to fall apart.

Osteoporosis involves a lack of calcium in the bones. It does not mean that there is a lack of calcium in the body or in the diet. To the contrary, much of the calcium leached from bone is not eliminated, it simply moves to other parts of the body. The real problem in osteoporosis is that the body is unable to synthesize a new structural bone matrix and to integrate calcium into it. Simply increasing the quantity of calcium in the body does not even begin to remedy this problem. The calcium simply deposits elsewhere in the body where there are no bone proteins.

In fact the evidence against adding calcium to the diet — in any form — is overwhelming (see Chapter 1). Excess calcium is a killer. It increases all-cause mortality by 250 percent and it dramatically increases vascular events, such as heart attack and stroke. It also increases the oxidative stress responsible for cancer initiation and aggressive cancer growth.

> *Excess calcium is a killer. It increases all-cause mortality by 250 percent.*

Perhaps the added death and disease risk might be worth bearing if there were substantial offsetting benefits. There aren't. While there can be some marginal improvement in bone density readings (this will be addressed later), there is really no concrete evidence that increased dietary and supplemental calcium deliver any real health benefit. That leads us to our next myth...

Myth #2: "You cannot get enough calcium in your diet without dairy products."

This myth has two parts:
1) the amount of calcium actually required in the diet, and,
2) whether that quantity can be reached without dairy products.

If the government's recommended daily allowance (RDA) of calcium — between 1,000 to 1,300 mg per day for most adults [1] — were correct, consumption of dairy products would be an easy way to reach that goal. However, as discussed in Chapter 6, this amount passes actual need by a mile. Not only is the government's RDA for calcium far too high, the idea that you can't get enough calcium without dairy products is patently false. Cultures that drink little to no milk all over the globe have a much lower incidence of osteoporosis than Americans.

It is true that dairy products are extremely calcium-rich. And if one legitimately needed to bolster calcium levels, ingesting more milk and cheese would be an easy way to do so. However, this myth assumes that everyone needs large amounts of dietary calcium while the truth is that virtually no one needs to deliberately increase the calcium content of their diets. The flaw in this argument was further addressed in the discussion of Myth #1.

To adequately know whether you need more calcium can't be answered until you know how much you actually need. This question is thoroughly discussed in Chapter 12. As you will see there, the average person has a small need that is more than adequately met when a balanced diet that includes meat, eggs, and vegetables is coupled with the maintenance of normal vitamin D levels. However, no dairy is required.

The concept of a general calcium deficiency assumes that a localized lack of calcium in the bones means that there is an overall lack of calcium in the body. In large part, this idea has been perpetuated by the dairy industry, but it is simply not true. If you want to consume dairy products that is certainly your choice. However, do not be misled into thinking that dairy consumption is essential, or that avoiding such products will result in an inadequate dietary intake of calcium.

Aside from extraordinarily peculiar and faddish diets that are focused on eating only a handful of different foods, deficient calcium assimilation will only result when your vitamin D levels are chronically low. Maintain normal circulating levels of vitamin D, eat a balanced diet without feeling compelled to eat dairy when you are not otherwise inclined to do so, and you will assimilate all the calcium your body needs. However, until you address your toxin exposures and your hormone deficiencies (to be discussed later), you will not prevent or resolve osteoporosis regardless of whether you are ingesting an appropriate or even elevated amount of dietary calcium.

Myth #3: "Everyone with osteoporosis has a calcium deficiency."

While not a completely incorrect statement, the complete truth is that all osteoporosis patients have calcium deficiencies in their bones. Throughout the rest of their bodies, however, they actually have excesses of calcium. The scientific evidence for this was addressed in great detail in Chapter 1. And even though much of the evidence demonstrating the chronic presence of excess calcium outside the bones is unequivocal and published in prominent medical journals, the mindset of both patients and their treating physicians continues to be that the obvious lack of calcium content in osteoporotic bones must mean that the body as a whole is depleted of calcium as well.

Ironically, it is the chronic loss of calcium from osteoporotic bone that fuels the excesses of calcium elsewhere in the body. Nevertheless, it is precisely this notion of a generalized "calcium deficiency" that has doctors and motivated laypersons alike always striving to supplement calcium or ingest more of it in their diets. Supplemental and excess dietary calcium does nothing good for the bones, while it decreases lifespan and increases the severity and symptomatology of virtually all chronic diseases

> *Ironically, it is the chronic loss of calcium from osteoporotic bone that fuels the excesses of calcium elsewhere in the body.*

before death finally occurs. And the scientific evidence for this is clear-cut as well.

Myth #4: "Calcium supplementation prevents fractures."

Admittedly, there are studies that report calcium supplementation is effective in decreasing the incidence of fractures in osteoporotic patients. Upon close examination, however, poor study designs leave more questions than answers. Osteoporotic fractures are not extremely common and often do not manifest until someone has had the disease for many years.

These realities make the size and duration of a fracture study very important. In some of the trials the number of subjects (cohort size) was very small, and in others the duration of the trial was very short. Additionally, some of these investigations were dependent upon the accuracy of the subject's self-observation and memory to determine the quantity and frequency of calcium supplement use. [2] Imagine having to remember (especially at an older age) how much calcium you've taken over the past ten years, or even one year. How accurate could that be?

Other studies failed to use methods to control patient and observer bias (such as double-blind placebo-controlled) where subjects and researchers are not allowed to know which subjects are using the tested therapy and which are simply using a non-active ingredient (a inactive pill or placebo). This prevents anyone, intentionally or otherwise, from swaying the results because of their own expectations or prejudice.

Nevertheless, placebo-controlled, long-term, large population studies that specifically investigate the isolated use of calcium and its impact on bone fractures in osteoporotic patients are decidedly lacking. However, many investigations involving the supplementation of calcium in tandem with vitamin D provide more than enough data to reliably conclude: Calcium supplementation does not prevent bone fractures.[3]

When properly analyzed the conflicting results from many calcium-vitamin D trials actually provide clear evidence that calcium alone does not reduce the incidence of fractures. Some of the trials concluded that vitamin D and calcium together did not reduce the risk of bone fracture while others produced a positive result. Closer examination of the data reveals that the success or failure of individual trials is dependent upon the amount of vitamin D used in conjunction with calcium supplementation.[4]

Three vitamin D studies, when evaluated with a statistical comparison of 12 others (a meta-analysis), further illustrate the singular importance of the vitamin D dosage administered. When 800 IU of vitamin D was given along with calcium to elderly women a significant reduction in bone fractures was observed.[5]

> *Calcium-vitamin D trials actually provide clear evidence that calcium alone does not reduce the incidence of fractures.*

A seemingly conflicting result was achieved in the much larger Women's Health Initiative study. However, these women were given calcium with only 400 IU of vitamin D. Even though a significant improvement in bone density was seen, no reduction in fracture incidence was demonstrated.[6] The meta-analysis of the dozen studies, some with and some without calcium supplementation, found that a daily vitamin D dose of 700 to 800 IU reduced fracture risk while a dose of 400 IU did not.[7]

Adequately dosed vitamin D supplementation, when investigated alone, has also repeatedly shown a decreased fracture risk.[8-10] A study on stress fracture incidence in female adolescents reached similar conclusions. Higher vitamin D intake produced lower stress fracture risk, while calcium intake demonstrated no clear link.[11]

While it might increase bone density, calcium does not decrease fracture risk.

Other studies have looked at women with and without previously diagnosed osteoporosis. It was found that the fracture rate was not related to the amounts of calcium consumed, high or low.[12,13]

Also, calcium supplementation does not prevent new fractures in elderly patients who have previously experienced a fracture — that was the finding of a randomized and placebo-controlled study.[14] Another study found no association between calcium ingestion and hip fracture risk in women, even when the calcium ingested was from milk.[15]

Collectively, these studies provide three powerful conclusions:

1. Any reduction in bone fractures attributed to calcium is actually due to the inclusion of adequately-dosed vitamin D.
2. Vitamin D plays a leading role in promoting normal bone physiology and formation in addition to its ability to increase calcium assimilation from the diet or from calcium supplements.
3. And finally, while it might increase bone density, **calcium does not decrease fracture risk.**

There's an important caution, however: Even though many vitamin D studies show that the minimal daily dose of vitamin D needs to be somewhere between 400 and 800 IU in order to reduce fracture risk, this still does not indicate that such an amount of vitamin D supplementation is the optimal or appropriate amount. That will be discussed later.

Myth #5: "Increased bone density always means stronger bones."

A bone density test, or bone densitometry, will reliably reflect the content of calcium in the bone being studied. When a younger person who has not been taking calcium supplements or ingesting large amounts of dietary calcium has a normal reading on such a scan it can reasonably be assumed that there is no significant osteoporosis present and it can also be assumed that the bone is of normal strength with a normal resistance to fracture. This is because the normal calcium content in the bone in a young healthy individual is also a reflection of normal amounts of related structural components in the bone as well.

However, when a higher score relative to a lower earlier score results following the extended administration of large amounts of calcium supplementation, it is only a reflection of increased calcium content in the bone, not of a normal structural matrix in the bone. Such bone only looks good, test-wise, but it has no greater resistance to fracture than the diseased bone before the new calcium deposition.

There is no question that baseline bone density tests are quite useful in the diagnosis of osteoporosis. Osteoporosis has lowered bony calcium content and this decline in calcium content (along with the other components of the structural bony matrix) will always reflect a lowered bone density.

However, when osteoporosis is being treated with increased calcium intake the bone density can legitimately increase, but the quality of the bone does not improve unless other important factors are addressed. Also, lower amounts of calcium supplementation might only reduce the rate of bone density decline rather than increase it outright,[16] but this still does not mean the calcium alone has helped in any way to prevent deterioration of the underlying structural bone integrity.

The increased density resulting from calcium supplementation is a cosmetic improvement only.

With regard to the underlying osteoporosis, then, the increased bone density resulting from calcium supplementation is a cosmetic improvement only (just like the fresh coat of paint on the rotten fence metaphor mentioned earlier). There continues to be no clear evidence that calcium supplements alone reduce fracture risk regardless of what effect they might have on bone density.[17]

When the calcium supplementation is accompanied by some degree of vitamin D supplementation, as noted above, fracture risk can be positively impacted depending on the amount of vitamin D being supplemented. It is also important to note that increased dietary calcium results in a higher bone density when vitamin D levels are quite low.

When vitamin D levels reach only the minimally deficient point, further increases of calcium in the diet no longer relate to increased bone mineral density[18] since the increased calcium uptake facilitated by the minimal amounts of vitamin D present is all that is needed.

Adequate vitamin D supplementation by itself results in increased bone mineral density and a lessened chance of fracture. This is further evidence that calcium intake, with or without supplementation, should never be increased for the purposes of bone health (or even general health, for that matter). Such supplementation offers no bone benefits and has many significant side effects, including an increase in all-cause mortality.

Myth #6: "The biggest danger faced by someone with osteoporosis is disability or death following a fracture."

When a person who has osteoporosis fractures a bone it's serious business. There is no doubt about that. Such an event can immediately incapacitate and it often leads to death in a relatively short period of time. However, dying or suffering from a heart attack, from any of a variety of cancers, or even from a stroke is not a desirable alternative to sustaining a fracture.

Nevertheless, this is exactly what often happens. A groundbreaking study made it very clear that a fracture is not the major concern for a majority of osteoporosis patients. A large study followed nearly 10,000 postmenopausal women with documented low bone mineral density over roughly a three-year period. It was found that there was a 60% increase in the risk of death in individuals with the lowest quintile (20%) of bone density compared to those individuals in the highest quintile. Most of the deaths, however, did not relate to a fracture. [19]

> *Low bone mineral density was associated with a 60% increase in the risk of death...most of the deaths, however, did not relate to a fracture.*

The likely reason for this is straightforward. Substantial data indicates a correlation between atherosclerosis and osteoporosis. [20] The more advanced the osteoporosis, the more calcium has been released from the bones over time. This release literally showers all the other tissues and organs of the body with a chronic excess calcium exposure.

Consistent with this concept, it was found in another prospective study on postmenopausal women that the less dense the bone was the greater the chance of sustaining a stroke. It was also noted that the inverse relationship to bone density was strongest for intracerebral hemorrhages and occlusions, events that would be promoted by calcium deposition in the arteries.[21]

> The chronic release of calcium from osteoporotic bone not only accelerates heart disease, but all diseases.

Another study showed that low bone mineral density was related to atherosclerosis in a group of postmenopausal women.[22]

In a group of **pre**menopausal women with Takayasu arteritis, a chronic inflammatory condition, it was found that severe arterial calcification was consistently associated with low bone mineral density. Furthermore, it was found that a longer disease duration was seen in those individuals with severe arterial calcification.[23] This also strongly supports the concept that arterial calcification and atherosclerosis are substantially fed and worsened by mobilization of calcium from osteoporotic bones with the contribution being significantly greater the more advanced and chronic the osteoporosis has been present.[24-27]

Perhaps the clearest indication that the most advanced degrees of osteoporosis seed the most calcium throughout the body comes from a study that correlated bone mineral density to death from all causes. In a study that tracked 3,501 adults over a period of up to 22 years, a total of 1,530 deaths occurred. A significant inverse relationship to all-cause mortality was found in black men and women as well as in white men with decreased bone mineral density. This decreased bone density also predicted death from all non-cardiac causes in the entire group.[28] It was shown as well that postmenopausal women with cardiovascular disease have increased risk of osteoporotic fracture.[29]

It is clear, then, that the chronic release of calcium from osteoporotic bone to the rest of the body not only accelerates heart disease, but all diseases, resulting in significantly decreased longevity. Increased vascular calcification in general has been shown to be associated with increased all-cause mortality.[30] Even though with current technology calcium is often quantified and tracked in the coronary arteries, its accumulation there pretty much means it is accumulating in many different areas of the body at the same time, thereby worsening all chronic diseases in the process. This means that the osteoporosis disease process is life-shortening far beyond the chance of osteoporotic fracture and potentially eventual death secondary to that event.

Older women with osteoporosis are already fighting an uphill battle. They should not have to deal with the toxic challenge of supplemental calcium.

As calcium excess in the body has been found to increase all-cause mortality and to literally be the most significant marker for increased cardiac risk (coronary artery calcium score), this should come as no surprise. What should be taken from this is that older women with osteoporosis are already fighting an uphill battle against diseases caused and aggravated by excess calcium released from their own bones. They should not have to deal with the additional toxic challenge of supplemental calcium and increased dietary calcium that have been assumed to be positive interventions in the treatment of their disease. It is especially difficult for patients who are being told to increase their calcium ingestion by healthcare providers who continue to ignore an increasingly large body of evidence on the long-term toxicity of such calcium intake. No patient is comfortable having to ignore the direct advice of his or her physician.

Vitamin D does much more than increase calcium absorption; it plays many roles in the metabolism of virtually all the cells of the body.

Myth #7: "Vitamin D just serves to increase calcium absorption."

This continues to be a pretty common misconception even though it has been established to be wrong for a long time now. Data has been accumulating since the 1980s on the presence of vitamin D receptors outside of the bone, kidney, and intestine where it had already been established to play a prominent role in calcium metabolism. [31-36] It is now well-documented in a very large body of scientific data in many different scientific journals that vitamin D has receptors throughout the body. Furthermore, vitamin D is now known to have a direct effect on about 200 genes with indirect effects on as many as 2,000 genes. [37-39]

So even though vitamin D does play an essential role in regulating and modulating calcium absorption and metabolism via its interactions with the bones, gut, and kidneys, it plays many additional vital roles in the metabolism of virtually all the cells of the body, as the widespread presence of so many vitamin D receptors would indicate. Receptors only exist if there is a purpose for their being bound to something. Many of these other functions are itemized in Chapter 8.

Unfortunately, and even a bit amazingly, many doctors still approach vitamin D as being essentially only another way to "supplement" calcium, in spite of the enormous amount of clear scientific evidence to the contrary. What is also true is that vitamin D not only facilitates the absorption of calcium from the diet, it will also reliably "overdose" that absorption when foods with high-calcium content (usually dairy) have vitamin D artificially added to them. When vitamin D is simultaneously supplemented along with any forms of specific calcium supplementation or just increased dietary calcium intake, the "overdose" absorption effect comes even more into play as well.

Just as vitamin D plays an essential role in the proper incorporation of calcium into newly generated bony mineral matrix, it is also essential that it be allowed to naturally regulate the amount of calcium coming in from the diet for an optimal calcium homeostasis to be reached. Only the poorest of diets do not have enough calcium in them for normal circulating levels of vitamin D to absorb and utilize all that is needed for bone and body health.

There really is no clearly defined syndrome of a primary calcium deficiency in man, although there is an age-related gradual loss of bone and bony calcium content that is unrelated to dietary calcium intake.[40] One of the reasons many think that such deficiencies exist is that they can be readily induced in laboratory animals on severely calcium-restricted diets. Such animals then develop significant bone loss.[41] However, no diets eaten by man are so restricted. And because there is no primary calcium deficiency syndrome the many factors involved in the abnormal physiology of bone aging, osteopenia, and osteoporosis need to be addressed comprehensively instead of just simplistically putting as much calcium inside the body as possible. When vitamin D levels are optimized, there is no longer an issue of inadequate calcium intake.

Myth #8: "You get all the vitamin D you need from the sun."

This statement would be true if someone actually spent a minimum of 30 to 60 minutes a day in the sun with enough skin area exposed, and in a part of the world close enough to the equator so that adequate vitamin D-generating ultraviolet light was penetrating the atmospheric barrier. The more accurate assertion would be that persons who receive enough skin exposure to the sun in the right areas of the world might be able to get all the vitamin D they need. However, the truth is that the modern way of living is very effective in shielding most people from the sun so completely that even a large percentage of individuals living in tropical climates are chronically deficient in vitamin D.[42,43] This truth is even more valid for the dark-skinned populations,[44] as the increased melanin in the skin further screens out so much of the vitamin D-generating ultraviolet light that even the 30 to 60 minute daily sun exposure goal mentioned above would generally be insufficient under otherwise optimal circumstances. Therefore, for nearly everyone on the planet, vitamin D supplementation is a must in order to get its blood levels in the range now known to support optimal bone health and general health.

CHAPTER 4

The Truth About Osteoporosis

The Real Reason Bones Become Brittle and Calcium Deficient

Osteoporosis (literally: "porous bones") is defined as a deterioration of the structural matrix of the bone associated with a continuous migration of calcium out of the bone along with an increased risk of fracture that worsens as the disease progresses. As demonstrated in the previous chapter, adding dietary and/or supplementary calcium does not diminish fracture risk. And while the root cause of this disease remains unaddressed and more and more calcium is leached from the bones, bone strength decreases and fracture risk increases.

Unfortunately it is the persistent fear of fracture that motivates increased calcium intake with little regard for the far greater health risks that result from such intake. A failure to address the fact that osteoporotic bone tissues have lost the ability to incorporate calcium and structural proteins into the bone matrix can be deadly. Since the body's ability to excrete excess calcium is limited, all remaining amounts accumulate in other parts of the body. Such depositions are directly linked to a significantly increased risk of heart disease, cancer, high blood pressure, stroke, and many other chronic degenerative diseases as well.

Truly, calcium migration from bone is quite serious. Nevertheless, it is not the cause of osteoporosis, but rather a symptom of it. The steady loss of calcium from osteoporotic bone is only evidence that the disease is evolving, it is not the disease itself. Giving calcium to bones already ravaged by osteoporosis makes as much sense as giving the cardiac enzymes released during a heart attack back to the patient. Just as the calcium will not restore the complex structural matrix of the bone, the enzymes will not magically grow new heart muscle.

> *Calcium migration from the bone is not the cause of osteoporosis, but rather a symptom of it.*

Unfortunately, traditional medicine often takes the "treat-the-symptom" approach with every degenerative disease. This is certainly the case with osteoporosis. Giving large amounts of calcium will eventually result in a small amount of it filling in pores in osteoporotic bones. However, it cannot be emphasized strongly enough that this approach is simply cosmetic. It will make the bones look somewhat better on a bone density test, but it does no more to improve bone strength than blowing finely ground chalk into the cracks of an earthquake-damaged building will restore its structural integrity. (Similarly, a fresh coat of paint on a rotting wooden fence will never make the fence stronger.) And such is precisely the case with osteoporotic bone. The cause has to be addressed, not the appearance. Successful prevention and reversal of osteoporosis must involve the elimination of the underlying cause of calcium migration from the bone.

The Root Cause of Osteoporosis

Bones perform four vital roles. Three of these — structural support, organ protection, and the production of blood cells — are commonly acknowledged. A fourth, as important but less celebrated function, is the storage of minerals for on-demand use by other parts of the body. These minerals include magnesium and phosphorus, but by far, the most plentiful of these warehoused minerals is calcium.

Blood levels of calcium are tightly regulated, perhaps one of the most strictly controlled processes in the body.

The best way to visualize this storage role of bones is to think of them as a mineral "bank." As previously noted, blood levels of calcium are tightly regulated, perhaps one of the most strictly controlled processes in the body. When calcium blood concentrations start to fall below the base level, calcium can be "withdrawn" from the bones. On the other hand, as calcium blood concentrations begin to approach the upper limit in a healthy individual, it is often "deposited" in the bones.

The process of withdrawing calcium from bones is called resorption, whereas the reincorporation of calcium back into the bone matrix is called absorption. These two processes, absorption and resorption, are constantly changing the shape and structure of the bone in a cycle that is called bone remodeling.

In addition to maintaining mineral blood levels (homeostasis), bone remodeling has many purposes. As children grow into adulthood, there are bones that fuse together (as in the skull), and others that must grow in length and girth. The change in load bearing needs during pregnancy also call for a remodeling of some of the bones to meet that need. Exercise forces bone remodeling as muscles grow and require more skeletal support. Additionally, the normal stresses of life cause micro- and mini-fractures in bone tissues that normally go unnoticed but ultimately weaken structural strength. Bone remodeling is the process the body uses to shape and heal these fractures.

Under certain conditions resorption (withdrawal of calcium from the bones) is abnormally high and absorption (deposition of calcium in the bones) is abnormally low. When calcium withdrawals in the bone continually exceed deposits, the calcium deficit results in osteoporosis.

Several factors contribute to an osteoporotic condition but there is one that is responsible for the lion's share of calcium loss. It initiates and severely worsens an imbalance in the bone remodeling (absorption-resorption cycle) and it prevents incorporation of calcium into the bone matrix. In clinical terms, the major cause of osteoporosis is a focal scurvy of the bones.

A large body of scientific evidence shows that reversing the focal scurvy improves bone density, reduces fracture risk, and greatly lowers all-cause mortality. The remedy is inexpensive, wildly effective, and totally safe. And yet, hardly anyone in mainstream medicine talks about it or is even aware of it. Quite simply, scurvy (severe vitamin C deficiency), whether general or localized (focal), can be prevented, cured, and reversed with appropriate dosing and administration of vitamin C and other important nutrients. (Recommended vitamin C protocols are discussed in specific protocol chapters and Appendix B.)

Vitamin C, Bones, and Osteoporosis

The creation of the structural matrix essential for the development of strong bone requires special cells called osteoblasts [literally bone seeds or bone makers]. Osteoblasts are the key players in the production of new bone.

They produce an organic material called bone matrix that contains Type 1 collagen. Bone matrix is the mortar that captures and incorporates calcium and multiple other minerals into the network of interconnected collagen fibers to make the final product of hard bone tissue. Another type of special cell, the osteoclast [bone eater] literally dissolves crystalline bone tissue in the resorption process. Just as osteoblasts create new bone, osteoclasts destroy existing bone.

In healthy children, the balance between bone-making osteoblasts and bone-dissolving osteoclasts favors the osteoblasts in order to meet the needs of growing bones. As we age the balance between them progressively shifts toward increasing osteoclast activity, setting the stage for the onset and the evolution of osteoporosis. Vitamin C's involvement in maintaining a healthy osteoblast/osteoclast balance is well documented. [1,2]

A focal bone scurvy initiates a severe loss in bone-building cells and an unchecked increase in bone-dissolving cells.

In the absence of vitamin C, bone-making osteoblasts fail to form. At the same time, since vitamin C impedes the creation of bone-dissolving osteoclasts, a focal scurvy inside the bones will allow them to multiply in an uncontrolled manner, thus initiating the imbalance that results in a detrimental breakdown of the bone integrity, along with calcium loss. [3,4] This scurvy-caused imbalance has been tested and observed in vitamin C-deficient laboratory animals. [5] By itself the fact that a focal bone scurvy initiates a severe loss in bone-building cells and an unchecked increase in bone-dissolving cells qualifies it as the cause of osteoporosis. However, vitamin C's involvement in the production/destruction balance in the bone is far more extensive.

A deficiency of vitamin C in the bones also directly increases the oxidative stress there. Oxidative stress is a destructive process that greatly impairs the production of healthy bone matrix, and it even prevents that production when the bony vitamin C deficiency/oxidative stress excess is sufficiently pronounced. It occurs when highly aggressive oxidizing compounds attack cellular structures causing damage and even death of the cell.

A vitamin C deficiency results in weaker bones.

Whether these aggressive, pro-oxidant molecules are byproducts of normal metabolism or toxins from outside sources, they increase in quantity in the absence of neutralization from sufficient vitamin C.

Increased oxidative stress can cause damage wherever it occurs, including outside of the cells in the bone as well. The presence of oxidative stress in the bones inhibits normal bone metabolism while directly resulting in greater bone resorption and destruction.

Studies in cell cultures, animals, and humans have confirmed the role of oxidative stress in the cause and development of osteoporosis.[6] The neutralization of bony oxidative stress by the antioxidant properties of vitamin C is another way in which vitamin C can prevent or lessen the evolution of osteoporosis.[7]

There is yet another way that vitamin C is foundational in the formation of healthy, fracture-resistant bone tissue. As mentioned above, osteoblasts use Type I collagen in combination with various minerals to form bone matrix. A ready supply of vitamin C is essential for the synthesis of collagen, and also for creating the fibrous interconnecting of collagen strands (cross-linking) required to optimize the physical strength and resilience of the bones.[8,9] Consistent with these effects, a vitamin C deficiency results in weaker bones.[10]

To recap, vitamin C's foundational roles in the formation and maintenance of healthy bone tissue include but are not limited to:

- Creation of bone-building osteoblasts
- Suppression of bone-dissolving osteoclasts
- Prevention of bone-destroying oxidative stress
- Synthesis of collagen
- Formation of bone-strengthening collagen cross-links

Vitamin C Prevents Bone Loss and Fractures

The clinical manifestations of generalized scurvy, the ultimate vitamin C deficiency, include decreased calcium deposition in bone tissues. It is also characterized by an increase in calcium excretion and/or calcium deposition into various non-bone tissues similar to the calcium depositions observed in atherosclerosis when vitamin C is profoundly depleted in the arterial walls.[11]

The clinical manifestations of scurvy, the ultimate vitamin C deficiency, include decreased calcium deposition in bone tissues.

A female's loss of estrogen production quickly results in osteoporotic calcium loss. Experimenting with mice that had their ovaries removed, research demonstrated that vitamin C supplementation compensates for this bone calcium loss.[12] Greater bone mineral density has also been reported in postmenopausal women who take vitamin C supplements.[13] A similar finding showed that women between the ages of 55 and 64 years of age who had taken vitamin C supplements for 10 years or more but who had NOT taken estrogen (an agent strongly supportive of healthy bone), had a higher bone mineral density than those who did not. [14]

Several clinical studies demonstrate the importance of vitamin C supplementation in the prevention of bone loss. [15-20] In contrast with dietary intake alone the need for and benefits of aggressive vitamin C supplementation was shown in a 17-year bone-fracture study with nearly 1,000 subjects between the ages of 70 and 80. The researchers reported that dietary vitamin C intake alone, without additional supplementation, provided no protection from fracture risk. In contrast, subjects who took vitamin C supplements showed a significant decrease in fracture risk in proportion to the amount of vitamin C supplemented — the higher the dose, the lower the risk of fractures. [21] This study also reinforces the fact that the true benefits of vitamin C cannot be realized by any amount of dietary vitamin C, but requires regular, significantly-dosed supplementation.

A dramatic rise in bone fracture risk accompanies low vitamin C levels, while increased vitamin C levels accompany clear decreases in fracture risk.

The significance of vitamin C's protective role in bone health has also been shown in blood level studies. A dramatic rise in bone fracture risk accompanies low vitamin C levels, while increased vitamin C levels accompany clear decreases in fracture risk.

"Significantly lower" blood concentrations of vitamin C were found in elderly patients who fractured their hips when compared to those who had not sustained such a fracture. [22] In the Framingham Osteoporosis Study, the subjects with the highest intake of vitamin C had significantly fewer hip and non-vertebral fractures compared to those with the lowest intake. Researchers also noted that intake of vitamin C limited to dietary sources alone had no statistically significant reduction of fractures; vitamin C supplementation was required to realize a decrease in risk.[23]

A similar conclusion comes from a study of individuals who had sustained low-energy fractures. Those of matched gender and age who had sustained fractures were found to have lower vitamin C levels.[24] Similarly, patients who had already sustained a recent hip fracture were found to have significantly low serum levels of vitamin C.[25] Consistent with these findings is the fact that mice with induced vitamin C deficiencies demonstrate increased spontaneous bone fractures.[26]

Patients with the higher intakes of vitamins C and E had lessened risk of osteoporotic fractures compared to those with lower intakes.

Not surprisingly, other antioxidants along with vitamin C appear important for good bone health as well. Researchers reported that the levels of not only vitamin C, but also other important antioxidants were found to be "markedly decreased" in a group of elderly women with osteoporosis.[27] In a different investigation, patients with the higher intakes of vitamins C and E had a lessened risk of osteoporotic fractures compared to those with lower intakes.[28]

Vitamin C Deficiency, Osteoporosis, and Coronary Heart Disease

The relationship connecting a chronic vitamin C deficiency, excess calcium, and osteoporosis becomes a self-perpetuating degenerative process that is responsible for far more than increasing bone fracture risk.

As previously mentioned in Chapter 1, non-bone depositions of calcium can initiate and contribute to degenerative disease conditions. Research continues to reveal the dangerous synergy between excess calcium and vitamin C deficiencies as these two are frequently found together at the tissue sites associated with different chronic degenerative diseases. We already know that calcium deposits contribute to oxidative stress. And it is also well-established that oxidative activity can continue unchallenged in a chain reaction of damage and destruction in the absence of vitamin C and/or other antioxidants.

Even though unchallenged oxidative stress has already been linked to virtually every disease known to man it is certainly not the only disease mechanism imposed by the combination of excess calcium and focal scurvy. These additional mechanisms are particularly visible in the progression of coronary heart disease. Just as a focal scurvy in the bones initiates a depletion of calcium stored there, a focal scurvy in the coronary arteries creates a magnet for the deposition of that mobilized calcium.

The mechanisms for this are developed more fully in my books, **Primal Panacea**, and even more thoroughly in **Stop America's #1 Killer!** For this discussion it is sufficient to understand that arterial lesions are initiated by a localized deficiency of vitamin C in the inner lining of those vessels. And just as the body's compensatory response to an open wound in the skin produces a scab, the body's response to an area of progressive weakness in a coronary artery wall produces calcium-rich arterial plaque. Calcium in the blood serves as a ready source for plaque growth. Then as calcium is pulled from the bloodstream it is replenished by more calcium released from osteoporotic bones, as well as any excess ingested calci-

Relationship Between Vitamin C and Osteoporosis

With Optimal Vitamin C Levels

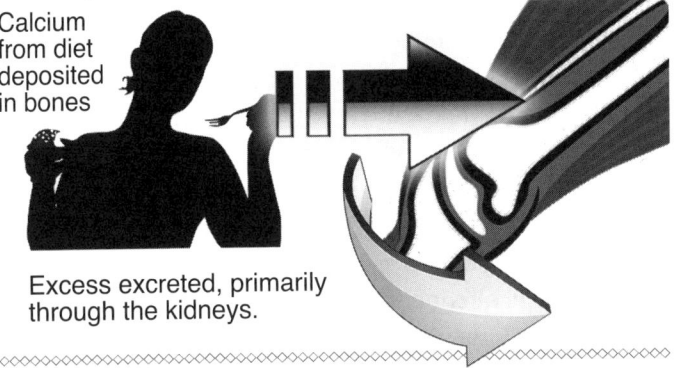

Calcium from diet deposited in bones

Excess excreted, primarily through the kidneys.

Deficient Vitamin C Levels / Focal Bone Scurvy

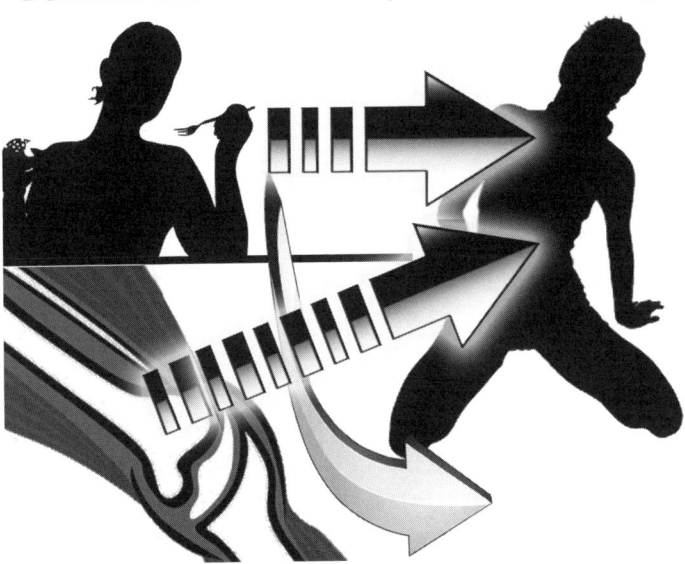

Calcium from diet PLUS calcium pulled from bones increases excess in blood. Some excess calcium in the blood is excreted, remaining calcium is deposited into cells and non-bone tissues throughout the body (e.g. brain, prostate, breasts, coronary arteries).

um. In this manner, a chronic vitamin C deficiency — both focal or generalized — sets the stage for a continuous mobilization of calcium from bones to evolving plaques in the coronary arteries.

As reported earlier, over a third of Americans over the age of 45 have evidence of arterial calcification.[29] Over half of all Americans over 50 have or will develop full-blown coronary heart disease. The calcification of arteries is so intrinsically related to coronary disease that the measurement of calcification in these vessels is a very accurate and useful tool in assessing the development and progression of the disease.[30,31]

The logical conclusion is simple: The elimination of vitamin C deficiencies and their causes is a required first step in preventing and treating both osteoporosis and atherosclerosis. These and other factors will be more fully addressed in subsequent chapters.

SECTION TWO:

Agents for Reversing Osteoporosis

CHAPTER 5

Building a Fracture-Resistant Frame

Vitamin C: The Foundation and Cornerstone of Strong Bones

Nothing in this book is intended to minimize the debilitating and even potentially fatal consequences of advanced osteoporosis. Bone fracture arising from osteoporosis is serious business!

Researchers are predicting that the annual incidence of osteoporotic bone fractures will top three million by 2025. In today's terms treatment of these fractures will cost over $28 billion.[1] According to the U.S. Surgeon General, nearly one in four women over age 50 fall once a year and by age 85 roughly half of women experience an annual fall. For men in the same age range the corresponding figures are about one in six climbing to over one in three falls per year.[2-4] Of course not every tumble results in a fracture, but each holds that potential.

As we have already seen, neither increased dietary calcium nor calcium supplementation lowers fracture risk. Despite the research showing the ineffectiveness of calcium therapies and the overwhelming evidence showing their toxicity and danger, it remains almost universally accepted that the best approaches to treating osteoporosis should always feature calcium supplementation.

The measuring stick and main goal of such therapy is the improvement of bone density tests. The scientific literature reveals that this approach produces nothing more than a cosmetic cover-up.

Vitamin C exhibits unparalleled protective and even curative effects in nearly every infectious disease and toxin exposure known to man.

If osteoporosis is actually a focal scurvy of the bones (as seen in Chapter 4), it is only natural that a reversal of the disease would require bringing vitamin C levels up to normal — in the bones as well as the rest of the body. Although vitamin C exhibits unparalleled protective and even curative effects in nearly every infectious disease and toxic exposure known to man, it's role in the physiology of bone synthesis and maintenance extends far beyond its antioxidant and antimicrobial properties.

Vitamin C: Essential in Bone Physiology — From Start to Finish

As discussed in the previous chapter, the physiology of bone involves an ongoing interplay of the following factors:

1. Bone formation (absorption), which includes the uptake and incorporation of minerals, including calcium, into the bony matrix
2. Bone destruction (resorption), where minerals are released from the bone, including calcium
3. Oxidative stress (modulation), with low levels favoring healthy bone formation and high levels favoring bone destruction and calcium release

Vitamin C is a key player in each of these processes. It is so important in the formation and maintenance of strong, resilient bones that osteoporosis can justly be blamed on a focal bone scurvy. To the degree that this vitamin C deficiency exists there will be a corresponding failure to effectively prevent or treat osteoporosis and the subsequent increase in fracture risk.

To the degree that vitamin C deficiency exists in the bone, there will be a corresponding failure to effectively prevent or treat osteoporosis.

The proliferation of osteoblasts (these bone-forming cells are discussed in more detail in Chapter 4) is essential for sufficient creation of new, strong bone material. Vitamin C stimulates the bone stem cells [mesenchymal cells] to produce osteoblasts [5,6] as well as simulating the proliferation of the stem cells themselves.[7] And vitamin C also is essential for the formation of Type III collagen, which is required for the accelerated growth of osteoblasts.[8]

Conversely, and just as importantly, vitamin C inhibits the proliferation of osteoclasts (these bone-destroying cells are also discussed more fully in Chapter 4).[9] Therefore, when a vitamin C deficiency is present osteoclasts proliferate and bone resorption increases.[10] When vitamin C levels get sufficiently low in the bone structure new bone cell formation declines, bone destruction increases, and overall bone loss accelerates.[11] All of this results in the release of the osteoporosis marker, calcium, from the bony matrix.

Vitamin C is also required for the formation and maintenance of healthy collagen. This protein imparts tensile strength to bones and everywhere else it is found. Collagen comprises about 90% of the bony matrix protein.

Whenever vitamin C availability falls there is a corresponding drop in the quality and quantity of the collagen produced. Insufficient and/or inferior collagen negatively impacts bone micro-architecture, resulting in increased bone fragility and decreased bone strength.

Of note, this increased fragility is largely independent of bone density. That is especially true when the increased bone density was the result of vigorous calcium supplementation instead of measures designed to reverse the physiological cause of the osteoporosis.

There are commonly used agents that can legitimately result in the preservation of bone or synthesis of new bone, such as estrogen, bisphosphonates, calcitonin, and/or parathormone. As useful as these agents can be they must still be combined with a vigorous antioxidant therapy led by vitamin C or they will simply increase bone density **without** significantly restoring bone quality. To be physically strong and resilient the collagen-dominated matrix of the bone **must have** a continual, generous supply of vitamin C.

Another important part of that resilient strength in bone involves cross-linking. Cross-linking is a chemical process that forms a powerful fibrous net interconnecting the collagen fibers. Vitamin C strongly supports this physiological process as well. [12,13] In summary, even if a particular drug therapy is improving bone mineral density test scores, vitamin C is still essential in restoring strength and resilience to bones.

> *To be physically strong and resilient, the collagen-dominated matrix of the bone must have a continual, generous supply of vitamin C.*

Vitamin C: Frontline Defender Against Oxidative Stress

The same array of toxic (pro-oxidant) insults to the body that initiate and fuel osteoporosis cause cancer, heart disease, and other chronic degenerative diseases. How and which diseases manifest in any particular individual is determined by a combination of genetic predisposition and the nature of the toxic insult. As more oxidative stress is generated in the bone tissue the vitamin C and other antioxidants inside the bone matrix are de-energized (oxidized). At the point where levels of energized (reduced) antioxidants are outnumbered by a continuing influx of toxins and/or increasing oxidative stress a focal scurvy begins.

Increased oxidative stress is always accompanied by decreased antioxidant presence in affected tissues.

With very few exceptions a large and steady toxic insult (such as is generated from root canal-treated teeth) will produce some degree of increased oxidative stress throughout the body. It will be the unique biological susceptibilities of the individual that determine whether the infectious and/or toxic exposure will first result in a heart attack, breast cancer, an osteoporotic fracture, or something else consistent with underlying conditions and genetic predispositions.

Increased oxidative stress is always accompanied by decreased antioxidant presence in affected tissues. Low or absent antioxidant levels allow oxidative stress to begin or to become more severe. In fact, if oxidative stress in the bones is held to normal levels by the presence of sufficient antioxidants osteoporosis cannot develop or evolve.

Elevated levels of oxidative stress are frequently accompanied by the increased presence of C-reactive protein, which is a well-established laboratory test correlating with body-wide inflammation. High levels of C-reactive protein reliably predict increased chances of osteoporotic fracture in elderly women.[14] High doses of vitamin C have been shown to significantly reduce levels of C-reactive protein and the other molecules [cytokines] that signal the presence of inflammation.[15] In addition, a strong relationship has been reported between the increased fracture risk resulting from osteoporosis and chronic degenerative diseases with observable inflammation.[16]

> *Bone density in individuals with substantially more vitamin C intake than is possible via dietary sources was found to be significantly higher at all sites tested.*

Unless oxidative stress in the bony matrix is normalized very early in the development of osteoporosis, however, such normalization by itself is generally not sufficient to allow the regeneration of a healthy bone structure. Nevertheless, failure to address increased oxidative stress in the bone will limit, and even prevent, healthy new bone synthesis.

Vitamin C Supplementation Increases Bone Density

Research demonstrating the strong relationship between vitamin C deficiency and osteoporosis includes some bone density studies. One such study found that postmenopausal women with higher dietary intakes of vitamin C had greater bone mineral density, but only in the lumbar region of the spine.[17] However, in those who supplemented with vitamin C — individuals with substantially more vitamin C intake than is possible via dietary sources — bone mineral density was found to be significantly higher at **all sites** tested. The increased density was particularly seen at the femoral neck, the typical site for most hip fractures.[18]

In an animal study, investigators demonstrated that large doses of vitamin C could actually compensate for the bone loss associated with a complete cessation of estrogen production.[19] This finding is extremely significant since the incidence of osteoporosis in women is frequently related to the drastic, menopausal reduction of estrogen production. Complete compensation for a loss of critical hormone function by a vitamin, particularly in a part of the body that is strongly dependent on that hormone to maintain normalcy, is very impressive!

Investigators demonstrated that large doses of vitamin C could actually compensate for the bone loss associated with a complete cessation of estrogen production.

Vitamin C Supplementation Lowers Fracture Risk

Even though little attention has been paid to some remarkable research on osteoporosis and vitamin C, it has been clearly established that supplemental vitamin C alone lowers the risk of osteoporotic fractures in elderly patients.[20] The Framingham Osteoporosis Study also found that the individuals with the highest levels of vitamin C supplementation had significantly fewer fractures than those with the lowest levels. Additionally, this study found that dietary vitamin C intake alone had no association with fracture risk.[21] These findings demonstrate the importance of dose and the relatively small amounts of vitamin C that are typically ingested by any dietary regimen in the absence of supplementation.

Consistent with these findings, elderly patients who had already sustained an osteoporotic fracture were found to have significantly lower blood levels of vitamin C compared to elderly patients who were fracture-free.[22] It has also been reported that elderly, osteoporotic women have markedly lower plasma levels of vitamin C and other antioxidants when compared to those of similar age without osteoporosis.[23]

Individuals with the highest levels of vitamin C supplementation had significantly fewer fractures than those with the lowest levels.

Vitamin C Supplementation Accelerates and Improves Quality of Bone Healing

Studies demonstrate that vitamin C accelerates and improves the quality of the bone healing in animals. In one study, vitamin C-supplemented rats with fractures of the tibia healed more rapidly.[24] In another study, vitamin C supplementation also produced accelerated healing in rats with fractures. Interestingly, that healing was not much affected by vitamin E, further suggesting that vitamin C's importance in bone healing extends beyond its antioxidant properties.[25]

Mechanical resistance/strength of the healing fracture area (callus) was shown to improve in elderly rats supplemented with vitamin C.[26] Vitamin C is so essential for fracture healing that a sufficient deficit in it can result in the failure of a fracture to heal.[27-29] Not only does vitamin C accelerate the bone healing process *per se*, it is also important to the:

1) Formation of non-collagen bone matrix proteins,[30]
2) Differentiation of mesenchymal stem cells into bone cells (osteocytes),[31] and

3) The regulation of cartilage-forming cells in the bone.[32]

Collectively, all these studies indicate vitamin C contributes substantially to both the speed and the quality of healing in fractured bones.

Vitamin C Supplementation Protects Against Dangerous Calcifications

Vitamin C is intimately involved in the calcium metabolism of the body. In scurvy, the ultimate deficiency state of vitamin C, irregular calcium deposits are scattered throughout the affected tissues. Furthermore, it appears that a significant vitamin C deficiency also facilitates the mobilization of calcium from the bone and its increased excretion in the urine.[33] This mobilization of calcium out of the bone to non-bone tissues or to the kidneys for elimination is basic to the evolution and worsening of osteoporosis.

Vitamin C also prevents calcification and calcium depositions by keeping calcium in a dissolved state. Calcium carbonate, one of the most insoluble of substances and the form most commonly found in abnormal calcium deposits throughout the body, can be rapidly put into solution by vitamin C. In fact, it takes strong hydrochloric acid to dissolve calcium better than vitamin C.[34,35] There is even some evidence that vitamin C can exert some calcium channel blocker-like activity, which is always desirable in treating diseases of calcium excess.[36,37]

Animal studies have demonstrated the necessity of adequate vitamin C for the support of normal bone

Vitamin C is so essential for fracture healing that a sufficient deficit in it can result in the failure of a fracture to heal.

metabolism and for incorporation of calcium into bone matrix, as well as for the formation of high quality bone. In a guinea pig study, adequate dietary calcium was unable to be deposited into bone to any significant degree while there was a vitamin C deficiency. Conversely, it was then demonstrated that the restoration of adequate vitamin C into the diet facilitated a rapid incorporation of calcium into the bone.[38] Other researchers also observed that while the total prevention of bone formation by an associated vitamin C deficiency in guinea pigs was not absolute, it was very clear that any new bone formation was limited and of poor quality.[39]

> *A vitamin C deficiency sets the stage for abnormal calcium deposition outside of the bone.*

Just as adequate vitamin C is necessary for calcium deposition in the bone, a deficiency of vitamin C sets the stage for abnormal calcium deposition outside of the bone. Men with the lowest plasma vitamin C levels had a significantly increased prevalence of coronary artery calcium deposition compared to those men with the highest plasma levels.[40]

Vitamin C Supplementation Protects Against Calcium-Laden Kidney Stones

Another manifestation of abnormal calcification in the body is seen in the formation of kidney stones. While the popular press and strongly opinionated, uninformed physicians have accused vitamin C of initiating these calcium oxalate stones, nothing could be further from the truth. Much continues to be made over the fact that vitamin C can contribute to the synthesis of oxalate in the urine. Many healthy foods and substances also contribute to the synthesis of oxalate, but oxalate does not cause kidney stones anymore than iron causes rust. Calcium oxalate crystals do not precipitate out of urine unless certain conditions exist — primarily the presence of oxidative stress. As you will soon see, rather than cause or support this precipitation, vitamin C actually fights against it.

If the synthesis and presence of oxalate were the sole cause of kidney stones, we would see a high incidence of these stones in pregnant women. A super-saturation of calcium oxalate in the urine — to the same degree observed in women who are predisposed to stone formation — is a common observation in pregnant women. And yet, normal pregnancies are **not** associated with increased calcium oxalate stone formation. [41]

> *Much evidence makes it clear that vitamin C, rather than being a cause of kidney stones, actually protects against their formation.*

Oxalate crystal formation is the necessary step before a stone can develop. In a cell epithelium study designed to closely simulate natural conditions in the kidney, vitamin C actually decreases the chances of calcium oxalate crystal formation. The primary predisposing factor for stone formation appeared to be the presence of oxidative damage to the cells. When adequately dosed, vitamin C would actually be expected to inhibit or even prevent this causative oxidative stress. [42]

In a similar type of study on kidney cells, antioxidant therapy prevented calcium oxalate precipitation. It was also noted that when calcium oxalate crystals began to form, their formation always occurred in an environment deficient of vitamin C and other antioxidants. [43] These observations indicate that oxalate stone formation is dependent upon a level of oxidative stress sufficient to damage the epithelial cells lining the kidney's interior.

This level of oxidative stress is prevented by vitamin C, not caused by it.

Much evidence makes it clear that vitamin C, rather than being a cause of kidney stones, actually protects against their formation. The ingestion of large doses of vitamin C in ten healthy males did not affect the principal risk factors associated with calcium oxalate stone formation in the kidneys.[44] In another study, urine specimens from a group of healthy male volunteers were compared with men who had recurrent calcium kidney stones. In the normal specimens, vitamin C had no effect on calcium oxalate crystal formation, while it actually inhibited crystal formation in the urines of the recurrent stone formers.[45]

> *Every 1.0 mg/dL increase in the serum vitamin C level was independently associated with a 28% decrease in the prevalence of kidney stones.*

Large prospective studies further acquit vitamin C of causative blame in the formation of stones in people with normal kidney function. In a Harvard study following 45,251 men between 40 and 75 years of age, no association was found between vitamin C and stone formation, even when vitamin C was consumed in high doses.[46]

A similar study looked at the risk of kidney stones in 85,557 women relative to vitamin C intake, and again no association with risk was found. In fact, the researchers advised that routine restriction of vitamin C intake to prevent stone formation was not warranted.[47] In another large study, the Harvard Prospective Health Professional Follow-Up Study, the individuals with the highest quintile (upper fifth) of vitamin C intake, greater than 1,500 mg daily, were found to actually have a lower risk of kidney stones when compared to those individuals in the lowest quintile (lower fifth) of vitamin C intake.[48]

In an even more conclusive study, the relation of serum levels of vitamin C to the incidence of kidney stones was examined. There was no indication that greater vitamin C levels increased the incidence of stones. Quite the contrary, in the men studied, every 1.0 mg/dL increase in the serum vitamin C level was independently associated with a 28% decrease in the prevalence of kidney stones.[49]

Observers report that administration of vitamin C actually dissolved and/or resolved preexisting stones in man and animals.[50,51] Although this observation is anecdotal, it is consistent with the calcium-dissolving properties of vitamin C described earlier.

Higher vitamin C intake resulted in fewer deaths from all causes, including deaths from coronary artery disease and cancer.

Vitamin C Supplementation Lowers All-Cause Mortality

The studies examining the relationship between vitamin C and death from all causes are very compelling. This is especially true of the relationship between vitamin C and death from heart disease or cancer. One study that looked at dietary intakes of vitamin C examined the differences in mortality between groups of men ingesting a average of 66 mg versus an average of 138 mg of vitamin C daily. Even at these low intakes of vitamin C a clear survival advantage for the group ingesting more daily vitamin C was demonstrated. The researchers reported that higher vitamin C intake resulted in fewer deaths from all causes, including deaths from coronary artery disease and cancer.[52] Another study that looked at dietary vitamin C intake also found only relatively small increases in dietary intake resulted in a substantial lessening of all-cause mortality.[53]

In fact, no toxic level of vitamin C has ever been found.

Dietary studies are always vulnerable to criticisms concerning the accuracy of intake measurement and therefore their conclusions are frequently suspect. Plasma level studies, however, leave little to no room for such criticisms. Several studies have looked at the relationship of plasma vitamin C levels and all-cause mortality. In every case the conclusion was the same: The higher the vitamin C level in the plasma, the lower the chances of death from cardiovascular disease and from all causes.[54-59]

In the subset of chronic kidney disease patients on hemodialysis, it has also been shown that the patients with the lower plasma vitamin C levels die sooner, typically from cardiovascular causes.[60,61]

These findings provide an inescapable conclusion: The more vitamin C you can get into your body, the less your chances of death from any cause.

Safety of Vitamin C Supplementation

The track record of safety for vitamin C has been well documented. Even when administered intravenously in doses as high as 200 grams (200,000 mg) at a time and given to the sickest of patients, such as for cancer and advanced infections, vitamin C has never been linked to any adverse side effect. In fact, no toxic level of vitamin C has ever been found. Except for individuals with a significant loss of kidney function, no consideration needs to be given to the possibility that too much is being supplemented. In kidney failure, however, vitamin C, or just about any other water-soluble agent that is excreted in the urine, must be dosed with consideration.

In 2007, vitamin C was the most widely sold single vitamin in the United States, a further testament that no previously unreported side effects are yet to occur.[62] As already noted above, the continued attempts to link vitamin C with kidney stones have never been founded on quality science. In fact, vitamin C reduces the incidence of kidney stones in regular supplementers.

Why so much effort should continue to be expended in undermining the enormous utility and safety of vitamin C is truly perplexing. When considering the overall safety of vitamin C, it should be realized that water would have to be considered an agent with vastly more potential toxicity than vitamin C. It has been shown that when too much water is ingested too quickly, as much as two gallons, osmotic brain edema with hyponatremia can result, and seizures leading to coma and death can result.[63] Yet, no one would ever consider water to be a toxic substance. Nevertheless, too much of it can kill. Not so with vitamin C.

Supplementing with Vitamin C

Vitamin C can be dosed over a very wide range and provide substantial benefits at any of the doses given. However, for most conditions, the optimal benefits of vitamin C will be realized at the highest levels of supplementation. As with all nutrient supplements, vitamin C must be administered appropriately to derive optimum benefit. Along with the vitamin C, the more quality antioxidants ingested, the better. Newly ingested antioxidants support and recharge the oxidized forms of the others.

Like any other supplementation or even prescription medications, long-term dosing is best determined with the help and follow-up of a healthcare practitioner who has experience with the utilization and benefits of highly-dosed antioxidant agents.

Competent clinical monitoring in combination with appropriate regular laboratory testing can be invaluable. This not only makes finding and maintaining the appropriate dosing of vitamin C and other antioxidants easier, it also allows the healthcare practitioner the opportunity to see whether to add or continue prescription drug therapy is appropriate.

While many osteoporosis prescription drugs have risks of substantial negative side effects and should only be added to a treatment regimen as a last option, many other prescription drugs are not only clearly beneficial, they also pose little to no risk for the conditions being treated. Many high blood pressure, anti-angina medications, and prescription calcium channel blockers are good examples of drugs that can be employed without reluctance.

Since the goal of vitamin C supplementation is to get vitamin C in as many areas of the tissues in the body in as high a concentration as possible, it is generally a good idea to supplement different forms of this vitamin in order to achieve this goal. General recommendations for the supplementation of vitamin C in regard to osteoporosis are covered in Chapter 16. Appendix B provides an even more extensive and practical guide for the optimal administration of vitamin C.

Almost all medical conditions (not an exaggeration) will respond positively, very positively, or even clinically resolve if vitamin C is optimally dosed and regularly administered in an optimal manner. When no significant improvement is seen in a given condition after a treatment protocol that includes vitamin C, one should always look to the guide provided in Appendix B before concluding that vitamin C is of little or no benefit.

Summary

Here's a recap of vitamin C's health-promoting properties:

- Osteoporosis is primarily a scurvy, or severe deficiency of vitamin C and other supportive antioxidants in the bone.
- Vitamin C is essential in every aspect of bone physiology.
- Vitamin C is a frontline defender against oxidative stress.
- Supplemental vitamin C results in greater bone density.
- Supplemental vitamin C lowers fracture risk.
- Supplemental vitamin C accelerates and improves quality of bone healing.
- Supplemental vitamin C protects against dangerous calcifications.
- Supplemental vitamin C protects against calcium-laden kidney stones.
- Supplemental vitamin C lowers all-cause mortality.
- Supplemental vitamin C is non-toxic and safe.

Osteoporosis is a chronic degenerative disease invariably caused by, and intimately associated with, increased oxidative stress throughout the body but especially in the bones. A wealth of scientific literature clearly documents the fact that vitamin C is deficient in the bones of all osteoporosis patients and that this deficiency is the primary factor in the causation and evolution of osteoporosis. As such, osteoporosis is a chronic focal scurvy of the bones. The medical literature further indicates that sufficient vitamin C is vital to maintaining good bone health, although restoring bone to a normal state from an osteoporotic state requires more than just vitamin C.

Many different factors can be involved in causing osteoporosis, but they all involve increased toxin exposure and decreased antioxidant levels in the bones, highlighting the fact that a vitamin C deficiency in the bones is the final common denominator in the causation of osteoporosis. Restoring antioxidant levels, especially that of vitamin C, to normal levels, requires that all significant ongoing toxin exposures be properly addressed in order for a quality program of supplementation to have optimal impact on the ability of the vitamin C to restore and maintain quality bone.

The studies collectively show that vitamin C is vital for both regaining and maintaining good bone health. In fact, it is doubtful how successful any osteoporosis treatment protocol could be if vitamin C is omitted completely. The studies also show that while vitamin C is the most critical of the antioxidants to take correctly, supplementing as many other quality antioxidants as can reasonably be afforded is definitely money well spent in the pursuit of good bone and general health. Much of the positive impact of the other anti-osteoporosis agents to be discussed — magnesium, vitamin K, vitamin D, essential fatty acids, estrogen, testosterone, thyroid hormone — results from the increased antioxidant impact they ultimately have in the bones and the rest of the body. Although not classically viewed as antioxidants, these agents nevertheless collectively comprise an important part of the overall antioxidant matrix in the body. Even though some positive benefits would likely accrue from administering only these agents to the osteoporotic patient, there is no good reason not to accompany them with vigorous vitamin C supplementation in order to gain maximal benefits.

CHAPTER 6

Nature's Calcium Channel Blocker

Magnesium: Its Importance and Life-Saving Power

Magnesium has long been regarded as a physiological, or naturally occurring, calcium channel blocker, with many different established clinical applications. Supplemental magnesium has been shown to be beneficial in: [1-9]

- Asthma
- Tetanus
- Inflammation
- Atherosclerosis
- Acute myocardial infarction
- Myocardial protection during heart surgery
- Prevention and treatment of heart rhythm abnormalities
- Eclampsia and preeclampsia
- Migraines
- Hypertension
- Stroke
- Prevention and treatment of convulsions
- Osteoporosis

Many of the effects of magnesium in the body simply parallel the effects of calcium channel blocker drugs.

The Calcium-Magnesium "Tug-o-War"

Magnesium and calcium can largely be characterized as biological antagonists. This adversarial relationship enables magnesium to function as a natural calcium channel blocker. Their antagonism toward each other excludes the possibility of having elevated levels of both minerals simultaneously. A state of calcium excess actually assures that a state of magnesium deficiency is present as well.

The average dietary intake of magnesium has been reported to be roughly 70% of the RDA, a number that is always exceptionally conservative.

The average dietary intake of magnesium in women has been reported to be roughly 70% of the recommended daily allowance (RDA), a number that is always exceptionally conservative. Even using the admittedly low RDAs for magnesium, this finding suggests that a very large percentage of older women are substantially deficient in magnesium. The presence of calcium excesses in nearly all older women further assures that there exists magnesium deficiencies comparable in degree to those calcium excesses.

As discussed previously, calcium excesses appear to be a common denominator among individuals with osteoporosis and other chronic degenerative diseases. Therefore, raising bodily concentrations of magnesium to normal or even slightly supranormal, in an effort to alleviate and possibly eliminate calcium toxicity appears to be universally advisable. Regular supplementation with bioavailable forms of magnesium, then, is of the utmost importance in the treatment of osteoporosis and chronic degenerative diseases in general.

The Calcium-Related Importance of Magnesium Supplementation

Many studies demonstrate the need for magnesium supplementation with regard to its calcium-related biological effects.

Biological Properties of Magnesium (as related to calcium):
- Dissolves calcium deposits and keeps them in solution. [10]
- Decreases intracellular oxidative stress by decreasing elevated intracellular calcium levels.
- Regulates active calcium transport. [11]
- Increases bone density and decreases fracture incidence. [12,13]

Magnesium Deficiencies (as related to calcium) contribute to:
- Excess calcium deposition. [14-17]
- Increased intracellular calcium levels. [18,19]
- Promotion of prostate cancer cell proliferation. [20]
- Initiation of osteoporosis.

The Biological Importance of Magnesium Supplementation

Additional important biological effects of magnesium that may or may not directly involve its interaction with calcium include the following:
- Regulates insulin action and insulin-mediated glucose uptake; magnesium deficiency is an important aspect of insulin resistance. [21]

- Helps prevent metabolic syndrome; magnesium deficiency is associated with a significantly increased risk of this syndrome, [22] which increases risk of heart disease.
- Supplementation blocks the atherosclerosis induced by excessive vitamin D in pigs. [23]
- Supplementation suppresses bone turnover, a major factor in age-related osteoporosis. [24,25]
- Possibly improves brain function and learning. [26]
- Required cofactor in more than 300 enzymatic reactions. [27]

Magnesium Deficiencies contribute to:
- Induction of inflammation and increased oxidative stress; [28-31] this magnesium deficiency-induced inflammation can be lessened by the additional induced deficiency of calcium, [32] further indicating that it is a relative excess of calcium to magnesium that determines the presence of inflammation and increased oxidative stress.
- Prevention of cellular release of nitric oxide. [33]
- Induction of endothelial dysfunction. [34]
- Acceleration of the aging process when deficiency is chronic. [35]

Magnesium Supplementation Lowers All-Cause Mortality

The effects of magnesium outside of the bones deserve as much consideration as its effects in stabilizing and regenerating healthy bone in osteoporotic patients.

This is especially true in light of the substantial negative side effects of most traditional osteoporotic treatments.

The side effects of magnesium are really all side benefits, and very significant ones at that. Substantial evidence indicates that magnesium decreases the incidence and the severity of heart disease. Much of this evidence also indicates that magnesium decreases all-cause mortality, not just from heart disease.[36-41] These mortality-reducing observations are completely consistent considering what is known about calcium:

A single treatment with any substance that provides several years of lowered all-cause mortality is nothing short of astounding!

1) Excess calcium increases heart disease.
2) Excess calcium increases all-cause mortality.
3) Calcium's mortality-increasing effects are countered by magnesium's calcium channel blocking properties.

Impressively, even short-term applications of magnesium can positively impact mortality for an extended period of time. This effect was demonstrated in a study where suspected myocardial infarction patients were given a loading dose of magnesium followed by a 24-hour intravenous infusion of it. Both cardiac mortality and all-cause mortality over an average follow-up period of about three years were significantly reduced.[42] In another investigation myocardial infarction patients deemed ineligible for thrombolytic therapy received a 48-hour infusion of magnesium. A similar drop in mortality was seen during an average follow-up period of about five years.[43]

A single treatment with any substance that provides several years of lowered all-cause mortality is nothing short of astounding! Magnesium's ability to produce such positive long-term effects powerfully demonstrates its importance in healthy cellular metabolism.

Magnesium also appears to play a positive role in lessening the chances of different types of cancer. This is certainly consistent with its documented positive effects in decreasing mortality from all causes, as noted above. As mentioned earlier, increased intracellular calcium levels result in increased intracellular oxidative stress. And calcium-induced oxidative stress frequently precedes and accompanies the malignant state. Because of the biological antagonism between calcium and magnesium higher levels of magnesium would be expected to reduce the incidence of cancer. To explore this very relationship, researchers looked at the ratio of serum calcium to serum magnesium and cancer.

> *Studies have demonstrated that higher magnesium intake appears to be associated with a lessened risk of colon, rectal, and lung cancer.*

One study showed that this calcium/magnesium ratio was higher in post-menopausal women with breast cancer than in post-menopausal women without breast cancer.[44] A few other studies have also demonstrated that higher magnesium intake appears to be associated with a lessened risk of colon, rectal, and lung cancer.[45-47]

No large prospective studies examining the effect of substantial magnesium supplementation on cancers of any kind could be found. However, it should be anticipated that greater amounts of magnesium in the body — especially relative to calcium levels in the body — would reliably lessen any increases in oxidative stress both inside and outside the cells. This should substantially lessen the chances of malignant transformation across the board.

Safety of Magnesium Supplementation

The medical literature seems to be devoid of any clinical magnesium toxicity syndrome in humans with normal kidney function. With that said however, magnesium, unlike a completely harmless nutrient like vitamin C, can become toxic when administered too vigorously. When too much is given intravenously,[48,49] or in aggressive non-oral administrations (such as by injection or enema), or orally (as with an overdose of magnesium-containing antacid),[50] magnesium has the potential of becoming toxic. Generally, the most common oral magnesium supplements will induce diarrhea well before causing a magnesium excess to the point of toxicity.

As a practical consideration, then, **dietary** and **supplemental** sources of magnesium will simply not induce a state of magnesium toxicity. Additionally the widespread nature of calcium excess in the older population makes it extraordinarily unlikely that a chronic excess of magnesium could ever replace the excess of calcium. As long as calcium excess is present, especially inside cells, magnesium will only act to counterbalance this state, not replace it with a state of magnesium excess.

While it is true that magnesium does have toxicity when administered in excessively high doses, it is important to realize that a chronic deficiency of magnesium is the common state. Of far more concern than the potential for short-term magnesium toxicity is the negative health impact of long-term magnesium deficiency. Practically speaking, chronic magnesium toxicity can never be present in an individual with normal kidney function. In most

> *In most older individuals and virtually all osteoporosis patients, the state of excess calcium almost guarantees a relative state of magnesium deficiency.*

older individuals and virtually all osteoporosis patients the state of excess calcium almost guarantees a relative state of magnesium deficiency. As long as kidney function remains normal, magnesium supplementation will never turn the pronounced calcium excess into a state of relative calcium deficiency.

The monitoring physician may recommend anywhere from 100 to 800 mg of magnesium glycinate daily.

The typical clinical goal is to supplement enough magnesium to minimize the impact of the excess calcium. Just as with prescription calcium channel blockers, the calcium channel blocking effects of magnesium have the potential to temporarily induce low blood pressure. In the rare event that unexpected hypotension follows the administration of magnesium, supplementation should be temporarily suspended until normal blood pressure is restored. Supplementation can then be resumed at a reduced level.

Important Magnesium Supplementation Considerations

In supplemental form, magnesium is always paired with other molecules [anions]. Although there are many of these molecules, common anions are chloride, carbonate, citrate, glycinate, and phosphate. The best forms of supplemental magnesium are combined with anions that have nutritious value in their own right. Independent of magnesium these anions need to be free from toxic effects. Obviously magnesium fluoride or magnesium cyanide would never be an option because of the highly toxic nature of the two anions, fluoride and cyanide.

Magnesium glycinate, the form recommended in the osteoporosis treatment protocol in Chapter 15, is a good example of this. Glycine is an amino acid with a wide variety of uses and also virtually without toxicity at any dose. Relative to other magnesium preparations, it is especially well absorbed, and it is less likely to provoke the diarrhea/laxative effect.

Depending on bowel sensitivity and the information obtained in clinical/laboratory follow-up the monitoring physician may recommend anywhere from 100 to 800 mg of magnesium glycinate orally daily. The typical dosage range is 100 to 400 mg but the physician may recommend 600 to 800 mg daily if well tolerated by the patient.

Without question magnesium is a valuable tool for preventing and treating osteoporosis.

Summary

Here's a recap of magnesium's health-promoting properties:

- Magnesium inhibits abnormal calcification outside of the bones.
- Magnesium helps dissolve preexisting abnormal calcifications.
- Magnesium helps prevent metabolic syndrome, lessening susceptibility to coronary artery disease.
- Magnesium increases bone density and decreases the incidence of fracture.
- Magnesium lessens abnormal increases in intracellular calcium levels.
- Magnesium is a natural (non-pharmacological) calcium channel blocker.
- Magnesium is a natural (non-pharmacological) anti-cancer agent.
- Magnesium decreases the incidence of some cancers.

- Oral magnesium supplementation is virtually devoid of any toxicity.
- Magnesium decreases all-cause mortality.
- By itself, very short-term intravenous dosing of magnesium can decrease the chances of death from all causes over at least the following 3 to 5 years.

Without question magnesium is a valuable tool for preventing and treating osteoporosis. Considering its vast nutritional value and the fact that excess calcium ensures a magnesium deficiency, supplementation of magnesium is also recommended for general health and longevity.

CHAPTER 7

Ignored Yet Essential Weapon Against Osteoporosis

Vitamin K: Dissolves Unwanted Calcium Deposits, Reduces Fracture Risk

Mainstream medicine in the United States makes little use of vitamin K in the treatment of osteoporosis. This is in spite of an enormous amount of scientific evidence documenting its important role in bone physiology, in the reduction of osteoporotic fractures, and in the mobilization/dissolution of abnormal calcifications.

It is, however, an important part of osteoporosis therapy in Japan. Not surprisingly then, much of the most significant literature and clinical studies on the benefits of vitamin K in the treatment of osteoporosis have come from Japan, as can be seen in the references cited in this section.[1]

Just as with vitamin C, the scientific literature reveals numerous, clear-cut applications for vitamin K. And while the evidence is overwhelmingly in favor of both nutrients, articles about them frequently end with the suggestion that while the nutrient proved to provide substantial benefit, more research needs to be performed before any recommendations can be made. This is particularly astounding for two reasons:

1) Vitamin K (like vitamin C) has no established toxicity at any dose.
2) Nearly all the traditional osteoporosis therapies have questionable benefit with definite toxicity.

Unfortunately, millions of patients pay the incalculable price for this nearly universal reluctance to employ non-prescription agents like vitamin C and vitamin K in treatment protocols.

Multiple Members of the Vitamin K Family

Vitamin K actually refers to a family of structurally similar fat-soluble molecules that include phylloquinone (K1), menaquinones (K2), and menadione (K3). The only commonly supplemented forms of vitamin K are the K1

The Vitamin K Family

Form	Chemical Name	General Description
Vitamin K1	Phylloquinone	Derived from degradation of MK-4, this is the least active form. The body converts a variable percentage of vitamin K1 into the MK-4 form of vitamin K2
Vitamin K2	Menaquinone-4	With regard to bone metabolism, this is the most active form of vitamin K
	Menaquinone-7	Some valuable functions in bone metabolism. Can degrade into MK-4 and/or vitamin K1
Vitamin K3	Menadione	Valuable in cancer treatment and also helps to regulate bone calcification

and K2 forms, while K3 has demonstrated very positive results in the killing of cancer cells when partnered with vitamin C.[2-5] Because of the limited scope of this chapter only K1 and K2 will be discussed.

Vitamin K Supplementation and Blood Coagulation

Discovered in 1929, vitamin K was first noted to play an important role in blood coagulation. Some years later the anticoagulant warfarin was discovered, and its role as a vitamin K antagonist became established. Even today, vitamin K remains the primary antidote to warfarin toxicity, or to the excessive anticoagulation effect from warfarin.[6] It is very important to note, however, that while vitamin K can neutralize the blood-thinning effects of warfarin, it can only normalize the thinned-out blood-clotting mechanism. Vitamin K cannot make the blood prone to abnormal clotting at any dose.[7]

Vitamin K cannot make the blood prone to abnormal clotting at any dose.

Vitamin K Supplementation Inhibits and Reverses Abnormal Calcification

Seventeen vitamin K-dependent proteins have now been identified. Two of them that have been especially well researched, osteocalcin and matrix Gla protein (MGP), are known inhibitors of abnormal calcification in the tissues outside of bone. Vitamin K plays a critical role in preventing and reversing such calcifications, along with promoting bone strength because of its ability to activate [carboxylate] these inhibitors.[8,9]

In osteoporosis patients the normal calcification process in the bones is not taking place. At the same time abnormal calcification outside of the bones [ectopic calcification) commonly occurs. This double dysfunction is called the "calcification paradox," especially since the ectopic [abnormal] calcification process is known to have multiple similarities with bone metabolism. Nevertheless, adequate amounts of vitamin K will dissolve ectopic calcifications while simultaneously preventing the dissolution, or calcium mobilization, from the bones.

> *Vitamin K plays a critical role in preventing and reversing [unwanted] calcifications, along with promoting bone strength.*

The anticoagulant warfarin, which is a vitamin K antagonist that inhibits the activation [carboxylation] of MGP, rapidly leads to arterial calcification in rats.[10] Mice given warfarin demonstrated similar effects, including calcification leading to some destabilization of atherosclerotic plaques.[11] But when warfarin-treated rats were given a high dietary intake of vitamin K, aortic calcification actually reversed and arterial elasticity began to normalize.[12]

Vitamin K is also essential to normal bone physiology, acting as a positive controlling [modulating] agent in bone remodeling. In addition, it is vital to the complex communication process that governs and organizes cellular activities [cell signaling], programmed cell death [apoptosis], cellular response to the presence of certain chemicals [chemotaxis], and in lessening inflammation.[13]

Since vitamin K is necessary for the MGP to be activated [carboxylated] and have its inhibitory effect on vascular calcification,[14] decreased levels of vitamin K should be seen in individuals with greater degrees of ectopic calcification. This turns out to be the case. A study on 36 hypertensive patients compared total calcium scores from combined readings on the carotid arteries, the coronary arteries, and the abdominal aorta. These total calcium scores were positively correlated with levels of inactive [uncarboxylated] MGP, indicating deficient vitamin K levels.[15] In another study, heart patients (angioplasty and aortic stenosis) and kidney patients (hemodialysis and calciphylaxis) were found to have decreased levels of uncarboxylated MGP relative to healthy subjects. Of note as well, the uncarboxylated MGP is known to accumulate at sites of vascular calcification, a reason for it's depleted levels in the blood.[16]

An increased dietary intake of vitamin K2 has been associated with a lesser incidence of coronary heart disease.[17] Consistent with this finding, individuals with the highest dietary intakes of K2 also had lesser amounts of coronary artery calcification.[18] In addition, vitamin K1 supplementation has been shown to slow the progression of coronary artery calcium scores over time,[19] even in relatively low doses.

An increased dietary intake of vitamin K2 has been associated with a lesser incidence of coronary heart disease and lesser amounts of coronary artery calcification.

Vitamin K Supplementation Lowers All-Cause Mortality

Increasing coronary artery calcium scores have now been shown to be associated with increases in all-cause mortality in addition to increased coronary heart disease risk.[20,21] In fact, increasing thoracic aortic calcification predicts increased all-cause mortality and heart attack [myocardial infarction].[22] A meta-analysis of thirty different articles found vascular calcification in general to be associated with an increased risk of cardiac events and mortality from all causes.[23]

In dialysis patients greater aortic calcification predicted a greater chance of death from all causes.[24] In conditions where MGP is undercarboxylated (under-activated), a clinical situation synonymous with vitamin K deficiency, all-cause mortality was increased as well.[25,26] All of these studies make it very clear that vitamin K supplementation should decrease all-cause mortality, especially when correcting a vitamin K deficiency. Finally, in a prospective study that followed 4,807 older men and women over a period of about seven years it was clearly demonstrated that the dietary intake of vitamin K2 was inversely related to all-cause mortality.[27] It appears to be a reasonable assertion that anything that will reliably reverse existing ectopic calcification will not only decrease the chances of heart attack, it will also lessen the chances of dying from any cause or disease.

Vitamin K Supplementation and Cancer Prevention

Not surprisingly then, considering the role that calcium plays in malignancy, vitamin K has been shown to have a positive effect in the prevention of some kinds of malignancies.[28] Multiple studies have reported on the positive effects that vitamin K2 (MK-4) at a dose of 45 mg daily, has in preventing the initial development of hepatocellular carcinoma in patients with viral cirrhosis. This dose also helps prevent recurrent hepatocellular carcinoma in such patients after curative treatment.[29-31]

MK-4 suppressed the proliferation and motility of hepatocellular carcinoma cells in culture.[32] It has demonstrated the ability to induce differentiation in a number of human myeloid leukemia cell lines, effectively lessening the degree of malignancy.[33]

In cell culture, vitamin K2 has also induced cell-cycle arrest and cell death in hepatoma cells.[34] Myelodysplastic syndrome, which frequently leads to acute myeloid leukemia, was successfully treated in an 80-year old woman with 45 mg of vitamin K2 daily. After a little more than a year, she no longer required regular transfusions due to impaired blood production, and she stopped the K2. Red cell production again dropped, and recovery was again realized when K2 administration was resumed.[35]

Multiple studies have reported on the positive effects that vitamin K2 has in preventing the initial development of hepatocellular carcinoma.

Vitamin K Supplementation and Bone Health

A major way in which vitamin K contributes to bone health is through its role as a cofactor in the carboxylation, or activation, of the bone formation marker osteocalcin.[36] A low degree of osteocalcin carboxylation in the body has been related to osteoporosis.[37] In a randomized, placebo-controlled, double-blind study, postmenopausal women with osteopenia (a state of reduced bone density that easily leads to osteoporosis) were given either 5 mg of vitamin K1 or a placebo daily. Even though the study was aimed at following the age-related decline in bone mineral density, additional significant observations were made. The researchers noted that although the age-related decline in bone mineral density was not affected, an increased percentage of osteocalcin was carboxylated indicating a lessening of osteoporotic activity. Furthermore fewer women in the vitamin K1 group had fractures, and fewer had cancers.[38] Note was also made that the K supplementation was well-tolerated. Although the design of the study was not to look at fractures and cancers, this data further supports the many other studies supporting the benefits of vitamin K1, as well as of vitamin K in general.

> *Fewer women in the vitamin K1 group had fractures, and fewer had cancers.*

In the treatment of osteoporosis, vitamin K supplementation will refer primarily to vitamin K2, and to a lesser degree, vitamin K1. Menaquinone-4 [MK-4] is the most biologically active form of vitamin K in appropriately controlling the increase or decrease in substances involved in bone metabolism.[39] Researchers use these substances as markers of osteoblast [bone-makers] and osteoclast [bone-breakers] activity. Although MK-4 is a form of vitamin K2, a variable percentage of K1 converts to MK-4 as well.[40] In addition, both vitamin K1 and MK-4 can be synthesized from the degradation of MK-7.[41] While direct supplementation with vitamin K1, MK-4, or MK7 might have different immediate measurable effects in a given study, it is important to know that they are all interrelated as well.

In a study on rats it was shown that vitamin K2 improved the quality of bone to the point that vertebral fractures were prevented even though bone mass was not increased.[42] In another study vitamin K2 (MK-4 and MK-7) prevented the bone loss that would otherwise develop from the loss of hormone production in rats subjected to removal of the ovaries.[43] In another study with rats without ovaries, vitamin K2 administration resulted in significantly improved bone strength and less susceptibility to fracture.[44]

In a group of rats with ovaries intact, the administration of MK-7 blocked the ability of parathyroid hormone to mobilize calcium from the bone. MK-7 supplementation also caused significant elevation of the activated form of osteocalcin in female rats with and without ovaries.[45] Osteocalcin is an important regulator of the calcium uptake needed for normal bone mineralization.

Rather than simply increasing bone density without improving bone structure, as is seen with calcium supplementation, all of this data clearly indicates the importance of vitamin K2 in maintaining and restoring quality bone architecture.[46] Unfortunately improving density test scores is the only goal for many osteoporosis-treating clinicians.[47] In contrast, the ultimate clinical goal in the treatment of osteoporosis should be to decrease fracture incidence. And of course, therapies used to reach this goal should not increase the incidence of other diseases or worsen the severity of existing ones.

> *All of this data clearly indicates the importance of vitamin K2 in maintaining and restoring quality bone architecture.*

Interestingly, vitamin K1 was shown to increase the bone mineral density in rats while vitamin K2, as noted above, did not affect this parameter even though it does have a protective effect against fractures.[48] This further emphasizes the lack of reliability in sole dependence on an improved bone mineral density test score as a validation of appropriate osteoporosis therapy. A better score might follow a positive intervention, but it can also follow calcium supplementation, which does nothing to prevent fractures. Understanding the physiology of what supports optimal physical strength in bone is of paramount importance in the proper clinical management of osteoporosis.

On the other hand, when bone density tests improve in the absence of calcium supplementation it is actually a reliable indication that the quality of the bone has been improved. That's because the increase in density is not from random cosmetic deposition of excess calcium into porous bone, but rather indicates a replacement of less dense porous bone with new healthy bone.

In another rat study vitamin K2 had a protective effect against the loss of the structural integrity of bone induced by removal of the sciatic nerve.[49] In hemodialysis patients K1 deficiency was the strongest predictor of vertebral fractures, while vitamin K2 (MK-4 and MK-7) deficiency most reliably predicted vascular calcification.[50] Taken together then, this indicates that vitamin K1 can increase bone density as a true reflection of bone integrity, while vitamin K2 increases bone quality and mobilizes ectopic calcifications. Clearly both of these forms of vitamin K should be a part of any osteoporosis treatment protocol.

Low blood levels of vitamin K, as well as of vitamin D, were found to be significant and independent determinants of osteoporosis and bone fracture risk.

In humans low intake of vitamin K, or low blood levels of vitamin K as well as of vitamin D were found to be significant and independent determinants of osteoporosis and bone fracture risk. Furthermore this risk was found to be independent of any generalized malnutrition.[51-54]

Low-dose (180 micrograms daily) of vitamin K2 (MK-7) over a three-year period was found to decrease bone loss in postmenopausal women.[55] In a randomized, double-blind, long-term study, this same small dose of MK-7 given to patients for a year following lung and heart transplantation positively impacted lumbar spine bone mineral density.[56]

Studies on diabetic patients have shown that their bone quality is generally poor even though bone density tends to be normal, but that vitamin K2 can improve the strength of such bones in a number of ways, including improved collagen cross-linking.[57]

Treatment with a pharmacological dose (45 mg daily) of vitamin K2 (MK-4) effectively prevents osteoporosis fractures while sustaining bone mineral density.[58] Consistent with this outcome this same dose of MK-4 also elevates significant bone formation markers.[59] Bone quality is also improved by MK-4, probably by increasing collagen quantity and the degree of cross-linking in the collagen.[60] A 45 mg daily regimen of MK-4 caused improvement of pertinent bone-related laboratory parameters in multiple cases of pregnancy-associated osteoporosis with multiple vertebral fractures.[61]

Treatment with 45 mg daily of vitamin K2 (MK-4) effectively prevents osteoporosis fractures while sustaining bone mineral density.

Lesser amounts of MK-4 supplementation have also been shown to be of clear benefit to healthy bone metabolism. In a randomized, double-blind, placebo-controlled trial, only four weeks of supplementation with 1.5 mg of MK-4 daily showed significantly improved carboxylation [activation] of osteocalcin.[62] Obviously the trial was not long enough to make any assertions of the benefit of this dose of MK-4 on the incidence of fractures.

In a rat study MK-4 was also shown to improve the mechanical strength of bone weakened by a deficiency of magnesium.[63] This is important since it emphasizes the need for a multi-faceted approach to osteoporosis in which all of the anti-osteoporosis agents being discussed should be utilized. It should not be surprising that individual agents that effectively treat osteoporosis would provide additive and even synergistic benefits when used together.

The Synergistic Power of Vitamin K and Other Anti-Osteoporotic Agents

The metabolic roles of vitamin K and vitamin D have considerable overlap, and substantial evidence has been presented that indicate their synergistic action in benefiting bone and the cardiovascular system.[64] One study looked at the net effect of combined agents in the treatment of osteoporosis. Vitamin D, vitamin K (MK-4), and prescription bisphosphonates (alendronate or risedronate) together were found to have a protective effect against hip fractures in elderly Parkinson's disease patients.[65]

Used together vitamin D, vitamin K, and prescription bisphosphonates were found to have a protective effect against hip fractures in elderly Parkinson's disease patients.

A synergistic effect in the inhibition of ectopic calcification in cultured smooth muscle cells was also seen with the administration of vitamin K2 and a bisphosphonate, pamidronate.[66] Treating mice with MK-4 followed by risedronate therapy prior to removal of the ovaries produced significantly increased femur strength. The improvement was substantially better when both were given together or the risedronate preceded the MK-4.[67] It would appear the MK-4 helped "set the stage" to optimize any benefit of the risedronate.

While bisphosphonates may be of benefit to some patients, they should be reserved for patients who are not responding adequately to the entirety of the recommended osteoporosis protocol in Chapter 15. Unnecessary exposure to the potential side effects of this class of drugs should be avoided if at all possible.

In a study examining bone metabolism and bone mass, the most positive changes seen in postmenopausal women consuming dairy products fortified with vitamin D occurred when vitamins K1 or K2 (MK-7) were part of the fortification.[68] In a study examining hip fracture incidence and the dietary intake of magnesium, vitamin D, calcium, and vitamin K, the greatest incidence in hip fracture occurred in Japanese men and women with the lowest vitamin K intake, more so than related to poor intake of magnesium, vitamin D, or calcium.[69] It would appear that vitamin K is not just an important part of an osteoporosis treatment regimen, but a mandatory one.

It would appear that vitamin K is not just an important part of an osteoporosis treatment regimen, but a mandatory one.

Also of interest is the potential relationship of vitamin D toxicity to a vitamin K deficiency. Animal studies indicate that high levels of vitamin D induce the production of proteins that require vitamin K for activation. As a result

Best Vitamin K Dosing
(Based on Studies Previously Cited)

Vitamin K1	5 mg daily
Vitamin K2 (MK-4)	45 mg daily in three separate 15 mg doses
Vitamin K2 (MK-7)	At least 200 micrograms daily

it appears that these vitamin D-induced proteins will use up increasing amounts of available vitamin K resulting in a vitamin K deficiency as vitamin D levels rise. This deficiency of vitamin K would explain many of the symptoms of vitamin D toxicity. It has also been suggested that vitamin A helps to protect against a toxic effect of excess vitamin D by decreasing the expression of these same proteins that need vitamin K for activation.[70] The bottom line is that a broad spectrum of vitamins and nutrients should be supplemented.

> *Vitamin K2 also has demonstrated no known toxicity or undesired side effects when administered to newborns or pregnant women.*

Safety of Vitamin K Supplementation

The lack of toxicity of vitamin K is nearly as impressive as its effectiveness in decreasing the incidence of osteoporotic fractures, preventing new ectopic calcification, and dissolving existing ectopic calcification. In an attempt to determine a toxic level of MK-7 ingestion, mice were given 2,000 mg/kg, the equivalent of roughly 140,000 mg (140,000,000 micrograms) for a 150-pound person. Clinical observations and data from ophthalmology, clinical pathology, gross necropsy, and histopathology found no toxicity attributable to the MK-7 form of vitamin K2 even at these astronomical amounts.[71] The amount given to these mice was well over one million times the amount of MK-7 that is commonly supplemented (100 micrograms). Vitamin K2 also has demonstrated no known toxicity or undesired side effects when administered to newborns or pregnant women.[72,73]

Vitamin K Supplementation Considerations

Currently, Glakay® produces 15 mg capsules of MK-4. These are manufactured by Eisai in Japan, and they are probably available if the physician in charge is willing to submit a prescription to an international pharmacy that can obtain it.[74] A good vitamin K product available in the United States is "Super K with Advanced K2 Complex," available from Life Extension Foundation (www.lef.org). One softgel contains 1,000 micrograms of K1, 1,000 micrograms of MK-4, and 200 micrograms of MK-7). Any good osteoporosis treatment regimen should include at least one of these softgels three times daily if the 15 mg MK-4 product from Japan cannot be obtained. And even with the product from Japan, it would be a good addition due to the K1 and MK-7 content.

Summary

Vitamin K reliably:
- Inhibits abnormal calcification outside of the bones.
- Helps dissolve preexisting abnormal calcifications.
- Neutralizes the anticoagulant warfarin, which promotes abnormal calcifications.
- (K2) lessens susceptibility to coronary artery disease.
- (K1) may increase bone density but definitely decreases fracture risk.
- (K2 as MK-4) prevents fractures, sustains bone density, and improves bone quality via increased collagen content and collagen cross-linking when administered in pharmacological doses.

- (K2 as MK-4) can compensate for the bone weakening induced by magnesium deficiency.
- Can prevent and/or effectively treat some forms of cancer.
- (K2 as MK-4) can augment the positive bone effects of bisphosphonates.
- (K2) decreases cardiac mortality as well as all-cause mortality.

IMPORTANT: Vitamin K1 and K2 have never been found to have definable toxicity at any dose level.

There is absolutely no sound scientific reason to deny any osteoporosis patient the benefits of regular oral vitamin K (K1 and K2) supplementation. The lack of toxicity of vitamin K, along with its enormous benefits in osteoporosis and in the reduction of all-cause mortality, should make it a mandatory part of any anti-osteoporosis treatment regimen. Just its positive effects as a therapy for heart disease and different forms of cancer are enough to warrant its routine supplementation in nearly everyone.

CHAPTER 8

Needed: An Immediate Divorce

Vitamin D Works Wonders When Separated from Calcium Supplementation

"Always together." The assumed marriage of calcium supplementation and vitamin D supplementation makes it difficult to view them separately. Relatively few osteoporosis studies investigate the properties of calcium and vitamin D individually. Instead, most clinicians and researchers treat them as a single supplement. As a result of this unhealthy union the dangers of excess calcium are greatly amplified while the benefits of vitamin D supplementation are severely diminished.

One need look no further than the words "Fortified with Vitamin D" printed on nearly every milk container in the country to see the prime example of the dangerous calcium-vitamin D marriage. Previous chapters have sufficiently warned of the serious health and life threats posed by excess calcium — whether obtained through supplementation, from calcium-rich dairy products, or both. In this chapter the reason these two nutrients must be separated will be explained and the advantages of vitamin D supplementation without calcium will also be presented.

Why Calcium and Vitamin D Should Not be Consumed Together

Here's the problem: Vitamin D significantly *increases* calcium absorption from the gastrointestinal tract. If excessive calcium were never an issue a calcium-vitamin D combination would not pose a health risk and might even offer benefits.

The dangers of combining vitamin D supplementation with excessive calcium ingestion in older adults are quite clear.

However that's not the case! Previous chapters have shouted the warnings against excessive calcium intake! For any who missed it: **Excessive calcium ingestion, from food and/or supplementation, is greatly hazardous to life and health.** The high incidence of atherosclerosis, high blood pressure, cancer, and osteoporosis in the United States demonstrates the massive scale and severity of an excessive calcium intake. **The last thing anyone suffering from these diseases needs is an improved mechanism for pumping more calcium into their already-calcifying bodies!**

Although the dangers of combining vitamin D supplementation with excessive calcium ingestion in older adults are quite clear, these risks have not been adequately studied or determined in younger adults and children. Caution is always appropriate in the consumption of calcium-rich, vitamin D-fortified foods and calcium supplementation for everyone.

Vitamin D and Bone Health

The important role of vitamin D in decreasing the chances of osteoporotic fractures has been clearly established. When adequate vitamin D has been supplemented a significant reduction in fracture risk has resulted.[1-3] Another fracture risk study that looked at vitamin D blood levels found that women in the lowest quintile [lowest 20%] with serum levels less than 20 ng/cc had double the fracture risk compared to women in the upper quintile with levels of 40 ng/cc or more. The upper quintile had an average of 50 ng/cc, with levels as high as 112 ng/cc.[4]

Other studies have long established the important relationships between vitamin D levels, calcium, and bone. These include the following:

- Vitamin D deficiency is a cause of osteoporosis.[5]
- Vitamin D deficiency is associated with an increased risk of fracture in children,[6] in adults,[7] and in patients with osteoporosis.[8]
- Vitamin D excess increases bone resorption, worsens osteoporosis, and causes ectopic calcification throughout the body.[9-11] Bone loss secondary to vitamin D excess rebounds quickly when vitamin D levels return to normal.[12]
- Correcting a vitamin D deficiency after menopause suppresses resorption of bone and loss of bony calcium,[13,14] and in osteoporotic bone, it results in a rapid recovery of bone mineral density.[15]
- Vitamin D status is a key determinant of bone mineral density in children and adolescents.[16]

The Biological Importance of Vitamin D Supplementation

Vitamin D plays a large role in regulating calcium metabolism and optimizing the correct assimilation of calcium into a renewed, healthy bone mineral matrix. Its contribution is of vastly greater importance than merely supplying increased amounts of calcium to osteoporotic bone. As discussed previously, proper supplementation with vitamin D increases bone density with a decrease in the incidence of fractures. Calcium, on the other hand, can only produce a cosmetic increase in bone density without affecting bone quality and structural integrity.

> *Vitamin D administered without calcium demonstrates the same degree of fracture protection seen in studies where vitamin D and calcium are used together.*

In fact, the only studies in the literature concluding that "calcium supplementation" lessened the incidence of fractures were those that combined vitamin D supplementation with the supplemented calcium. The critical factor was the dose of the vitamin D. When 800 IU of vitamin D was used a significant reduction in fractures was observed. When the dose of vitamin D was dropped to 400 IU the calcium/vitamin D combination provided no protection against fracture.

Vitamin D administered without calcium demonstrates the same degree of fracture protection seen in studies where vitamin D and calcium are used together. And as already noted, when calcium is tested without vitamin D there is no fracture protection. Clearly, calcium supplementation does not reduce the incidence of fractures,[17] and calcium supplementation does not help vitamin D provide such protection.

While a detailed discussion of the following is beyond the scope of this chapter, it is important to note the many and important functions of vitamin D beyond its effects on calcium metabolism and the maintenance of healthy bone. Although there is much we do not know about vitamin

D, its importance to health is becoming more evident all the time. In fact, this nutrient is so essential that vitamin D receptors have been identified in nearly all the organs and tissues of the body. We now know that vitamin D affects the expression of hundreds, and perhaps as many as 1,000 to 2,000 genes. [18]

Recent findings indicate that vitamin D plays a beneficial role in:

- Autoimmune diseases [19,20]
- Cell differentiation and proliferation [21]
- Male reproduction [22]
- Skeletal muscle [23,24]
- Multiple sclerosis [25]
- Immune function [26]
- Cancer regulation [27,28]
- Asthma [29]
- Ankylosing spondylitis [30]
- HIV infection [31]
- Diabetes, hypertension, atherosclerosis, and inflammation [32-34]

Vitamin D is so essential that vitamin D receptors have been identified in nearly all the organs and tissues of the body.

Optimal dosing of vitamin D has also proven to be extremely effective in reducing the incidence of a wide array of diseases and medical conditions. These include cancers, coronary artery disease, as well as some bacterial and viral infections. [35]

Vitamin D Lowers All-Cause Mortality

The regulation of calcium metabolism with agents that tightly control its absorption and deposition can be expected to have many more positive effects than just stabilizing or reversing osteoporosis. The positive effects of vitamin D on a large number of other chronic degenerative diseases is further evidence of this fact.

In a study of 1,006 adults over more than six years, those in the highest quartile [highest 25%] of vitamin D levels (>26.5 ng/cc) had a significantly decreased all-cause and cardiovascular disease mortality compared to those individuals in the lowest quartile of vitamin D levels (<10.5 ng/cc).[36] A similar outcome resulted from a study on 3,408 individuals followed for more than seven years.[37] Other researchers came to similar conclusions in large, long-term studies.[38-45]

> *Optimal dosing of vitamin D has also proven to be extremely effective in reducing the incidence of a wide array of diseases and medical conditions.*

The Importance of Maintaining Vitamin D Levels in the Normal Range

Over time, sufficiently abnormal elevations of vitamin D in the blood will always lead to excess calcium assimilation. As a consequence the clinical manifestations of vitamin D excess mirror the effects of calcium excess. By increasing resorption, sufficiently elevated abnormal levels of vitamin D pull calcium out of the bone and dump it into the blood. Simultaneously, vitamin D is increasing calcium uptake from diet and supplements. Working in tandem these processes further worsen the detrimental calcium excess in the rest of the body. This well-established effect of excess vitamin D has been demonstrated in tissue cultures,[46] animals,[47] and healthy male subjects.[48]

An excess vitamin D-induced loss of calcium from the bones makes such levels of vitamin D an additional cause, or aggravation, of osteoporosis. Yet it is clear that vitamin

D deficiency also results in a loss of calcium from the bones, making it a contributing factor to the development of osteoporosis as well.

When low vitamin D levels are normalized in patients with calcium-poor bone, bone mineral density recovers quickly.[49] Conversely, the bone mineral density lost as a result of vitamin D intoxication also rebounds promptly when the levels are allowed to return to normal.[50]

Given these facts it is vital that vitamin D levels be maintained in the normal range. Both vitamin D excess and vitamin D deficiency promote bone resorption, with much of the calcium loss from the bone contributing to excess calcium elsewhere in the body.

It is vital that vitamin D levels be maintained in the normal range, since both vitamin D excess and vitamin D deficiency promote bone resorption.

Vitamin D excess results in increased levels of calcium in both the intracellular and extracellular spaces. The most advanced forms of vitamin D excess result in a picture of calcium deposition throughout the body. When this calcium deposition occurs it can show up in any of a number of different tissues and organs of the body.[51]

Such widespread calcification occurs whenever calcium levels, vitamin D levels, or phosphate levels get high enough for a long enough period of time. And when more than one of these levels elevate the tendency toward calcification is even more pronounced.

Excessive intake of vitamin D also tends to have long-lasting effects, as it can be stored in the fatty tissues, liver, and muscles for many months.[52] These tissue stores result in a continued slow release of vitamin D for an extended period after regular vitamin D intake has been terminated. In one case study a patient was reported to have elevated vitamin D levels for 22 months after discontinuing vitamin D intake.[53]

Safety of Vitamin D Supplementation

Unlike the remarkable safety seen in the dosing of vitamin C, vitamin K, magnesium, and the essential fatty acids, vitamin D can become toxic if blood levels remain elevated for too long. Arguably, chronic vitamin D excess is as bad for the health of the bones as a chronic vitamin D deficiency, especially for those with osteoporosis. Excess vitamin D results in excessive calcium assimilation and thereby promotes detrimental calcifications throughout the body. As previously discussed at length, this calcium excess will aggravate and accelerate virtually all of the diseases that vitamin D would normally help. However, potential toxicity should not dissuade individuals from supplementing with this vital nutrient. The benefits of vitamin D supplementation can be enjoyed and the toxicity easily avoided through relatively infrequent monitoring of vitamin D blood levels.

Important Vitamin D Supplementation Considerations

As noted above, vitamin D is vital to bone health, and it must be present within an optimal range to have its optimal effects. Too much or too little vitamin D is bad for the bones and the general health. Blindly supplementing with a large daily dose is not wise. To ensure proper dosing, vitamin D blood levels **must be** regularly monitored early in the course of supplementation. Currently the available scientific literature would indicate that a good target level of vitamin D in the blood would be between 40 and 80 ng/cc. Some advocate higher levels, but only a few advocate lower levels.

Within this range a level of between 50 and 60 ng/cc would probably be the best for long-term maintenance. The best vitamin D blood tests measure 25-hydroxyvitamin D. This is the direct precursor to the active form of vitamin D. Good ***starting*** doses, based on blood levels are as follows:

If the level is...	*The starting vitamin D3 dose should be*
Under 10 ng/cc	7,000 to 10,000 IU daily
10 to 20 ng/cc	5,000 IU daily
20 to 30 ng/cc	2,000 to 4,000 IU daily
30 and 40 ng/cc	1,000 to 2,000 IU daily

Recheck the vitamin D level every 2 to 3 months, and adjust accordingly. Once an acceptable level has been reached it would be a good idea to recheck it every six months or so.

Summary

Assuming the maintenance of optimal blood levels, here's a recap of the health-promoting benefits of vitamin D supplementation:

- Helps prevent osteoporosis.
- Lowers risk of bone fracture.
- Suppresses resorption of bone and loss of bony calcium.
- Produces rapid recovery of bone mineral density.
- Decreases the incidence of many cancers.
- Boosts the immune system.

- Beneficial in the treatment of multiple diseases including hypertension, atherosclerosis, cancer, asthma, diabetes, and inflammation.
- Vitamin D decreases all-cause mortality.

Properly-dosed vitamin D is essential in maintaining healthy calcium metabolism, and it has many other health and longevity benefits as well. However, periodic monitoring of vitamin D3 blood levels is essential in the supplementation of this extremely valuable nutrient.

CHAPTER 9

Stronger Bones and More Calcium Channel Blocking

Omega-3 Fatty Acids Further Indict and Combat Calcium Toxicity

The health-promoting properties of the omega-3 form of essential fatty acids (EFAs), found abundantly in fish oil, have been widely celebrated for the last two decades. Few if any who care about nutrition have not heard of their benefits for heart and brain as well as for defense against degenerative diseases.

Why do EFAs exhibit such positive health effects? EFAs inhibit cellular uptake of calcium. It is very reasonable that a lion's share of their health-promoting abilities can be traced to this inhibitory activity. The effects of such a calcium-blocking mechanism is yet another indictment against the disease-causing effects of excess calcium.

What Are Essential Fatty Acids?

Fatty acids are comprised of straight carbon-hydrogen strings that have a carboxyl (carbon-oxygen-oxygen-hydrogen) group on the front end. They are called fatty acids because of their fat-like properties. But unlike fats that the body uses for fuel, essential fatty acids are used for biological processes in the body. Depending on the number of carbons that are chained together, EFAs can be short-, medium-, or long-chain. The last carbon on the end of the chain is called the omega carbon (named from the last letter of the Greek alphabet).

Whether a fatty acid is designated as an omega-3 or an omega-6 depends of the location of the first carbon double bond from the omega end of the chain. An omega-3 has a double bond between the third and fourth carbons from the last carbon in the chain, whereas an omega-6 has a double bond between the sixth and seventh from the end.

Essential fatty acids, which are normal constituents of every membrane in the body, are fatty acids that must be obtained from the diet.

Essential fatty acids (EFAs), which are normal constituents of every membrane in the body, are fatty acids that must be obtained from the diet.[1]

Generally, of these diet-derived fatty acids, the omega-3 fatty acids are the most important ones for helping to sustain healthy bones and good health in general. These are also known as omega-3 long-chain polyunsaturated fatty acids (PUFAs).

An important source for supplemental omega-3 PUFAs is fish oil, which contains substantial amounts of the omega-3 PUFAs known as eicosapentaenoic acid (EPA) and docosahexaenoic acid (DHA).[2] Both EPA and DHA have proven to be especially important in conferring health benefits for the heart, the brain, the immune system, the bones, the treatment of cancer, the lessening of inflammation, and the lowering of elevated triglyceride levels.[3-18]

Researchers have demonstrated the calcium channel blocking, or calcium inhibiting function of DHA.[19] In endothelial cell cultures pretreatment with DHA significantly reduced cellular uptake of calcium.[20]

Omega-3 Fatty Acids and Bone Health

In growing male rats given controlled diets, one group was given corn oil and the other tuna oil (EFA-rich). Those in the tuna oil-fed group all showed significantly higher calcium absorption, bone mineral density, and bone calcium content relative to the corn oil-fed group.

The long-term increased intake of EFA improved the mechanical properties of bone.

In particular the DHA content of the red blood cell membranes correlated significantly with bone density and bone calcium content.[21] A study on mice showed that the long-term increased intake of EFA improved the mechanical properties of bone.[22]

Another animal study, this time on hens, showed that supplementation with alpha-linolenic acid, an omega-3 fatty acid similar to EPA, resulted in a 40% to 60% reduction in keel bone (sternum) fractures that commonly occur during egg laying.[23] It should also be noted that alpha-linolenic acid can be converted to EPA and DHA in the body.[24]

Consistent with the preceding animal studies, animals deficient in EFAs develop severe osteoporosis along with significant calcification in the kidneys and the arteries. EFAs, and EPA in particular, play a vital role in the regulation and prevention of undesirable, abnormal [ectopic] calcifications.[25]

Conversely, omega-3 fatty acid supplementation in rats clearly decreased these abnormal calcifications of the aortas and kidneys.[26] In rat studies where calcification in the kidneys was induced by abdominal injections of calcium gluconate, adequate doses of EPA were highly effective in reducing it.[27]

Other animal studies have shown that diets high in omega-3 fatty acids result in several positive effects on the bone. Most notably, researchers have reported improved calcium balance, increased osteoblast (bone-forming cell) activity, and a reduction of inflammation as evidenced by an inhibition of cytokine activity.[28] Cytokines are a class of molecules that regulate different processes in the body, usually in reaction to a particular condition such as increased inflammation.

> *Men with the top 20% DHA concentrations appeared to have better protection from loss of bone mineral density compared to all the other subjects..*

Supplementation with omega-3 fatty acids (EPA and DHA) has also been shown to decrease both urinary oxalate excretion and the risk of calcium oxalate crystallization in the urine of healthy subjects.[29] In other studies that looked at individuals who were already known to be stone formers, omega-3 fatty acid supplementation resulted in significant decreases in urinary calcium and oxalate excretion.

These are factors that should result in decreased stone formation, suggesting a protective role of EPA in the development of kidney stones.[30,31] A significant reduction in urinary calcium excretion by calcium-regulating agents, such as EPA and DHA, often means that there is less chronic mobilization of calcium from the bones.

A number of human studies support the conclusions of these animal studies, although large long-term studies investigating the impact of high-dose supplemental (versus dietary) omega-3 fatty acids on osteoporosis could not be found.[32] Of the studies that have been done, many are small in size and with substantial differences in the protocols. One group reviewed 10 randomized controlled trials and found either positive effects or no effects for omega-3 fatty acids on osteoporosis patients.[33]

In a study looking at plasma levels, men with the top 20% DHA concentrations appeared to have better protection from loss of bone mineral density compared to all the other subjects.[34]

Other researchers suggest that DHA supplementation decreases bone turnover and significantly increases bone mineral density. Their conclusions were based on the evaluation of favorable markers of bone formation and degradation using DHA as part of an osteoporosis treatment regimen.[35]

Higher levels of DHA and EPA in the red blood cells was associated with less osteoporosis and greater bone mass.

A study in postmenopausal Korean women found that higher levels of DHA and EPA in the red blood cells were associated with less osteoporosis and greater bone mass.[36]

Another study found that greater dietary intake of omega-3 fatty acids, and PUFAs in general, was associated with increased bone density measured at the lumbar spine.[37] It is highly likely that a large, long-term trial with highly dosed EPA and DHA would demonstrate improved bone health and lessened fracture risk in osteoporosis patients.

There is no evidence that omega-3 fatty acids produce any adverse effects in osteoporosis patients. Considering the many well-documented positive effects and the decreased all-cause mortality associated with them, supplementation with omega-3 fatty acids is clearly justified.

It should be noted that combining different positive agents to treat osteoporosis or any other chronic degenerative disease, usually provides additive, and frequently synergistic, benefits. In a small randomized, placebo-controlled, and double-blind study, 70 patients were given either calcium only or a product containing genistein (a phytoestrogen with antioxidant properties), vitamin D3, vitamin K1, and a polyunsaturated fatty acid ester containing EPA and DHA. After only six months, the control group demonstrated a significant decline in bone mineral density while the supplemented group maintained bone density.[38]

Omega-3 fatty acids were effective in preventing coronary events, including cardiac death, especially in persons with a high cardiovascular risk.

Omega-3 Fatty Acid Supplementation Lowers All-Cause Mortality

Increased dietary and supplemental omega-3 fatty acid intake has demonstrated impressive results in decreasing the chances of death from heart disease, cancer, and even all causes. The effects on all-cause mortality clearly indicate that this group of nutrients, like magnesium and vitamins C, D, and K, play an important role in helping to optimize the metabolism of all the cells in the body, in addition to the role they play in calcium metabolism in general.

In a review of studies looking at the dietary and/or supplemental intake of the omega-3 fatty acids DHA and EPA, the conclusion was that these nutrients were effective in preventing coronary events, including cardiac death, especially in persons with a high cardiovascular risk.[39]

A retrospective study that looked at the effect of taking supplemental omega-3 fatty acids in patients after myocardial infarction [heart attack], both with and without diabetes, resulted in a lessened all-cause mortality.[40]

Another retrospective study on 36,003 Chinese found that those individuals consuming the most fish (a source of much DHA and EPA) on a regular basis also had lower all-cause mortality.[41] A small prospective study with supplemental omega-3 fatty acids also demonstrated a clear tendency to reduced all-cause mortality.[42]

Another study that examined DHA levels in the red blood cells of hemodialysis patients found those levels to be an independent predictor of all-cause mortality. Those patients in the highest tertile (1/3) of DHA levels were less likely to die relative to those patients in the lowest tertile.[43]

In the most definitive prospective study on omega-3 fatty acids and all-cause mortality, nearly 1,000 patients with stable coronary artery disease were followed over a six-year period. The blood levels of EPA and DHA were found to be inversely related to total mortality.

It was also noted that the findings were independent of standard and emerging cardiac risk factors and unaffected by any adjustment for age, sex, ethnicity, or even inflammatory markers. These investigators were able to conclude that above-average blood levels of omega-3 fatty acids had a lower risk of death relative to patients with lower levels. They also concluded that a reduced blood omega-3 level is an independent risk marker for death from any cause in coronary heart disease patients.[44] Another omega-3 fatty acid product studied conferred an additional 20% reduction in all-cause mortality in a group of post-myocardial infarction patients.[45]

> *Patients with the higher EPA and DHA intakes had both a lessening of new breast cancer events and a decrease in all-cause mortality.*

EPA and DHA intake from diet and supplements in a group of 3,081 women with early stage breast cancer were analyzed. Patients with the higher EPA and DHA intakes, compared to lowest tertile of intake, had both a lessening of new breast cancer events and a decrease in all-cause mortality. [46] Omega-3 fatty acids have actually been shown to slow growth and induce cell death in a variety of cell lines derived from human cancers of the colon, pancreas, prostate, and breast. [47]

Safety of Omega-3 Fatty Acid Supplementation

EFA supplementation, typically from fish oil or other marine source oil, is generally safe and tolerated very well. Although no clear toxic effects are known to be associated with the intake of EFAs, undesirable side effects from very high dosing can manifest as gastrointestinal discomfort and/or diarrhea. One research group found the maximum tolerated dose of EFAs from fish oil to be 0.3 g/kg, meaning a 150-pound person can take as much as 21 grams daily, having a content of roughly 13 grams of EPA and DHA. [48] In a review of the literature examining the safety of EFA supplementation, no severe adverse effects were reported. The minor adverse effects reported generally related to gastrointestinal discomfort. [49]

Probably the main concern with EFA supplementation from fish oil is the need to purchase a high enough quality of fish oil so that there is no significant contamination with heavy metals like mercury and other environmental toxins. One particular recommendation, while not the only quality fish oil supplement available, is made in Chapter 16.

Omega-3 Fatty Acid Dosing Considerations

The overall suggested dosing range of EFA from fish oil would be between 1 gram and 4 grams of total EPA and DHA content daily, although higher dosing short of causing gastrointestinal upset is acceptable and can provide additional benefits. Along with the other supplementation recommended, most individuals will do well on a dose between 1 and 2 grams daily.

Summary

The human studies on osteoporosis, bone quality, and fracture risk relative to EFA intake are consistently suggestive of a positive effect, but not nearly so dramatically as is seen with vitamin C, vitamin K, vitamin D, magnesium, and the sex hormones. However, the effects that EFAs have on calcium metabolism and calcification in general, along with the evidence that EFA intake also decreases all-cause mortality, still makes the recommendation to include omega-3 EFA supplementation in an osteoporosis treatment regimen a good one.

CHAPTER 10

Bone Health: The Hormonal Component

Estrogen, Testosterone, and Thyroid

Resisting the physiological changes that occur as hormone production declines over time with hormonal replacement is an additional powerful therapeutic tool for optimizing bone health. The fight against osteoporosis and the other chronic degenerative diseases that ensue as calcium mobilizes from the bones to other parts of the body is much more effective when deficient hormone levels can be skillfully returned to normal levels. This requires prescription medication from a healthcare practitioner experienced in dealing with hormone replacement to carefully monitor its effects over time.

Deficiencies of estrogen in women, testosterone in men, and thyroid hormone in men or women can profoundly limit the degree of positive response seen with all of the other measures discussed. All too frequently today, testing for these hormones is still not routinely performed, and a great deal of the potential benefits from other good treatments are being lost by many people for a wide variety of medical conditions. Although not an exhaustive review of these three hormones, what follows will present much of what you and your physician will want to consider as you treat any of these hormone deficiencies in order to improve bone health and/or general health.

> *Seven to eight years of estrogen therapy in postmenopausal women was found to substantially inhibit calcium deposition in the coronary arteries.*

Estrogen

Estrogen plays a big part in the metabolism of virtually all the cells of the body. It wields far greater influence than its well-established role in maintaining the health of the reproductive and sexual organs and in determining the appropriate secondary sex characteristics in women. The major focus of the following information is the reality that osteoporosis is strongly promoted by a deficiency of estrogen in women.

Estrogen Therapy Inhibits Abnormal Calcification

Estrogen has its own positive effects in lessening, preventing, and probably reversing abnormal calcification in the body. It has been found to inhibit the ability of a bone metabolism protein to promote vascular calcification.[1] In rabbits that lost their estrogen production due to removal of the ovaries a fourfold increase in vascular calcification resulted.[2]

Seven to eight years of estrogen therapy in postmenopausal women was found to substantially inhibit calcium deposition in the coronary arteries. This randomized clinical trial was conducted with women who were between 50 and 59 years at the beginning of the trial.[3] Similar results were obtained in a study looking at women aged 50 to 80 years.[4] An investigation of serum estradiol levels in postmenopausal women found that the women with the higher levels had the lower coronary artery calcium scores, independent of age and other coronary artery risk factors.[5]

Estrogen and Bone Health

It is well established that the postmenopausal decline in estrogen levels seen in women is a major factor in the development and evolution of osteoporosis. Even in osteoporotic men the prevalence of an estrogen deficiency exceeds that of testosterone deficiency.[6] It has also been shown that bone mass density in postmenopausal women tends to decline as serum markers of oxidative stress increase.[7] This is fully consistent with the theory that a significant antioxidant deficiency — especially vitamin C — in the bones initiates, and over time worsens, osteoporosis.

The postmenopausal decline in estrogen levels seen in women is a major factor in the development and evolution of osteoporosis.

The greatest loss of bone in postmenopausal women occurs closest to menopause and declines thereafter.[8] This is important to remember when considering how to dose estrogen in hormone replacement therapy. Lower estrogen levels in premenopausal women also produce a lesser decline in bone mineral density followed by a precipitous density decline at menopause.[9] Since estrogen is important to bone health at any age, correction of an estrogen deficiency will have its greatest impact when started early after menopause or at the first indication of a significant decline in estrogen levels.

Even if the prime time for estrogen therapy is missed, it will still arrest bone loss years after the onset of menopause. The low levels of estrogen seen late in menopause continue to exert a restraining effect on healthy bone turnover and lead to a further deterioration of bone health. [10] Starting the therapy relatively late will just have a less substantial impact on the overall prevention of fractures.

Hormone replacement therapy reduces the incidence of all osteoporosis-related fractures in postmenopausal women.

An estrogen deficiency increases the production of pro-inflammatory signaling molecules [cytokines], which will also use up antioxidant stores. [11] The longer and the more pronounced the production of such cytokines, the greater the loss of antioxidants. Bone loss initiated by estrogen deficiency occurs with a simultaneous increase in pro-oxidant cytokine production, resulting in a compounding effect. Postmenopausal women with the highest receptor levels for pro-inflammatory cytokines — indicating elevated inflammation and decreased antioxidant levels — had the most hip fractures. [12]

It has now been established that hormone replacement therapy (HRT) reduces the incidence of all osteoporosis-related fractures in postmenopausal women, even in those who are at low risk of fracture. [13] In contrast, discontinuation of postmenopausal HRT has been found to dramatically increase the chances of hip fracture by 55% when compared to women who continued such therapy. [14,15] Furthermore, an animal study showed that when fracture did occur in the presence of estrogen deficiency, poor healing took place. [16] Estrogen therapy has been established to increase bone mineral density in postmenopausal women compared to a placebo group that lost bone mineral density during the three-year trial period. [17]

Estrogen, like vitamin D, is a double-edged sword. Too little is bad and too much is bad. However, the fear of aggravating other conditions such as heart disease with too great an estrogen effect should not stop the physician from trying to find the appropriate form and (small) dose of estrogen to best benefit the patient.

The optimal approach to estrogen therapy varies greatly with each patient so individual adjustments are essential. Some patients might also benefit from some progesterone support as well.

Hormone replacement therapy always requires a regular monitoring of laboratory tests. These tests should watch for indicators of increased inflammation, track factors associated with increased cardiac risk, and monitor for signs of metabolic syndrome. Decisions to continue or discontinue a given therapy, changes in dosages, change in form, and even decisions to discontinue therapy should be made in response to these test results. The other aspects of the suggested treatment protocols in Chapter 15 may occasionally have enough positive impact on the bones and the blood work to minimize or even eliminate the indication for estrogen therapy.

> *The optimal approach to estrogen therapy varies greatly with each patient so individual adjustments are essential.*

Estrogen Therapy Side Effects and Impact on Mortality Risk

How estrogen replacement therapy is administered is of the utmost importance. Results of specific estrogen protocols can and do vary on an individual basis. Doing things the wrong way will often cause significant adverse side effects. Some hormone replacement regimens have even produced an increase in heart disease, cancer, and stroke.[18] Understanding why undesirable side effects occur allows an approach to hormone replacement therapy that is virtually devoid of problems while resulting in substantial benefits.

It has been established that women with low estrogen levels have greater all-cause mortality.[19] Estrogen deficiency also promotes metabolic syndrome,[20-22] which typically involves at least three of the following: abdominal obesity, increased triglycerides, low HDL lipoproteins, high blood pressure, and an elevated fasting blood sugar. The presence of metabolic syndrome is associated with an increased risk for the development of heart disease and diabetes mellitus.

> *Studies have shown that hormone replacement therapy can lower all-cause mortality.*

Transdermal estrogen administration, discussed at greater length below, has been shown to have a protective effect against the risk factors of the metabolic syndrome in women following the removal of the ovaries or the ovaries plus the uterus [surgical menopause].[23] Recent animal studies also indicate that properly administered estrogen can improve or reverse metabolic syndrome.[24,25] However, standard-dose oral estrogen appeared to increase coronary heart disease events when metabolic syndrome was present at the start of therapy.[26]

Additionally, studies have shown that hormone replacement therapy can lower all-cause mortality. A 10-year follow-up study showed that two to three years of hormone replacement therapy in postmenopausal women decreased all-cause mortality compared to women not taking hormones.[27] Similarly, a Swedish study following 23,346 postmenopausal women also found hormone replacement therapy to significantly reduce all-cause mortality over a follow-up period of eight to nine years.

The therapy showed a reduction of deaths in each of the 12 major cause-of-death categories in the study.[28]

It is also important to remember that all of the potential side effects of aggressive hormone replacement therapy are secondary to mechanisms of increased oxidative stress. The therapeutic approaches recommended in this book feature robust antioxidant support. Mainstream therapeutic protocols, for the most part, completely ignore the importance of protective antioxidant administration. While the ultimate decision on modifying or discontinuing estrogen therapy will rely on clinical evaluation with the serial monitoring of appropriate laboratory tests, the concomitant intake of large amounts of vitamin C and other antioxidants will always lessen side effects and frequently eliminate them completely.

> *Mainstream therapeutic protocols, for the most part, completely ignore the importance of protective antioxidant administration.*

The Women's Health Initiative on hormone replacement therapy produced some additional noteworthy results. This study on healthy postmenopausal women was randomized and controlled. Even though the trial demonstrated increases in some cancers and in some cardiovascular events, the overall chances of death, or all-cause mortality, was not increased by the hormones. Estrogen was administered at a standard-dose amount, and progestin was given as well.[29,30] This widely published and reviewed study warned of an increased risk of thrombotic cardiovascular events seen during the trial. Awareness of this study induced a panic in women throughout the United States, and many of them discontinued their hormone therapy. Many physicians as well became reluctant to prescribe hormone replacement.[31]

Sadly, many of those women would have derived substantial benefit, including decreased all-cause mortality had they been treated with a lower-dose estrogen without the progestin. Although this adverse side effect was blamed on estrogen, it must be emphasized that virtually all of the women in this trial were supplementing calcium as well. Such supplementation, along with the progestin and the typically marginal magnesium intake in such a population of patients, are all factors that can cause the increased thrombotic cardiovascular events that were seen in this trial.[32]

> *Is there is a way to safely restore estrogen deficiencies, at least to some degree? The simple answer is yes.*

Estrogen Therapy Considerations

The compelling issue, then, is whether there is a way to safely restore estrogen deficiencies, at least to some degree. The simple answer is yes. However, multiple factors are involved and the prescribing healthcare practitioner must pay closer attention than when prescribing most drugs for most conditions. The factors involved include the following:

1) Dose
2) Types
3) Formulations
4) Other hormone administration
5) Routes of administration
6) Duration of administration
7) Timing of initial administration
8) Concurrent antioxidant administration
9) Serial clinical correlation
10) Serial laboratory testing

1) **Estrogen Dosing:** Side effects reliably increase in number and significance the higher the dose of estrogen used. Standard doses of estrogen have consistently demonstrated an increased stroke risk of about one-third in women older than 60 years of age.[33] A study in early postmenopausal women demonstrated that low-dose oral estrogen had a profile of positive effects on lipids and blood flow comparable to standard-dose estrogen with significantly lessened side effects such as vaginal bleeding and breast tenderness.[34] The same low-dose of oral estrogen that was compared to the standard-dose was also found to significantly increase bone density in the hip and spine of postmenopausal women over a 24-month period. Control patients, those who did not receive treatment, showed significant decreases in bone density in the hip and spine.[35]

2) **Estrogen Types:** Conjugated equine estrogen is commonly used in hormone replacement therapy, especially in the United States. Approximately 100 different estrogens are in this preparation, all naturally occurring in horses, with only a few forms naturally occurring in humans. Many estrogen formulations now available in the United States contain bioidentical estrogens which are molecularly identical to the naturally produced estrogens.[36]

Unfortunately much of the research looking at effects and side effects has utilized conjugated equine estrogen. One can reasonably conclude any good effects of this product will be shared by bioidentical estrogen, but it is not necessarily true that the side effects will be equally prevalent with the bioidentical product. Because of this much of the positive effect of estrogen and the true nature of its side effects profile have not been definitively documented. However a substantial amount of physiological data and many positive clinical outcomes have already clearly shown that bioidentical hormone use is associated with lower risks and is more efficacious than the use of their animal-produced and synthetic counterparts. [37]

3) **Estrogen Formulations:** These include pills, gels, emulsions, sprays, and injectables.

4) **Other Hormone Administration:** A two-fold increase in venous thromboembolism (blood clotting) has been seen with oral estrogen and progestogen combination hormone replacement therapy. However, no significant increase in this side effect has been seen with oral estrogen alone. [38] Also, oral estrogen alone reduces the incidence of breast cancer, while estrogen and progestogen together have been shown to increase the incidence of breast cancer. [39]

5) **Routes of Estrogen Administration:** Many routes of administration are available for the administration of hormones such as estrogen. These include oral, transdermal by patch, percutaneous by cream or gel, intramuscular, subcutaneous, sublingual, vaginal, and nasal.

Oral Estrogen. Oral doses of estrogen are more rapidly metabolized and undergo significant processing by the liver. [40]

Non-Oral Estrogens. Non-oral administrations of estrogen that do not pass through the liver from the intestine (transdermal, percutaneous, vaginal) have fewer or no side effects along with equal or better desirable effects. And this is achievable at equal or even smaller doses.[41-43]

Transdermal Estrogen. Low-dose transdermal estrogen has been shown to provide a high level of menopausal symptom relief and typically was very well-tolerated by the patients in one study.[44] Transdermal estrogen lessened the atherogenic profile in the plasma while oral estrogen aggravated it even though the oral estrogen did increase HDL cholesterol while lowering LDL cholesterol, considered desirable effects by themselves.[45] Appropriate blood tests must be monitored during hormone therapy, as transdermal estrogen had no significant effect on the inflammation parameter C-reactive protein (CRP), while standard-dose oral estrogen increased it significantly.[46] The increased CRP levels from the oral preparation are felt to be due to the obligatory processing of the doses through the liver, which does not occur with the transdermal preparation.[47]

In addition a comparison of the same two estrogen preparations found that the transdermal preparation was even more effective than the oral preparation in promoting bone growth in the spine in young girls with deficient endogenous estrogen production. These girls were otherwise destined to develop osteoporosis [Turner syndrome].[48] This result is consistent with the findings that transdermal estrogen, oral estrogen, and oral estrogen plus progestogen all had similar therapeutic value in the prevention of bone loss in postmenopausal women.[49] Even ultra-low-dose transdermal estrogen monotherapy has been shown to significantly increase bone mineral density and reduce the markers of bone turnover while having little to no side effects of consequence.[50] Slightly higher transdermal dosing is indicated in the women with very low to undetectable estrogen levels in order to reach optimal levels during treatment.[51] For patients with adverse skin reactions to transdermal estrogen preparations a very well tolerated lotion-like nanoparticle estradiol emulsion is available for use.[52]

6) **Duration of Administration**: The optimal duration of treatment has not been conclusively established. One thought is that estrogen therapy should be utilized for prevention of bone loss and fracture in the early postmenopausal period for about five years. A meta-analysis that reviewed a large number of studies found an association between estrogen use and breast cancer, more strikingly so for therapy given longer than five years. Unfortunately transdermal estrogen preparations were not differentiated from regular oral estrogen administration in this study.[53] Women deemed to be at low risk for adverse events such as venous thrombosis appear to be good candidates for continued therapy beyond five years.[54] However, regardless of the duration of therapy, the route of administration is especially important for women at high risk of venous thrombosis. In these cases transdermal

estrogen administration appears to largely eliminate this adverse event.[55,56]

7) **Timing of Initial Administration:** Some studies have shown that menopausal hormone therapy appears to increase the risk of cardiovascular disease when initiated late in menopause while having beneficial cardiovascular effects in younger women near the time of onset of menopause.[57,58] This finding is consistent with the observation that early estrogen therapy in rats with lack of estrogen due to removal of the ovaries prevented the development of oxidative stress that would occur otherwise, while late-onset estrogen therapy did not have this effect.[59]

8) **Concurrent Antioxidant Administration:** As demonstrated in previous chapters, keeping antioxidants and antioxidant nutrients at optimal levels in the body decreases all-cause mortality. As a reminder, all side effects are ultimately caused by, or inflict their damage through, pro-oxidant mechanisms. Therefore it is highly likely that judicious estrogen therapy, when accompanied by a high level of antioxidant support, would present few if any discernible side effects. When all the "side effects" of an antioxidant treatment protocol are decreased oxidative stress and increased longevity the inclusion of additional agents that do have a legitimate negative side effect profile in such a protocol rarely demonstrates any clinical or laboratory test downsides.

9) **Serial Clinical Correlation:** If an estrogen administration is appropriate the undesirable symptoms associated with menopause should be minimized and they should never be aggravated. A clinician should

never ignore negative patient feedback just because a given form and dose of estrogen is deemed necessary. There will be some patients, usually the most elderly, who will not require estrogen replacement in their osteoporosis treatment protocol as their clinical response to all other parts of the protocol will be sufficiently positive. Another key to determining proper dosing of estrogen relates to control of the vasomotor symptoms following menopause. Hot flashes correlate to lower levels of plasma antioxidants, increased cardiac risk factors, and a higher risk of aortic calcification. Prompt adjustment of form and type of estrogen therapy should occur when vasomotor symptoms are pronounced and estrogen therapy should be discontinued if such adjustments cannot readily control those symptoms and largely reverse any cardiac risk factors that had been exacerbated. [60,61]

10) <u>**Serial Laboratory Testing:**</u> This is essential to assure that a treatment protocol is completely beneficial and appropriate for a given patient. Parameters that reflect inflammation should generally improve or at least stay the same. Any estrogen administration that worsens such parameters should be discontinued or modified in dose or form so that the changes resolve. The same reasoning also applies to laboratory parameters that reflect general cardiac risk, such as the lipids like cholesterol and triglycerides. Few patients should ever have an estrogen-provoked poor outcome such as a stroke or a heart attack that was not heralded to some degree by a worsening of a number of blood tests during the course of the estrogen therapy. Properly administered

estrogen therapy should lessen the chances of a negative cardiovascular outcome (stroke, heart attack, venous thrombosis), the chances of a new cancer, and even the chances of new-onset diabetes. [62,63] Such therapy results in an improvement in critical serial blood tests.

Estrogen Summary and General Recommendations

Menopause develops in response to reduced estrogen production by the ovaries. Once menopause has occurred, some degree of estrogen deficiency is virtually assured. Prior to the commencement of hormone replacement therapy, the first and most important question to ask is how severe the deficiency is in a given patient. This can be established by determining how the deficiency is affecting critical laboratory tests and by evaluating overall clinical status. For both the osteoporosis patient as well any other patient with a significant chronic degenerative disease, this evaluation should be conducted a few months after all other aspects of the suggested protocol (See Chapter 16) have been initiated. If a completely satisfactory clinical and laboratory response has not been seen, then estrogen therapy should be considered.

Unless there are compelling reasons not to do so this replacement hormone therapy should be given transdermally in the lowest available dose and of a bioidentical type. Depending on further clinical and laboratory follow-up, the estrogen can be increased in dose, kept at the same dose, or even discontinued. All ten of the factors discussed above need to be kept in mind in order to arrive at the best estrogen replacement therapy for a given patient. This includes a possible determination that a given patient may be better off with no replacement therapy. The other recommendations in the suggested protocol can be reliably employed to substantially neutralize undesirable side effects that could occur from suboptimal estrogen administration.

Testosterone

Like estrogen deficiency in women, testosterone deficiency in men is a strong promoter of osteoporosis. Although long considered to be primarily a sex hormone, the scientific literature has now documented testosterone to have many different biological functions with effects on virtually all of the tissues and organs of the body.[64] It has especially pronounced effects on the general metabolism, the integrity of bone and muscle, the cardiovascular system, and the brain.

> *It is estimated that testosterone deficiency is present in at least 30% of men aged 40 to 79 years.*

A substantial and prolonged deficiency of testosterone results in impaired glucose metabolism, increased bone turnover, weakness in the muscles, lessened cognitive function, and generalized fatigue and lethargy. Correcting or lessening the degrees of significant testosterone deficiency will do far more than arrest or help to reverse osteoporosis. As with estrogen, an appropriate protocol for hormone administration needs to be followed to assure optimal benefits and minimal risks.

The negative effects of testosterone deficiency have resulted in a substantial public health burden,[65] as a very large number of men are being found to have low testosterone levels and only a relatively small number of them are being diagnosed and given any hormone replacement therapy at all. It is estimated that testosterone deficiency is present in at least 30% of men aged 40 to 79 years.[66]

Roughly this same percentage of diabetic men were evaluated and found to have testosterone deficiency as well, with 17% felt to have severe deficiencies.[67] Above and beyond the role that testosterone deficiency plays in promoting osteoporosis, testing for deficiencies in older men should be taking place much more routinely than it is now.

Testosterone and Bone Health

Testosterone deficiency has been shown to be a clear risk factor for hip fractures in men.[68] This is an especially important point to realize since fully one third of hip fractures occur in men.[69,70] Furthermore, such hip fractures in men are associated with nearly twice the mortality of osteoporotic women with the same fractures.[71,72] And when men do have osteoporotic hip fractures, testosterone deficiency is present 50% of the time.[73]

Consistent with the increased fracture risk seen with testosterone deficiency, multiple studies have shown that lower bioavailable testosterone levels directly relate with lower bone mineral densities.[74-76] In a randomized placebo-controlled trial, osteoporotic men with low testosterone levels were treated with only 20 mg orally daily of testosterone undecanoate. Bone mineral density significantly increased and no significant effects were seen on PSA testing. Interestingly, the 20 mg dose was found to be equally effective as a 40 mg dose.[77] Another recent study showed that a long-acting injectable form of testosterone resulted in a significant increase in bone mineral density in men with low testosterone and metabolic syndrome.[78] This effect of testosterone on bone mass was also documented to occur in very young men with low testosterone

> *When men do have osteoporotic hip fractures, testosterone deficiency is present 50% of the time.*

levels.[79] In general, testosterone therapy should be a part of an osteoporosis protocol for men deficient in testosterone at the initiation of therapy. Therapy should be continued as long as regular blood testing verifies that critical blood tests are improving or stable.[80]

> *Studies have now shown that low testosterone levels independently predict increased cardiovascular mortality.*

Testosterone, Cardiovascular Health, and All-Cause Mortality

It has been clearly established that there is a high prevalence of low testosterone levels in men with coronary artery disease. This association is present regardless of patient age. Low testosterone is also a documented risk factor for metabolic syndrome, which fits well with its association with increased coronary artery disease.[81-83] Studies have now shown that low testosterone levels independently predict increased cardiovascular mortality.[84-87]

Most significantly, multiple studies have established that blood levels of testosterone are inversely related to death from all causes, not just heart disease. The effect appears to persist as long as the testosterone is low and one of the studies found that the men in the lowest quartile (25%) of testosterone levels had a 24% increased risk of all-cause mortality.[88-93] Consistent with these findings, low testosterone levels have also been directly linked to an increased risk of major adverse cardiovascular events in hypertensive patients.[94,95]

The risk of death appears to be especially increased when a vitamin D deficiency is combined with a free testosterone deficiency.[96] Furthermore, the judicious administration of testosterone in deficient men appears to reduce the risk of cardiovascular disease, as reflected in a lessening of risk factor-related laboratory tests.[97] This is further evidence of the importance of the effects of testosterone on all the cells of the body, since its deficiency increases the chances of death from anything. In other words, a testosterone deficiency is going to substantially worsen any underlying disease process regardless of the organ system involved.

Further support for this connection between low testosterone and death comes from the application of androgen deprivation therapy to men with prostate cancer. Androgen basically refers to testosterone, which is well known to stimulate prostate cancer cells to grow. Prostate cancer cell growth can be arrested and some such cells will even die when testosterone production is drastically lowered, stopped completely, or the effects of testosterone are blocked. However, the administration of androgen deprivation therapy, which is largely equivalent to the severe lessening or absence of testosterone effect in the body, has been shown to be associated with increased cardiovascular risk, including death.[98-100]

Testosterone has been found to have some calcium channel blocking effects similar to the calcium channel blocking effects of the drug nifedipine.

Testosterone has been found to have some calcium channel blocking effects similar to the calcium channel blocking effects of the drug nifedipine.[101-103] This is consistent with its ability to relax blood vessels and to decrease peripheral vascular resistance.[104] This importance of testosterone in decreasing all-cause mortality is also consistent with the known beneficial effects of other calcium channel blockers on all-cause mortality.[105-108]

The prevention of abnormal calcification is an important factor in longevity and the nonspecific lessening of the symptoms of all chronic degenerative diseases. Mobilization and dissolution of existing calcium deposits also produce these desired effects. The benefits of restoring testosterone levels are further reflected in the fact that bioavailable testosterone levels in men were found to be inversely related to the presence and degree of detectable coronary artery calcium.[109] Like vitamin C, magnesium, vitamin K, vitamin D, the essential fatty acids, and estrogen, testosterone also promotes the integration of calcium into normal bone formation while inhibiting its deposition elsewhere in the body — thus accounting for much of its ability to decrease death from all causes.

> *Testosterone also promotes the integration of calcium into normal bone formation while inhibiting its deposition elsewhere in the body.*

Testosterone Therapy Side Effects

Testosterone therapy for men with deficient levels can have significant side effects if the therapy is inappropriately administered. Nevertheless, following a protocol that uses low doses with attention to clinical response and any untoward changes in blood tests will much more often provide help rather than harm. Like estrogen, multiple factors come into play in the optimal administration of testosterone to a given patient. In treating a patient with osteoporosis it is very important to see how effective the rest of the recommended protocol (Chapter 16) is before proceeding directly to hormone replacement therapy.

In years past a great deal of concern had been raised over the relationship between testosterone administration and prostate cancer. However, recent research has indicated that although testosterone will certainly promote the growth of existing prostate cancer it is not associated with the development of new prostate cancer.[110,111] In fact the incidence of prostate cancer in testosterone-deficient men receiving hormone replacement therapy is lower than its incidence in a population of untreated men with normal baseline testosterone levels.[112]

Any persistent fear about testosterone and prostate cancer should be greatly tempered with the fact that prostate cancer is frequently associated with low testosterone levels.[113]

As long as a given patient is followed carefully an unexpected increase in a prostate-specific antigen (PSA) test after starting testosterone therapy can be considered a benefit. It simply means cancer will have been discovered sooner than it would have occurred otherwise, and the testosterone therapy can be promptly discontinued.

Any persistent fear about testosterone and prostate cancer should be greatly tempered with the fact that prostate cancer is frequently associated with low testosterone levels.

Like estrogen, vitamin D, and thyroid hormone, too much is bad and too little is bad. Intelligent administration of these agents is always indicated and except for rare cases, they should not be avoided completely when their levels are known to be low.

Concerns have also long existed regarding the relationship of testosterone to increasing prostate mass but not in a malignant manner (benign prostatic hypertrophy, BPH). A double-blinded study on middle-aged men showed that their mean prostate volume was increased by 12% over an 8-month period of testosterone treatment.

An oral dose of 160 mg daily of testosterone undecanoate, a significantly high dose capable of producing levels above normal, was given during this period. Currently, a standard dose of this form of testosterone is 40 mg daily. And in spite of the slight increase in prostate volume, it was also noted that there was not the development of any obstructive urinary symptoms during the treatment period.[114,115]

> *In general, lower doses and slower absorption forms of testosterone are largely free of any undesirable side effects.*

A much more recent study on men with low testosterone levels and moderate to severe lower urinary tract symptoms demonstrated that testosterone replacement therapy rarely worsened the symptoms. In fact, many of the men showed an improvement in symptoms. Of note, the testosterone administered was in just a topical or a topical plus subcutaneous pellet form, a much gentler way to supplement than with oral testosterone undecanoate.[116]

A study on testosterone-deficient rabbits with metabolic syndrome actually showed that testosterone administration protected the rabbits from the prostatic hypoxia, fibrosis, and inflammation that help to develop prostatic hypertrophy and obstructive lower urinary symptoms.[117] This finding is totally consistent with the preceding human study.

Testosterone Therapy Dosing Considerations

Like estrogen, there are many different ways to administer testosterone therapy in testosterone-deficient men. In general, lower doses and slower absorption forms are largely free of any undesirable side effects. In one study aggressive dosing resulted in increased cardiac side

Bone Health: The Hormonal Component

effects for some individuals even though desirable effects such as increased muscle strength were occurring as well. The subject cohort was older (average age of 74), however, and target testosterone levels were too high (500 to 1000 ng/dL). More of the treated patients had preexisting hypertension and cardiovascular disease and were on statin therapy, more had hyperlipidemia, and more had worsening triglyceride levels over time.[118]

Age is an especially important factor in the safety of testosterone therapy. In a study on 1,438 testosterone-deficient men ranging in age from 34 to 63, both clinical and laboratory parameters were substantially improved with long-acting injections of testosterone.[119]

It is the therapeutic goal to always keep blood levels of testosterone in the middle of the normal range.

Larger doses that periodically exceed the desired long-term blood levels will tend to be less well-tolerated. They also have the potential to worsen important blood tests rather than improve them or leave them unaffected. It is the therapeutic goal to always keep blood levels of testosterone in the middle of the normal range rather than at supra-normal levels for any period of time.

Testosterone can be effectively administered orally, by intramuscular injection, by transdermal patches or gels, by subcutaneous pellet placement, and by buccal bioadhesive tablets [buccal tablets are discs placed in the mouth, generally on the gums above the left or right incisor once or twice per day].[120]

Optimally, testosterone levels and important blood chemistries, such as those associated with metabolic syndrome, should be checked every 3 months the first year. Clear worsening of any cardiac risk factor laboratory testing should be a red flag to either discontinue testosterone or proceed with lower doses in a less aggressive form of administration, such as transdermal. As the clinical situation and the serial laboratory tests become clearly stable with no worsened results, testosterone levels and other blood tests can be checked at intervals of six months to one year. [121] In older patients even greater attention needs to be paid to non-aggressive dosing along with keener attention to cardiac risk factors, with less ambitious long-term goals than might be the case with younger patients.

In order to minimize any chances of significant side effects occurring the goal of testosterone replacement therapy should only be to restore the testosterone level to the low normal to mid-normal section of the normal range. In a randomized, double-blind, placebo-controlled trial of testosterone therapy in men over 65 years of age, the most significant bone mineral density increases were seen in men who went from subnormal levels of testosterone up to mid-normal levels. When men who started with low normal levels of testosterone were raised to mid-normal levels overall bone density did not increase. [122]

Two important points are strongly suggested by this trial:

1) No man who has low normal levels of testosterone should receive testosterone therapy for his osteoporosis, and
2) Men with clear testosterone deficiencies should never be pushed to testosterone levels beyond the mid-normal range.

The idea is to give the cells some metabolic support but not to over-stimulate them, especially when those cells are no longer young. When levels are pushed into the high normal section of the normal range testosterone benefits tend to be minimized, while the negative side effects are maximized. Jet fuel is for jets, not for Model-Ts. Only in cases where testosterone replacement is being very carefully monitored and abnormal blood tests are continuing to improve with testosterone levels higher than mid-normal, should such dosing be maintained.

Testosterone Summary and General Recommendations

Testosterone deficiencies are commonly present in older men and not uncommonly in many middle-aged men as well. Such deficiencies are associated with increased all-cause mortality and they will always substantially worsen any existing osteoporosis. They should always be addressed unless clinical symptoms and abnormal laboratory tests can be resolved with the remainder of the treatment protocol discussed in Chapter 16.

The most important factors to keep in mind when treating a testosterone deficiency is to go low in dose and aim for no more than low normal to mid-normal target levels of testosterone in the blood. Transdermal applications are especially good for avoiding significant side effects. Other preparations can be utilized effectively as well. However, it is important to completely avoid the presence of blood levels of testosterone that are ever higher than normal even for limited periods of time.

For osteoporosis a reasonable goal is to realize some increase in bone mineral density or at least no deterioration, while improving or leaving unchanged important laboratory tests, such as PSA and the risk factor tests associated with metabolic syndrome and an increased risk of heart disease.

Finally it should be realized that the entirety of the protocols recommended in Chapters 16 and 17 will reliably lessen and often eliminate any potential side effects of inappropriately administered testosterone. High doses of vitamin C, vitamin K, bioavailable magnesium, and essential fatty acids, along with properly-dosed vitamin D and other antioxidants should protect against the manifestation of any significant side effects.

Thyroid

Thyroid hormone is another very important hormone that has substantial effects on the metabolism of all the cells in the body.[123] Significant morbidity and mortality occur when thyroid hormone is either substantially deficient or when it is present in excess. As such it is important to address the thyroid status in a manner similar to that of vitamin D and the sex hormones. Do not just assume that the levels of these critical hormones are in the optimal range. The proper laboratory screening tests must be performed when a treatment protocol is planned.

As a practical point, however, thyroid deficiency is much more common than thyroid excess, and it will be primarily addressed in the rest of this section. As well, many cases of hypothyroidism, especially those that are subclinical in degree, are diagnostic challenges, while the clinical and laboratory picture of hyperthyroidism is not nearly as problematic.

In a general fashion, thyroid hormone can be regarded as the pacemaker of the metabolism of the body. The right amount of this hormone lets the body run at its healthiest pace. Excess hormone revs it up, and deficient hormone slows it down.

Thyroid and Bone Health

Thyroid hormone has an important role in the health of the bone. It is required for the proper initial skeletal development and the establishment of peak bone mass.[124] Overall bone quality is compromised by too little or too much thyroid hormone. In both hyperthyroidism and hypothyroidism the risk of fracture is significantly increased. [125,126] However, the pathophysiological changes in the bone resulting from excess thyroid hormone versus decreased thyroid hormone are significantly different.

Excess thyroid levels accelerate bone turnover and this has resulted in hyperthyroidism being an established secondary cause of osteoporosis. [127-129] Deficient thyroid hormone, however, slows bone turnover and does not appear to decrease bone density. [130,131] However, even though hypothyroidism does not result in classically osteoporotic bone it still results in weaker bone, with an increased risk of fracture.

Overall bone quality is compromised by too little or too much thyroid hormone.

While it is well-established that the effective treatment of hyperthyroidism allows the restoration of some of the bone density lost while the thyroid hormone was elevated, the traditional treatment of hypothyroidism has less clear-cut effects on overall bone structure and bone health. The treatment of hypothyroidism with levothyroxine (T4) can result in a reduction in bone density. [132,133]

Based on the bone health seen with variable levels of thyroid hormone it would appear that traditional laboratory testing for thyroid function falls short of the mark in defining a true range of normal. Postmenopausal women with thyroid function tests in the upper range of normal were found to have decreased bone mineral density and greater fracture risk compared to patients with tests in the lower range of normal. [134]

In postmenopausal women with overall thyroid function test results in the normal range the women with the lowest levels of thyroid stimulating hormone (TSH) were found to have a significantly higher prevalence of fractures compared to women with the highest levels of TSH. [135] TSH is the hormone produced by the pituitary to stimulate the thyroid gland to produce thyroid hormone. It has also been shown that higher TSH levels in postmenopausal women with technically normal thyroid function tests are less prone to fracture as long as the TSH level does not exceed the normal range.[136]

It now appears that thyroid stimulating hormone has a direct bone-protecting effect.

Like with so many other hormones, too little TSH is bad, and too much TSH is bad. Generally, a TSH level will be lowered by thyroid therapy. These levels can be:

- Very low and suppressed (<0.04 mU/liter)
- Low but not suppressed (0.04 to 0.4 mU/liter)
- Within the normal range (0.4 to 4.0 mU/liter), or
- Elevated (>4.0 mU/liter)

A study on 17,684 patients taking T4 replacement therapy followed over eight years was conducted. It showed that individuals with high or suppressed TSH levels (elevated or very low) had an increased risk of cardiovascular disease and fractures. However, individuals with low but not suppressed TSH levels were free of this increased risk.[137] Generally, effective thyroid replacement therapy will always lower the elevated TSH level present before therapy, but a dose should not be given that pushes the TSH level into the very low and suppressed range noted above.

TSH was long considered to be active on the thyroid gland but nowhere else. Animal studies have now shown that TSH has a direct effect on bone, suppressing bone remodeling and turnover.[138-141] Expressed differently, it now appears that TSH has a direct bone-protecting effect. As such it does not appear to be desirable to drop TSH levels into the very low range with thyroid replacement unless clinical and laboratory considerations other than bone effect are of concern.[142] This should be an unlikely scenario, however, as very low TSH levels were also associated with increased cardiovascular risk and this is never a desirable effect, regardless of whatever other positive effects the thyroid replacement therapy might be achieving.

Thyroid, Cardiovascular Health, and All-Cause Mortality

Not surprisingly, both overt hyperthyroidism and overt hypothyroidism are independent risk factors for death from all causes. Even more significantly, relatively subtle increases or decreases in thyroid function play very prominent roles in general health, as both subclinical hyperthyroidism and subclinical hypothyroidism have also been established as clear risk factors for increased mortality.[143,144] Subclinical hypothyroidism is present when thyroxine (T4) levels are normal but the TSH is elevated.[145,146]

Multiple studies have also confirmed that both high and low thyroid function are associated with increased death from all causes.

This highlights the importance of checking thyroid function routinely in the initial medical evaluation of any patient and not just someone with osteoporosis. Subclinical thyroid-related disease states are typically undetectable without the assistance of laboratory testing. Multiple studies have also confirmed that both high and low thyroid function are associated with increased death from all causes.[147-150]

Not surprisingly the effective treatment of subclinical hypothyroidism has been shown to lessen the chance of death from heart disease.[151] Similarly thyroid hormone replacement therapy in hypothyroid dialysis patients appeared to lessen the increased all-cause mortality otherwise seen in this group of patients.[152] Another study on chronic kidney disease patients found that the lowest levels of the T3 form of thyroid hormone predicted increased all-cause mortality as well.[153]

There is also a subset of individuals who have an increased risk of all-cause mortality even though their thyroid function laboratory tests fall completely within the range of normal. Thyroid stimulating hormone (TSH or thyrotropin) levels that are in the high normal ranges are associated with an increased risk of all-cause mortality compared to individuals with lower but normal TSH levels. Furthermore the lowest overall mortality was seen in those individuals with TSH levels in the midrange of normal.[154] Another study found that patients with higher TSH levels within the normal range were associated with an increased incidence of heart attack.[155] It would appear that truly accurate and well-defined laboratory parameters of normal thyroid function remain to be established.

Thyroid Therapy Side Effects and Dosing Considerations

There are multiple ways to approach thyroid hormone administration. The best protocols carefully follow both clinical response and important thyroid and non-thyroid laboratory tests. TSH levels, which are always elevated under the traditional diagnostic criteria for hypothyroidism, should end up between 0.04 and 4.0 mU/liter. As noted above, higher or lower levels are associated with increased cardiovascular problems. A greater assurance of the long-term safety of a given protocol will also be reflected in an improvement or a lack of change in any of a number of laboratory tests related to cardiac risk such as those seen in the metabolic syndrome.

Thyroxine, or T4, and triiodothyronine, or T3, are the most commonly administered forms of thyroid hormone. There are also many individuals who take dessicated thyroid extract. All of these forms can do the job. The need for attentive clinical and laboratory monitoring applies to any type of thyroid taken by the patient and dosing is highly individualized. One size does not come close to fitting all. [156]

Any degree of hyperthyroidism should be appropriately treated to bring thyroid hormone levels into the normal range. It is also important to monitor thyroid functions for extended periods of time to make sure the hyperthyroidism therapy does not eventually push the patient into a hypothyroid state.

Also, as with estrogen and testosterone, the additional elements of the protocol in Chapter 15 can be expected to prevent many side effects that would otherwise manifest themselves with suboptimal administrations of thyroid hormone.

Hormone Replacement Summary

In previous chapters it has been demonstrated that there are a number of powerful natural agents that very effectively halt and even reverse osteoporosis. These have documented abilities to lessen the risk of fracture, which is the ultimate parameter of whether something is benefiting the osteoporotic patient. What should be most impressive is that bioavailable magnesium, vitamin K, vitamin C, vitamin D, and essential fatty acids individually decrease all-cause mortality when properly dosed.

As discussed in this chapter, deficiencies of estrogen in women and testosterone in men, as well as high and low levels of thyroid hormone, also increase the risk of all-cause mortality. The only aspect of the protocol recommended in Chapter 16 that is shared with the recommendation of mainstream medicine is the use of estrogen.

The cumulative positive effects of the protocols for osteoporosis and chronic degenerative disease should prove to be enormously positive. Only the hormone, or hormone-like (vitamin D) agents need to be given with appropriate care to assure the proper level and not an overdose is reached in the body. All of the other agents have no significant toxicity at any dose. At the same time their collective antioxidant properties should prove to largely eliminate the potential side effects of hormone replacement even when suboptimally administered.

SECTION THREE:

What's Right with Calcium

CHAPTER 11

More Than Teeth and Bones

The Vital Roles of Calcium

Most of the information in this book springs from the reality that **excess** calcium presents a grave danger to health and life. This is an essential message that must be understood. However, in the effort to warn against this danger it is never intended that the reader reach the conclusion that calcium *per se* is toxic and that its role in normal physiology is not vital in all the cells of the body. Due to our modern diets and lifestyles, along with the many sources of toxins to which we are regularly exposed, it is almost impossible to induce a calcium deficiency in the body outside of the bones. As a result, you need never worry that following any of the protocols in this book will ever come close to inducing a calcium deficiency throughout your body. Nevertheless, calcium is a necessary nutrient. It simply must be obtained through dietary sources only and it must be ingested in appropriate amounts.

In this chapter some of the more significant physiological roles of calcium along with the more important hormones that regulate calcium will be discussed.

General Information about Calcium

Non-bone calcium is so important to human physiology that the body tightly controls plasma concentrations within very precise limits.

The average adult weighing about 150 pounds has between two and three pounds of calcium in his body. About 99% of it is found in the teeth and bones with the remaining 1% being distributed in cells and in extracellular fluids. By weight calcium comprises a little less than 33% of healthy bone tissue.

Until the bones reach peak mass, somewhere in the third decade of life, a large portion of the calcium consumed is used for bone growth. One's need for dietary calcium then substantially diminishes.

Non-bone calcium is critical to normal physiology and the body tightly controls plasma concentrations within very precise limits. When levels fall below the minimum, calcium is retrieved from calcium stores.

These stores are primarily in the bone but are also found in intracellular structures including mitochondria and the endoplasmic reticulum. As the blood concentrations of calcium inch over the upper levels of normal, excess calcium is returned to these stores, excreted, or when bodily chemistry is sufficiently out of balance it can start to deposit ectopically [abnormally] throughout the body.

Calcium is transported by the blood in three forms:
- About 40% is bound to proteins (mainly albumin and prealbumin)
- About 10% is found in sulfate, phosphate, or citrate complexes
- Roughly 48% is in the ionic form (unbound)

Calcium's Roles in Healthy Non-Bone Metabolism

Aside from its obvious and previously discussed role in bones calcium is critical in such vital functions as:

1) Transmission of nerve impulses
2) Contraction of muscles
3) Constriction of blood vessels
4) Increasing/decreasing the ability of certain molecules to pass through cellular membranes [permeability]
5) Coagulation and clotting of blood
6) Maintenance of balanced blood pH

Calcium performs an important messenger role in nerve cells [neurons], muscles, blood vessels, and in the fertilization process.

The first three functions listed above require signal transduction. Signal transduction allows individual cells to respond to environmental stimuli. Various receptor molecules are embedded in the membranes of cells. When a signaling molecule outside a cell activates a specific receptor a second messenger transmits the message inside the cell. Calcium performs this second messenger role in nerve cells [neurons], muscles, blood vessels, and in the fertilization process.

Calcium Homeostasis: Hormones that Help Keep Calcium Levels in Balance

Calcium homeostasis in the body strives to accomplish two results: enough calcium delivery to support ongoing healthy bone structure, and the maintenance of a normal level of freely ionized calcium in the blood within a tight range. Multiple hormones affect the regulation of calcium homeostasis, with prominent effects in the gastrointestinal tract, bone, and kidneys, but elsewhere in the body as well. These hormones include:

- Vitamin D
- Parathyroid hormone
- Calcitonin
- Stanniocalcin
- Estrogen
- Testosterone
- Thyroid hormone

A brief description of the role each plays in the regulation of calcium in the body follows.

> **Vitamin D:** It is very clear that vitamin D is essential for regulating both calcium uptake into the diet and its proper incorporation into a healthy bone mineral matrix. A major function of vitamin D as a calcium regulator is to increase calcium absorption from the intestine.[1] It is the main stimulator of active, energy dependent, intestinal transcellular calcium absorption. Some evidence also indicates that vitamin D can facilitate passive movement of calcium through the spaces between cells.[2] Although the direct effects of vitamin D on bone and its related calcium metabolism are not fully understood, vitamin D receptors have been identified in osteoblasts [bone-makers]. This indicates that the effects of vitamin D on calcium metabolism extend well beyond its effects on intestinal calcium absorption.[3,4]
>
> **Parathyroid Hormone:** This is secreted by the parathyroid glands, which are very sensitive to even minute changes in blood calcium levels. When the free calcium level drops sufficiently, parathyroid

hormone is secreted, and calcium levels are bolstered in the blood and extracellular fluid by at least three different mechanisms:

1) The stimulation of renal tubular reabsorption of filtered calcium, an effect that can occur within minutes of increased hormone secretion. [5]
2) The release of calcium via increased resorption of bone, an effect that can occur within minutes to hours (although bone *formation* can result from the intermittent administration of low doses of parathyroid hormone). [6]
3) The increased uptake of calcium from the intestine. This results from the stimulation of renal tubular conversion of active vitamin D from its precursor, an effect with a lag time of 12 to 24 hours. [7] When vitamin D levels are low, increased parathyroid hormone secretion ensues, resulting in a state of secondary hyperparathyroidism. [8]

Calcitonin: This is a 32-amino acid peptide hormone that is produced by the thyroid gland [9] and it is capable of exerting a potent hypocalcemic effect. It is released from the gland in response to elevations in blood calcium. Calcitonin interacts with specific receptors on the osteoclast [bone-breakers] to inhibit bone resorption, slowing the ongoing normal release of calcium from the bone. [10,11] Because of this ability to inhibit the release of calcium from the bone it has been widely used in the treatment of diseases with increased osteoclastic activity, such as osteoporosis and Paget's disease. [12,13]

Calcitonin effectively works in a fashion counter to the calcium release induced by parathyroid hormone-stimulated activation of osteoclastic [bone-dissolving] activity.[14] Basically the parathyroid hormone from the parathyroid glands works to increase blood calcium and the calcitonin from the thyroid gland works to lower blood calcium. Physiologically, calcitonin is best viewed as a hormone that works to prevent hypercalcemia [too much calcium] rather than to induce hypocalcemia [calcium deficiency]. Even though calcitonin and parathyroid hormone are antagonistic to each other in their effects on calcium, calcitonin has only a relatively weak effect on blood calcium levels compared to parathyroid hormone.

Stanniocalcin: This is another hormone with a hypocalcemic effect. Although originally identified in fish it has now been identified in humans.[15] Similar to calcitonin, the primary function of stanniocalcin appears to be the prevention of hypercalcemia although the physiological significance of this hormone is not as clearly defined as the other hormones discussed. Of note, increased vitamin D has been shown in the rat kidney to result in upregulation of stanniocalcin (stanniocalcin 1),[16] which works to limit the calcium-increasing effects of vitamin D. However, vitamin D also appears to suppress (downregulate) a second form of stanniocalcin (stanniocalcin 2), which has an *anti*-hypocalcemic effect.[17] Vitamin D's interaction with both forms of stanniocalcin work to prevent hypercalcemia. Parathyroid hormone has been shown to have the same kinds of influence over stanniocalcin as vitamin D in the rat kidney.[18]

Estrogen: A deficiency of estrogen has long been known to result in a negative calcium balance with a resultant bone loss in postmenopausal women.[19] This bone loss is associated with a rise in plasma and urinary calcium. The rise in plasma and urinary calcium has generally been ascribed to an increase in bone resorption. It has been suggested, however, that estrogen has a direct effect on the tubules of the kidney to increase calcium reabsorption, with an increased renal wasting of calcium when estrogen is deficient.[20]

Estrogen receptors have been identified in the duodenum, colon, and both the proximal and distal tubules of the kidney. In postmenopausal women the loss of estrogen at first causes an outflow of calcium from the bone into the extracellular fluid. This early movement of calcium results in a compensatory decrease in parathyroid hormone secretion.

As the estrogen loss becomes chronic the loss of the extraskeletal effects of estrogen on the intestine and kidneys leads to increased whole body loss of calcium resulting in a low serum calcium level. When this occurs parathyroid hormone secretion increases, and a state of secondary hyperparathyroidism is induced. This is in contrast to primary hyperparathyroidism, where a parathyroid tumor or an overactive parathyroid gland is continually secreting increased amounts of parathyroid hormone.[21,22]

While estrogen therapy is generally not effective in reducing the increased parathyroid hormone seen in elderly cases of secondary hyperparathyroidism,[23] a proper estrogen balance is vital for the optimal treatment of osteoporosis and the maintenance of bone integrity.

Testosterone: In addition to a host of other effects, testosterone plays a strong role in the maintaining of healthy bone as well in restoring healthy bone when a deficient level is restored to normal. Testosterone plays an active role in the regulation of calcium, as it has been determined to have properties of a calcium channel blocker.[24]

Testosterone also plays a definable role in lessening abnormal calcium deposition, a finding that is completely consistent with the relationship of increased coronary artery disease with decreased testosterone levels. In a human aortic vascular smooth muscle cell study, testosterone was found to inhibit calcification in a concentration-dependent manner.[25] In a study on men, increased levels of bioavailable testosterone were found to be inversely related to coronary artery calcification.[26] Both of these studies demonstrate the known relationship between the increased incidence of heart disease in the metabolic syndrome seen with decreased testosterone levels.

Thyroid Hormone: This hormone has long been regarded as having effects on calcium metabolism. Increased calcium levels in the blood have been repeatedly observed in humans and animals with abnormally high thyroid hormone levels. In keeping with these observations prolonged hyperthyroidism is associated with increased bone resorption. In a study on rats, it was demonstrated that thyroid hormone increased calcium reabsorption in the kidney.[27] The same researchers also demonstrated that thyroid hormone stimulated an increase in calcium uptake in rat intestines.[28] Interestingly, this effect was significantly increased in hyperthyroid animals and decreased in hypothyroid animals.

The elevation of thyroid hormone in hyperthyroid patients has also been reported to be associated with low plasma levels of vitamin D. In mice it was demonstrated that a hyperthyroid state is associated with "marked" decreases in plasma vitamin D with no observable changes in plasma concentrations of calcium or parathyroid hormone. It was found that thyroid hormone suppressed expression of the gene needed to convert vitamin D precursor into active hormone in the kidney.[29]

Vitamin D and parathyroid hormone are the two most important modulators of bone and calcium homeostasis.

Thyroid hormone also affects the production of stanniocalcin 1. Investigators showed in human skin fibroblasts that the gene for the production of stanniocalcin 1 was induced by thyroid hormone (T3-triiodothyronine).[30]

The effects of the seven different hormones discussed above were not exhaustively addressed by any means and they are certainly not the only factors that affect calcium homeostasis. However they are the primary ways in which the body manages its calcium metabolism. Of note as well is that vitamin D and parathyroid hormone are the two most important modulators of bone and calcium homeostasis.[31]

Dietary factors, including how much calcium is ingested and/or supplemented, are important as well.

Summary

Calcium is not only essential in the composition of bones and teeth, but it also plays essential roles in many vital aspects of non-bone metabolism. It is through the rise and fall of intracellular concentrations of calcium that it performs many of these functions. As demonstrated throughout this book, it is when concentrations of calcium chronically exceed normal limits that health problems ensue. Dietary calcium is essential but not nearly to the degree that most doctors and patients now believe. The important question now is: How much dietary calcium does a person need? That's the subject of Chapter 12.

CHAPTER 12

Getting Calcium in Balance

Where You Get It, How Much You Really Need

Calcium: What the Government Says You Need

The current recommended daily intake of calcium is largely the result of the massive marketing efforts of the dairy industry over the last half-century or so. Unfortunately persistent misconceptions about calcium metabolism among most healthcare practitioners and nutritionists have added support to these excessively high recommended daily allowances (RDAs).

In 1992, the U.S. Department of Agriculture published the "Food Pyramid." This chart recommends 6-11 daily servings of grains (breads, cereals, rice, and pasta) and 2-3 daily servings of dairy products (milk, yogurt, and cheese). It is important to realize that the primary purpose of the U.S.D.A. is to bolster the sales of U.S. agriculture, not to promote public health. Many nutrition scientists have commented on the Food Pyramid's unhealthful emphasis on grains and dairy. These marketing approaches to dietary standards have greatly contributed to American obesity and ill health.

In a scathing 2010 article in the medical journal *Nutrition*, the Dietary Guidelines for Americans Committee (the group that establishes U.S. Dietary Guidelines and that provided the recommendations for the food pyramid) was rightly taken to task for ignoring good science:

> "Although appealing to an evidence-based methodology, the DGAC Report demonstrates several critical weaknesses, including use of an incomplete body of relevant science; inaccurately representing, interpreting, or summarizing the literature; and drawing conclusions and/or making recommendations that do not reflect the limitations or controversies in the science... Lack of supporting evidence limits the value of the proposed recommendations as guidance for consumers or as the basis for public health policy. It is time to reexamine how US dietary guidelines are created and ask whether the current process is still appropriate for our needs." [1]

The U.S.D.A. food pyramid and the government's calcium RDAs have encouraged all of us to ingest toxic amounts of calcium at an incalculable cost to public health. If one considers the actual adult need for daily calcium intake, just the consumption of the recommended 2-3 servings of dairy or the ingestion of the 1,000+ mg RDA constitutes a veritable calcium overdose.

In response to requests by both the United States and Canadian governments the Institute of Medicine released its dietary reference intakes for calcium in November of 2010. Their published daily RDA for calcium is between 1,000 mg and 1,300 mg for individuals between the ages of 4 and 70, with upper level intake recommendations ranging from 2,000 to 3,000 mg. More specifically, females 51 years of age and older, the osteoporosis subset, had a

RDA of 1,200 mg of calcium and a recommended upper level intake of 2,000 mg.

There is no science for this! These recommendations do not reflect either the actual calcium needs of the body or the changes in these needs as patients grow older. Calcium intake should actually *decrease* with age, not increase. And just as importantly, the baseline RDAs need to start at a **much** lower level.

Calcium: What You Actually Need

While calcium can be considered a nutrient it is not a nutrient in the traditional sense of the word. In the bones a limited amount of calcium is needed to participate in the ongoing synthesis/breakdown cycle seen in healthy bone. However, outside of the bone the calcium content that plays a role in muscular contraction, blood coagulation, cardiac activity, and the general metabolism of all cells is not "released" from these sites in the same way it is released in active bone metabolism, osteopenia, or osteoporosis. While some calcium turnover occurs everywhere it is located in the body the areas outside of the bone do not need the significant ongoing replenishment/supply of calcium that the bones need.

Once bones reach their full size the actual need for calcium is limited to the replenishment of calcium lost in the sweat or urine plus an additional 30% because the digestive system only absorbs about 70% of the calcium ingested.

Children and young adults need about 80 to 100 mg daily to supply what is required for growing bones. After age 35 the bones have reached full size and there is no further calcium needed for this purpose. Most healthy individuals excrete approximately 170 mg of calcium per day in the urine and perspiration. Based on these actual needs, see the following table showing calcium intake requirements: [2]

Average Calcium Needs by Age
(Male and Female)

Age	Avg. Bone Growth Needs/Day	Avg. Excreted/Day	Total Avg. Daily Need	Total Avg. Ingestion Need*
15 to 35	~80 mg	~170 mg	~250 mg	300 to 400 mg
36 to 80	0 mg	~170 mg	~170 mg	200 to 300 mg

*More calcium must be ingested to compensate for the approximately 30% of calcium that is not absorbed by the digestive system

Based on actual daily replenishment requirements for calcium young adults need 300 to 400 mg. It is not uncommon for many young adults to drink a quart of milk every day. That's about 1,200 mg! When one adds the calcium-absorption-increasing vitamin D to the milk this literal overdose is massive. A single 8-ounce glass of milk meets the entire daily calcium requirement on its own, even without the added vitamin D.

STRONG RECOMMENDATION: Regular ingestion of milk as a beverage needs to be completely avoided.

Other dairy products can be consumed to a limited degree, even with the implementation of the osteoporosis protocol outlined in Chapter 16, but milk cannot be a regular beverage if you want to avoid the widespread calcification of your body as you grow older. And without question the time to curtail milk and dairy is as a young adult. Prevention of a calcified body is much easier and provides much greater health benefits than trying to decalcify it later.

The daily requirement for most older men and women, including those with osteoporosis, should actually be no more than 200 to 300 mg. This can be accomplished quite readily with a balanced diet completely devoid of dairy products, as long as normal blood levels of vitamin D are maintained (regulating the calcium absorbed from that diet). The regular ingestion of more calcium than this will progressively feed the calcium excesses discussed earlier. The more calcium taken in, the more deposited throughout the body and the more calcium inside the cells, which is the final common denominator to fueling all known chronic degenerative diseases, notably heart disease and cancer.

Milk and dairy products are actually "luxury" foods. The poorest countries and populations consume vastly

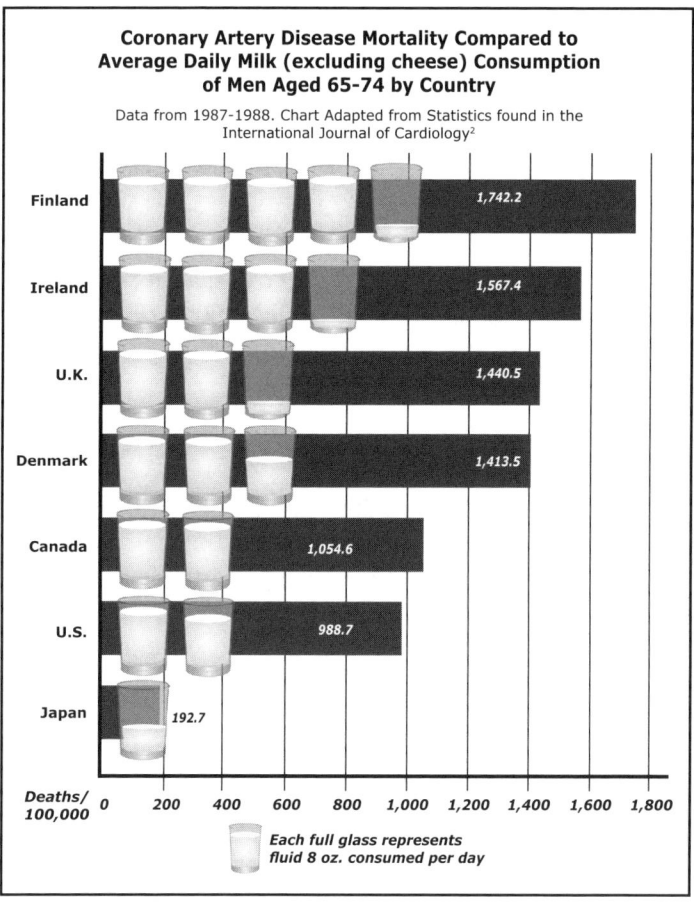

less than the United States and these populations have dramatically less mortality from heart disease as a result. A study on per capita milk consumption (excluding cheese) by nation provides a chilling picture of the danger of milk consumption (see chart). The nations included in the study were all industrialized countries in Europe, the U.S., Canada, New Zealand, Australia, and Japan. The coronary artery disease mortality for these countries demonstrates a nearly perfect correlation between milk consumption and death. [2]

Chapter 18 will discuss an approach to lessen the negative impact of consuming any dairy in the diet. Ultimately, however, motivated individuals will need to look at the evidence of calcium deposition in the body with serial coronary artery calcium scores to see if they are still accumulating calcium, staying unchanged, or actually mobilizing and excreting excess calcium, assuming they started with positive scores. At the very least you should know that ingesting any dairy, especially milk, impacts your health negatively in a cumulative manner over time. If dairy cannot be eliminated completely decrease it to a "special treat" status to minimize the negative impact it has on the calcium status in your body.

Dietary Sources of Calcium

The calcium content information available below is not inclusive of all foods. But it is a good starting point. Even so, figures can vary greatly. The following charts are not exhaustive and are only for relative comparisons only.

The first chart shows a list of foods in order of descending calcium content and the second chart is an alphabetical listing to aid in finding a particular food.

Since calcium is considered to be an essential nutrient packaged foods containing calcium must post the calcium content on the label. However this is usually only presented as a percentage of RDA rather than an actual amount. As a rule of thumb, multiplying the RDA percentage by 5 will provide a realistic percentage of your true daily requirement. Many places on the internet provide calcium content in grams for unpackaged produce.

Calcium Content of Selected Foods
Sorted by Highest to Lowest Content

Yogurt, plain, low fat	8 oz	415 mg
Cheese, ricotta, part skim	1/2 cup	337 mg
Sardines with bones	3 oz.	325 mg
Milk, nonfat	8 oz.	302 mg
Yogurt, soy, plain	6 oz.	300 mg
Rice milk	8 oz.	300 mg
Orange juice (calcium fortified)	8 oz.	300 mg
Soymilk, calcium-fortified	8 oz.	299 mg
Milk, whole	8 oz.	291 mg
Milk, buttermilk, lowfat (1% milk fat)	8 oz.	284 mg
Tofu, processed with calcium sulfate	4 oz.	276 mg
Yogurt, plain, whole milk	8 oz.	275 mg
Cheese, swiss	1 oz.	272 mg
Cheese, ricotta, whole milk	1/2 cup	257 mg
Black-eyed peas, boiled	1 cup	211 mg
Cheese, cheddar	1 oz. (1 slice)	202 mg
Cheese, gouda	1 oz.	200 mg
Cheese, mozzarella, part skim	1 oz.	183 mg
Salmon, pink, canned, solids with bone	3 oz.	181 mg
Salmon, canned	3 oz.	181 mg
Soybeans, cooked	1 cup	175 mg
Molasses, blackstrap	1 Tbsp	172 mg
Cheese food, pasteurized American	1 oz.	162 mg
Trail mix (nuts, seeds, chocolate chips)	1 cup	159 mg
Bok choy, cooked	1 cup	158 mg
Beans, baked, canned	1 cup	154 mg
String cheese	1 stick (1 oz.)	150 mg
Cheese, mozzarella	1 oz.	147 mg
Cheese, feta	1 oz.	140 mg
Parmesan cheese, grated	2 Tbsp.	138 mg
Hazelnuts	1 cup	135 mg

Artichoke, medium	1 medium	135 mg
Tahini	2 Tbsp.	128 mg
Collard greens, cooked	1/2 cup	125 mg
Milk, reduced-fat (2% milk fat)	8 oz.	121 mg
Almond butter	2 Tbsp.	111 mg
Collards, boiled	1/2 cup	110 mg
Almonds	1.5 oz. (36 nuts)	105 mg
Yogurt, frozen	1/2 cup	103 mg
Kale, raw, chopped, 1 cup	1 cup	100 mg
Turnip greens, boiled	1/2 cup	99 mg
Iceberg lettuce	1 head	97 mg
Kale, fresh, cooked, 1 cup	1 cup	94 mg
Green peas, boiled	1 cup	94 mg
Soymilk	1 cup	93 mg
Ice cream, vanilla, ½ cup	1/2 cup	84 mg
Okra, boiled	1/2 cup	77 mg
Trout, rainbow	3 oz.	75 mg
Chinese cabbage, bok choi	1 cup	74 mg
Bread, white, 1 slice	1 slice	73 mg
Ice Cream	1/2 cup	72 mg
Cheese, cottage 1% lowfat	1/2 cup	69 mg
Hummus	1/2 cup	62 mg
Navy beans, canned	1/2 cup	61 mg
Pudding	4 oz.	55 mg
Orange, fresh	1	52 mg
Mustard greens	1/2 cup	52 mg
Pinto beans, canned	1/2 cup	51 mg
Lentils	1 cup	50 mg
Eggs, boiled	2 eggs	50 mg
Crab, cooked	3 oz.	50 mg
Broccoli, chopped	1/2 cup	47 mg
Tortilla, corn	6" diamter - 1	46 mg
Squash, acorn or butternut	1/2 cup	45 mg
Chick peas, canned	1/2 cup	38 mg
Papaya, fresh	1/2 medium	36 mg
Figs	2	36 mg
Kidney beans, canned	1/2 cup	34 mg

Tortilla, flour	6" diamter - 1	32 mg
Sweet potato, baked	1/2 cup	32 mg
Sour cream, reduced fat, cultured	2 tbsp	31 mg
Bread, whole-wheat, 1 slice	1 slice	30 mg
Parsnips, boiled	1/2 cup	29 mg
Lentils, boiled	1/2 cup	29 mg
Haddock	3 oz.	28 mg
Raspberries, fresh	1 cup	27 mg
Lima beans, boiled	1/2 cup	25 mg
Black beans, boiled	1/2 cup	23 mg
Orange juice	8 oz.	22 mg
Peas, boiled	1/2 cup	20 mg
Kiwi	1	20 mg
Rice, white	1 cup	19 mg
Flour, wheat	1 cup	19 mg
Flour, rice	1 cup	16 mg
Cheese, cream, regular, 1 tablespoon	1 Tbsp.	14 mg
Cod, Atlantic	3 oz.	13 mg
Tuna, light, canned in water	3 oz.	10 mg
Sugar, brown	1 tsp	4 mg
Honey	1 Tbsp.	1 mg
Sugar, white	1 Tbsp.	0 mg

Here are a few highlights from the above chart that are worth noting.

1) Dairy foods are predominantly present at the top of the list, containing the most calcium.

2) A single serving from many dairy foods (or dairy substitutes) easily meets the daily calcium intake need.

3) Generally, the higher the fat content, the lower the calcium content of dairy foods.

4) The daily calcium intake requirements can easily be met without any dairy consumption at all.

Calcium Content of Selected Foods
Sorted Alphabetically

Food	Serving	Calcium
Almond butter	2 Tbsp.	111 mg
Almonds	1.5 oz. (36 nuts)	105 mg
Artichoke, medium	1 medium	135 mg
Beans, baked, canned	1 cup	154 mg
Black beans, boiled	1/2 cup	23 mg
Black-eyed peas, boiled	1 cup	211 mg
Bok choy, cooked	1 cup	158 mg
Bread, white, 1 slice	1 slice	73 mg
Bread, whole-wheat, 1 slice	1 slice	30 mg
Broccoli, chopped	1/2 cup	47 mg
Cheese food, pasteurized American	1 oz.	162 mg
Cheese, cheddar	1 oz. (1 slice)	202 mg
Cheese, cottage 1% lowfat	1/2 cup	69 mg
Cheese, cream, regular, 1 tablespoon	1 Tbsp.	14 mg
Cheese, feta	1 oz.	140 mg
Cheese, gouda	1 oz.	200 mg
Cheese, mozzarella	1 oz.	147 mg
Cheese, mozzarella, part skim	1 oz.	183 mg
Cheese, ricotta, part skim	1/2 cup	337 mg
Cheese, ricotta, whole milk	1/2 cup	257 mg
Cheese, swiss	1 oz.	272 mg
Chick peas, canned	1/2 cup	38 mg
Chinese cabbage, bok choi	1 cup	74 mg
Cod, Atlantic	3 oz.	13 mg
Collard greens, cooked	1/2 cup	125 mg
Collards, boiled	1/2 cup	110 mg
Crab, cooked	3 oz.	50 mg
Eggs, boiled	2 eggs	50 mg
Figs	2	36 mg
Flour, rice	1 cup	16 mg
Flour, wheat	1 cup	19 mg

Getting Calcium in Balance

Green peas, boiled	1 cup	94 mg
Haddock	3 oz.	28 mg
Hazelnuts	1 cup	135 mg
Honey	1 Tbsp.	1 mg
Hummus	1/2 cup	62 mg
Ice Cream	1/2 cup	72 mg
Ice cream, vanilla, ½ cup	1/2 cup	84 mg
Iceberg lettuce	1 head	97 mg
Kale, fresh, cooked, 1 cup	1 cup	94 mg
Kale, raw, chopped, 1 cup	1 cup	100 mg
Kidney beans, canned	1/2 cup	34 mg
Kiwi	1	20 mg
Lentils	1 cup	50 mg
Lentils, boiled	1/2 cup	29 mg
Lima beans, boiled	1/2 cup	25 mg
Milk, buttermilk, lowfat (1% milk fat)	8 oz.	284 mg
Milk, nonfat	8 oz.	302 mg
Milk, reduced-fat (2% milk fat)	8 oz.	121 mg
Milk, whole	8 oz.	291 mg
Molasses, blackstrap	1 Tbsp	172 mg
Mustard greens	1/2 cup	52 mg
Navy beans, canned	1/2 cup	61 mg
Okra, boiled	1/2 cup	77 mg
Orange juice	8 oz.	22 mg
Orange juice (calcium fortified)	8 oz.	300 mg
Orange, fresh	1	52 mg
Papaya, fresh	1/2 medium	36 mg
Parmesan cheese, grated	2 Tbsp.	138 mg
Parsnips, boiled	1/2 cup	29 mg
Peas, boiled	1/2 cup	20 mg
Pinto beans, canned	1/2 cup	51 mg
Pudding	4 oz.	55 mg
Raspberries, fresh	1 cup	27 mg

Rice milk	8 oz.	300 mg
Rice, white	1 cup	19 mg
Salmon, canned	3 oz.	181 mg
Salmon, pink, canned, solids with bone	3 oz.	181 mg
Sardines with bones	3 oz.	325 mg
Sour cream, reduced fat, cultured	2 tbsp	31 mg
Soybeans, cooked	1 cup	175 mg
Soymilk	1 cup	93 mg
Soymilk, calcium-fortified, 8 ounces	8 oz.	299 mg
Squash, acorn or butternut	1/2 cup	45 mg
String cheese	1 stick (1 oz.)	150 mg
Sugar, brown	1 tsp	4 mg
Sugar, white	1 Tbsp.	0 mg
Sweet potato, baked	1/2 cup	32 mg
Tahini	2 Tbsp.	128 mg
Tofu, processed with calcium sulfate	4 oz.	276 mg
Tortilla, corn	6" diamter - 1	46 mg
Tortilla, flour	6" diamter - 1	32 mg
Trail mix (nuts, seeds, chocolate chips)	1 cup	159 mg
Trout, rainbow	3 oz.	75 mg
Tuna, light, canned in water	3 oz.	10 mg
Turnip greens, boiled	1/2 cup	99 mg
Yogurt, frozen	1/2 cup	103 mg
Yogurt, plain, low fat	8 oz	415 mg
Yogurt, plain, whole milk	8 oz.	275 mg
Yogurt, soy, plain	6 oz.	300 mg

SECTION FOUR:

Osteoporosis and Toxins

CHAPTER 13

Toxin Exposure and Degenerative Disease

Eliminating Hidden Causes of Osteoporosis

We float in a veritable sea of pathogens and poisons. Fortunately many of us are protected from many of these hazards by a powerful immune system. Regardless of the source, all these pathogenic and toxic challenges to health and life have one thing in common: They increase oxidative stress in the body.

Oxidative stress plays a primary role in the initiation and evolution of **all** chronic degenerative diseases, including osteoporosis. At first blush this may seem to be rash overstatement. How could a single process be responsible for such a variety of disease manifestations? Is it possible that diabetes, atherosclerosis, osteoporosis, arthritis, Parkinson's, and Alzheimer's start and are intensified by the same mechanism? In a word, "YES!"

Oxidative stress is abundantly present in every disease process known to man. And in fact the references to oxidative stress in the medical literature of the last 30 years are almost as ubiquitous. This concept is so important that a complete discussion of the subject can be found in Appendix C. Since the theory is adequately defended there, for the purposes of this chapter it is sufficient to state the conclusion here:

The factors that create oxidative stress are the factors that ignite and fuel all chronic degenerative diseases.

The healthy human immune system, when regularly fed a wide array of antioxidant-rich foods, is well-equipped to handle the oxidative stress that arises from normal metabolism. A continual flood of toxins from external sources, however, can ignite increased oxidative stress that quickly overwhelms antioxidant and immune defenses and the onset of diseases begins. A combination of a person's genetic predispositions (weaknesses) and the location of the greatest oxidative stress is critical in determining the specific disease or diseases that manifest.

> *Molecule for molecule, toxins require electron donation from antioxidants such as vitamin C in order to be neutralized.*

This means there are two major factors that always need to be considered in evaluating and treating any disease:

1) The patient's chronic toxin exposures (type, source, quantity)
2) The patient's consistent antioxidant intake (type and quantity)

Conceptually these two factors address the majority of the issues involved in the diagnosis and treatment of any chronic disease process.

Many sources of toxin exposure are universally acknowledged. Generally these are environmental toxins that are present in the food, air, and water that are byproducts of our industrialized lifestyle. Then there are the rarer but well-known industrial toxin hazards that are usually associated with a particular type or place of work. Although both of these sources of risk are important, the purpose of this chapter is to consider toxin exposures that are common, continual, pose great risk, but seldom if ever are discussed.

Two major sources of this chronic toxin exposure are:

1) The digestive system (poor eating habits and poor digestion)
2) The mouth (in large part due to modern dental practices)

> *Chronically high toxin exposure makes it virtually impossible to have and/or to maintain a normal antioxidant status in the body.*

Molecule for molecule, toxins require electron donation from antioxidants such as vitamin C in order to be neutralized. The more toxicity present, the more antioxidants are needed for neutralization. Further antioxidant support is also needed to eventually mobilize and excrete accumulated toxins.

Chronically high toxin exposure makes it virtually impossible to have and/or to maintain a normal antioxidant status in the body. This is especially true of vitamin C, even with excellent supplementation and an optimal regimen of nutrition digested perfectly. When toxin levels are high antioxidant levels are low, and increased levels of disease-generating oxidative stress are present. Infections, even when not producing identifiable toxins, also relentlessly oxidize the areas they infect, further increasing oxidative stress at those sites.

1) Digestive Sources of Disease-Causing Oxidative Stress

A common, although little recognized, source of chronic toxin exposure comes from poor nutrition and poor digestion. A malfunctioning gut, an especially common problem in the elderly, presents the body with another chronic source of pathogens and pathogen-generated toxins aside from the mouth.

Many such individuals are plagued with constipation, which is a condition that facilitates a great deal of toxin exposure. When bowel function slows, putrefaction and rotting of food starts to compete more significantly with digestion and highly toxic anaerobic bacteria, such as those making up the genus *Clostridium*, begin to proliferate. The proliferation of such bacteria produces enormously potent exotoxins, some as or more toxic than botulinum toxin.

As a practical point, anyone who does not have at least one bowel movement daily (bowel transit time of 24 hours or less) faces a large added source of toxicity that keeps body antioxidant levels low. Optimally one should have two or more formed bowel movements daily to keep this source of toxicity at minimal levels, and normal bowel transit time from food intake to bowel evacuation should really average no more than 12 hours.

This is of paramount importance, since a gut that takes more than 24 hours to process a meal and proceed to elimination is always highly toxic. The pathogens that proliferate under such circumstances are similar and often identical to the highly toxic microbes found in an infected mouth. When everything else is corrected but the gut remains constipated, the toxicity of the pathogens and the toxins they generate can be roughly equivalent to leaving one or more root canal-treated teeth unextracted.

While there are multiple additional ways to make the diet more nutritious and ultimately less toxic, a practical outline of what to do to minimize gut toxicity includes the following:

1) Chew all food thoroughly.
2) Combine foods properly. For example, it is almost impossible to properly digest a sizeable quantity of protein when eaten together with a significant amount of carbohydrate. Much of the protein ends up putrified rather than processed appropriately. Combine low carbohydrate-containing vegetables with protein.
3) Minimize beverages with meals, including water.
4) Eliminate milk as a beverage. Not only is milk a source of excess calcium, but it substantially impairs good digestion when it is combined with nearly every other food. Milk also contains a large amount of protein.
5) Increase vegetable intake.
6) Decrease/minimize (but not eliminate) meat intake.
7) Minimize foods with a high glycemic index (generally refined carbohydrates); eliminate refined sugar as much as possible.
8) Minimize/eliminate highly toxic seafoods (such as tuna and swordfish)

And most individuals should supplement with quality digestive enzymes.

It should be noted that the suggestions itemized above are of significant importance in assuring proper digestion, especially the first six. Proper digestion involves normal gut motility with only a minimal window of opportunity for toxic gut microbes to proliferate. When the ingested foodstuffs proceed through the gut in a timely fashion a great deal of toxin exposure can be avoided.

It is also important to consume the best quality in foods, as many other toxins can be directly consumed if this consideration is ignored. However, it is important to emphasize that toxin exposure from the gut is much greater when digestion is poor rather than when dietary choices are poor. In other words, excellent, organically-grown food when poorly digested will produce a substantially greater new toxin challenge than a perfectly digested meal of "junk" foods. Obviously the best option is to consume a quality diet, following the principles noted above so that it is properly digested as well.

While eating a diet of optimal quality can be too expensive for many, a few simple considerations can still make a big difference in minimizing dietary toxicity. Fresh foods are always better than frozen foods, and both of these are always better than canned and packaged foods. As well, many fresh foods are actually less costly than their canned/packaged counterparts. The only reason not to eat fresh foods on a regular basis is the inability or unwillingness to shop more frequently and/or the inability or lack of desire to cook or prepare foods in a manner more involved than using the microwave.

2) Dental Sources of Disease-Causing Oxidative Stress

Modern dental procedures often employ toxic metals and chemicals. In addition, periodontal (gum) disease and root canal-treated teeth are accompanied by chronic infections and associated anaerobic microbial toxins. All these factors continuously pump high doses of pro-oxidant toxins throughout the body. This source of exposure is so great that the entire next chapter is devoted to the danger this poses and how it can be managed.

CHAPTER 14

Cleansing the Foul Mouth

The Overlooked Source of Infections and Toxins

The mouth is an extremely common site for both infections and toxin exposure. Modern dentistry regularly produces some exceptionally toxic assaults to the human body. These toxins, often the result of infections, ignite and fuel the oxidative stress that initiates and worsens chronic degenerative diseases, most notably heart disease and cancer. This happens in two basic ways:

1) Scientifically flawed dental procedures allow existing infections in the gums and teeth to continue and even morph into more toxic infections.
2) Toxic dental materials are used to fill, cap, and treat diseased teeth, providing a perpetual source of toxin exposure.

Dental infections and their associated toxins can overwhelm the immune system with an insurmountable drain on the body's antioxidant stores. A large antioxidant capacity in the body is the single most important protection the body has against diseases developing and taking hold. Therefore any positive intervention supporting good health will be severely limited in its effectiveness as long as dental infections and toxins remain unaddressed. And even though very many chronic degenerative diseases begin in the dental chair, this does not have to continue to be the case.

Root Canal-Treated Teeth: A Death Sentence

The root canal is arguably the most effective way to infuse a perpetual fountain of killer toxins into the human body. One root canal-treated tooth's ability to devastate the antioxidant capacity of the body cannot really be overstated.

Some individuals who allow root canal treatment on one or more teeth are fortunate enough to postpone the eventual decline in health that is nearly guaranteed by the procedure. The vigor of youth, a naturally strong immune system, and/or excellent nutrition coupled with a quality regimen of antioxidant supplementation may provide ten, twenty, or more years without the clinical appearance of disease. Eventually, however, the antioxidant-draining capacity of these toxic teeth will gain the upper hand. When a "healthy" man has his first heart attack at age 50 or when a woman of equal age first notices what turns out to be a malignant breast lump, the apparent good health in the years leading up to these events are exposed as having been anything but good.

While exceptions exist most chronic degenerative diseases, which include heart disease and cancer, take years to develop before they become clinically detectable. If you have a heart attack or discover cancer one day, how healthy do you really think you were the day, the week, the month, or the year before? As it turns out, the appearance of a deadly disease is not quite the random unpredictable event that many doctors and patients assume it to be.

Physiology of a Root Canal

A healthy tooth has a relatively soft interior known as the dental pulp. Comprised of connective tissue bearing an abundance of blood vessels and nerves, the pulp is always sterile in a normal and healthy tooth. The pulp-containing cavity extending to the root tips of the tooth is known as the root canal. It is never normal to find microbes of any kind in this area of the tooth, even though the mouth itself is normally teeming with microorganisms.

Calcium channel blockers have been used to effectively treat a myriad of diseases that have nothing to do with hypertension.

Basically, a root canal procedure is the evacuation, or routing out, of this dental pulp followed by the insertion of a dental material designed to fill that evacuated space. Most commonly, the term "root canal" refers to the tooth that has received the root canal procedure or to the procedure itself rather than as an anatomical term referring to the physical space housing the dental pulp.

Most commonly a root canal procedure is performed on a patient complaining of significant tooth pain. Such tooth pain is frequently, but not invariably, associated with an infection in the dental pulp. Ironically, and very inaccurately, modern dentistry typically maintains that doing such a procedure "cleans up" the tooth and eliminates the infection. Some dentists will even perform the root canal procedure on the premise that they want to "prevent" the tooth, often heavily decayed, from later becoming infected.

Nothing could be further from the truth!

All Root Canal-Treated Teeth Are Dangerously Toxic

A particularly disturbing fact about root canal-treated teeth is that they are all infected and highly toxic. Over 5,000 consecutive extracted root canal-treated teeth were analyzed and 100% of them were found to house any of a variety of highly potent toxins. This toxicity testing makes it clear that gambling that your root canal-treated tooth is not toxic would be like playing Russian roulette with a gun that has bullets in every chamber. The nature of the root canal procedure actually makes it impossible that any treated tooth could ever be nontoxic even one out of 5000 times. Ignore this scientific data only at your own grave peril.

All root canal-treated teeth continually produce toxins from the ongoing metabolism of the bacteria and other microbes proliferating inside them. It has been established that dental pulp infections, such as are found in root canal-treated teeth, harbor an incredibly large and diverse array of microbes and pathogens, including fungi, viruses, and over 460 different types of bacteria. [1]

In the 1950s when the root canal procedure was much less common than today, Dr. Josef Issels found that 98% of his adult cancer patients had "between two and ten dead teeth." Dr. Issels considered all root canal-treated teeth as dead, infected teeth. His protocol for advanced cancer patients who had been deemed to be incurable started with the extraction of all root canals and any other teeth that appeared infected. His cancer survival rates vastly exceeded any mainstream therapies then or now. [2]

The toxins isolated from extracted root canal-treated teeth have consistently blocked/poisoned the activity of several critical metabolic enzymes necessary in the production of energy in the body much more effectively than even botulinum toxin. Botulinum toxin, currently considered to be the most potent toxin known to man, is produced when *Clostridium botulinum* bacteria are trapped in an environment severely deprived of or completely devoid of oxygen. This results in the type of severe poisoning that occurs when food is contaminated with such bacteria and is subsequently vacuum-packed, losing all access to oxygen. Similarly, the bacteria inside the evacuated pulp chamber encounter little or no oxygen. Just like the bacteria deprived of oxygen inside a sealed can, the bacteria trapped in the oxygen-starved environment inside the root canal-treated tooth will readily and rapidly produce severely potent toxins.

How Root Canal-Treated Teeth Poison and Kill

Even if a root canal procedure was performed on a tooth that was not infected at the start it will always end up infected, or at least seeded with the microorganisms that will promptly lead to chronic infection by the time the procedure is completed. And for the exceptionally overconfident dentist who maintains that his or her root canal procedure was done in a technically perfect and completely antiseptic fashion, the nature of the root canal procedure will always result in an infected dental pulp that will remain infected as long as the treated tooth remains in the mouth.

The basic problem with the root canal procedure is that it is a fatally flawed technique by design. A living tooth has sophisticated mechanisms for fending off pathogens; the root canal procedure destroys this capacity. The pulp of the tooth is rich with nerves, connective tissue, and a blood supply that allows a continual access to the body's immune system cells and other immune factors. A root canal effectively reams out the core of the tooth and fills the empty space with any of a number of different dental materials. One, and only one, positive clinical result often springs from this removal of much of the nerve supply: a pain-free tooth.

However, the negative clinical consequences are substantial. Immune system agents must come in contact with their targets before they can neutralize and/or kill them. This access requires a physical pathway or a matrix. With the removal of the pulp the natural landscape required for the immune cells to reach any microbes present has been removed. It would be just as plausible for a man to leap across the Grand Canyon as for an immune cell to cross the evacuated pulp of the root canal-treated tooth in order to confront infecting microorganisms. The filling material used in the root canal provides absolutely no mechanism for immune cells to reach all parts of the tooth; in fact it serves to further help block those cells from gaining access.

If immune cells cannot physically reach the microbes harbored in a root canal-treated tooth, they have no chance at all of killing them or even of impeding their multiplication. Furthermore the same lack of a normal blood- and nerve-containing matrix inside the tooth prevents the proper mobilization and elimination of toxic waste products that will instead continue to accumulate. The root canal-treated tooth has literally had its heart removed, and although it can continue to function mechanically in the chewing of food it is dead physiologically. The dentist has effectively assumed the role of a taxidermist, except that the root canal-treated tooth remains mounted in the mouth rather than on the wall.

To make matters worse the anatomy of the tooth adds another hurdle that makes fighting a progressive infection over time even more implausible. The dentin is the hard portion of the tooth immediately surrounding the pulp. This dentin of each tooth contains miles of microscopic tubules scarcely larger in diameter than most common bacteria. These tubules extend away from the pulp in a near-perpendicular direction. Even before the root canal procedure is performed, a tooth that begins with an infection in the pulp will have innumerable bacteria and other microbes occupying much of the space in the dentin tubules. Sterilizing such a tooth inside the mouth is impossible, at least with currently known dental techniques.

But even if a root canal-treated tooth could be reliably sterilized after the procedure, the lack of immune competence inside the evacuated pulp would result in its prompt re-infection shortly thereafter. So no matter how "competently" the root canal procedure is performed, a state of chronic infection is assured after the procedure is completed.

Why Lasers Do Not and Cannot Eliminate Root Canal Infection

Currently many dentists maintain that such sterilization can readily be achieved with a dental laser. Any dentist believing this simply does not understand the basic principles of a laser.

When a laser of sufficient intensity irradiates a microbe directly in its path it is certainly capable of killing that microbe. However, remember that the microbe-harboring dentin tubules extend away from the line of the pulp chamber at nearly a 90-degree angle (perpendicular). A laser only inactivates or destroys something directly in its path; it cannot take a right- or left-turn. However, and this seems to be where the confusion lies, a tooth will noticeably glow when a laser is directed into its pulp chamber. This glow is comprised of scattered light, not direct laser light, and it has no more of an ability to kill a microbe than a desk lamp. The only outcome achievable by a laser directed into the pulp chamber is a temporary kill-off of resident microbes directly in the path of the laser beam.

The reappearance of these microbes would take place rapidly from both the microbes living in the dentin tubules and from the mouth. The dental crown often placed at the termination of the root canal procedure represents no significant obstacle to the renewed migration of mouth microbes into the now surgically evacuated pulp chamber. The material used to fill the evacuated pulp chamber may minimally slow the rate of re-infection. However it will never prevent it from taking place.

Root Canal-Treated Teeth: Efficient Toxin Pumps

The nature of chewing makes root canal-treated teeth especially well-designed delivery systems for toxins. Rather than just staying put inside the tooth, the toxins along with the pathogens that have produced those toxins are expressed directly into the lymphatic and venous blood drainage of the jawbone, much more so every time chewing takes place. The act of chewing generates extremely high pressures, making the increased extrusion of pathogens and microbes a natural outcome every time a significant meal is eaten (or gum is chewed).

Dental Research Recognizes the Danger of Root Canal-Treated Teeth

A surprising study — surprising because it was published in a mainstream dental journal — found that individuals with root canal-treated teeth were significantly more likely to have coronary heart disease than individuals without them.[3] An earlier study showed that x-ray evidence of infection in the dental pulp correlates with the more rapid appearance of coronary heart disease.[4]

Anytime the pulp of the tooth becomes infected, the long-term negative health consequences of that infection will approach, if not equal, that of a root canal-treated tooth as long as it stays in the mouth.

Despite the evident dangers an entire large branch of dentistry (endodontics) is dedicated almost solely to the performance and further development of this root canal procedure. Additionally many other dentists that do not specialize in this procedure perform it very frequently as well.

Relative to the bulk of other commonly performed procedures in dentistry, the root canal procedure is relatively simple, rapid, and generously reimbursed. While the endodontics industry is nowhere close to stopping or even minimally curtailing this life-shortening procedure it is now acknowledged in the mainstream endodontic literature that persons "presenting lesions of endodontic origin" or "pulpal inflammation" have an increased risk of coronary heart disease.[5]

Understandably the researchers are not admitting that there is always an increased risk of heart attack when root canal-treated teeth are present. However, they are acknowledging that some infections of the tooth pulp can seed the coronary arteries with pathogens and toxins.

A very recent study has shown that bacterial DNA "typical for endodontic infection" is present in over 75% of the thrombi (blood clots) aspirated from patients with acute myocardial infarction.[6] Yet another study clearly showed that patients who sustained heart attacks had more "inflammatory processes" in their root canal-treated teeth.[7] The cause-and-effect relationship between root canal-treated teeth and coronary heart disease is really very clear. It just continues to be ignored, denied, or just scorned by those who benefit most financially from doing root canal treatments.

Root-Canal Treated Teeth: A Final Appeal

Roughly 14 million root canal procedures are performed every year. Over a ten-year period the number of root canal procedures performed is roughly equivalent to 50% of the entire U.S. population. When viewed in terms of the totality of the public health the impact of this toxic procedure is enormous.

Based on the science and information already presented there is only one reasonable approach to be taken (assuming one's general health is more important than the anatomy of the mouth): The root canal procedure is simply a procedure that should no longer be performed on anyone. Ever. And the teeth that have already had this procedure should be properly extracted. Period. The heart attacks and cancers that begin their development after this procedure is performed are literally countless.

Patients must be the guardians of their own health. The prevalence of root canal procedures continues to grow. It is highly unlikely that any amount of scientific evidence is going to eliminate this enormously popular dental procedure in the near future, if ever. Even when frank abscesses [obvious collections of pus] develop in association with root canal-treated teeth, dentists frequently evacuate the abscesses and try to perform "repeat" root canal procedures, sometimes more than once, before even considering the extraction of the tooth.

Even when a root canal-treated tooth is finally extracted there is often substantial irreversible damage that has already been inflicted on the immune system and affected tissues of the body. Like the boxer who has taken 500 punches rather than five, recovery is less rapid and less complete the more pounding takes place. The body, and its immune system, do not have unlimited abilities to recover.[8]

Dental Cavitations: Perpetually Toxic Wells

A cavitation is the residual hole resulting from the incomplete healing of the jawbone after a tooth is extracted. Although much of mainstream dentistry is reticent to recognize their existence, they are extremely common. Nearly 90% of the time an exploring bit will find cavitations at the sites of healed-over wisdom teeth extraction sites — even decades after the extraction.[9] Once they form they stay there permanently unless and until they are properly repaired surgically and appropriate measures are taken to support new bone growth.

Physiology of a Cavitation

Every tooth in the mouth is undergirded by a dense connective tissue that physically separates the entire root of the tooth from the surrounding bone. This tissue is called the periodontal ligament. It not only anchors the tooth in its socket, it also acts as a natural "shock absorber" for the tooth, gums, and jaw during chewing. Without the periodontal ligament, chewing would be like driving a car on its rims. The ride would be rough just as the chew would be tough.

The routine dental extraction procedure makes no attempt to remove the periodontal ligament. Therefore, when the tooth is extracted much of the periodontal ligament typically remains in place. Most likely this failure to remove the periodontal ligament is the reason most cavitations form.

If all or part of the ligament still remains the bone cells in the jawbone that directly surround the tooth have no physiological awareness that the tooth is gone. It is only when this ligament is removed along with the tooth that the natural stimulus for the growth of new bone cells is present and healing can begin. As long as any part of the ligament remains the hole in the jawbone never completely heals.

The actual size of the cavitation depends upon the percentage of the ligament that is coincidentally extracted with the tooth. The greater amount of ligament left in the mouth the less bone is able to grow into the hole and the larger the resulting cavitation. When little or no ligament is removed when the tooth is extracted, bone growth only initiates at the top of the extraction site, where the ligament ends. Subsequently a thin cap of bone eventually grows over the extraction hole, equal roughly in size to the extracted tooth itself.

Even though the removal of the periodontal ligament at the time of extraction is not an involved or time-consuming undertaking modern dentistry still does not include it as a routine part of a dental extraction.

The Toxic Consequences of Cavitations

If a cavitation were nothing more than a hole in the jawbone it would have little impact on the overall health of the body. The only real consequence would involve a lesser ability to properly chew food due to the absent tooth. However the contents of cavitations are always highly toxic. The typical cavitation contains a putrid and usually foul-smelling sludge indistinguishable pathologically and chemically from wet gangrene. Typically a minimal presence of pathogens is seen, along with a large quantity of toxins like those found in the root canal-treated tooth. The bulk of the cavitation contents is necrotic [dead, decomposed] material along with a small sampling of different immune cells.

While the contents of the cavitation are consistently necrotic and very toxic, the clinical impact of one or more cavitations in the jawbone is highly variable. The clinical picture varies because of the health of the surrounding jawbone and the overall size of the cavitation. When a significant amount of the periodontal ligament is extracted along with the tooth a relatively small cavitation will usually form and the toxic contents largely stay in place, especially in a younger patient with a stronger immune system and relatively healthy surrounding bone. Healthy bone better resists the gradual spread or extension that is often seen with cavitations. Some individuals appear to resist the detectable spread of smaller cavitations completely.

However, older patients with generalized osteoporosis, decreased circulation in the jawbone, and compromised immune systems will often demonstrate a steady progression of the amount of necrosis in a cavitation. This amoeba-like spread can go in any direction in the jawbone, sometimes tunneling in a seemingly aimless, serpentine manner. Older individuals who have had all of their teeth extracted will often have relatively continuous, channel-like cavitations extending through much of the length of the jawbone. The overall volume of such a channel cavitation can sometimes approach the size of a small pencil.

Sometimes the larger cavitations can involve enough of the jawbone that the deeply seated alveolar nerves are surrounded by the progressive necrosis. Alveolar nerves branch into the trigeminal nerves that supply sensation to the face, teeth, mouth, and nasal cavities. The myelin sheath surrounding and protecting the nerve can be destroyed by the presence of the necrosis as well. Intense pain syndromes can result when cavitations extend this deeply. Accordingly, cavitation-associated pain syndromes can variably involve the jaws, face, head, and/or neck. When such a syndrome of pain is discovered to be associated with a cavitation the cavitation is referred to as Neuralgia-Inducing Cavitational Osteonecrosis [NICO].[10]

It should be emphasized, however, that having any significant cavitation-associated pain, either directly over the cavitation or in some referred pattern, is the exception rather than the rule. Most patients with cavitations are completely pain-free in their jaws and face. Being pain-free, however, does not mean that a significant amount of cavitation-related toxicity is not challenging the immune system and impacting the rest of the body.

As a practical point, root canal-treated teeth have a consistently greater negative impact on health than cavitations even though the involved toxins and pathogens are essentially the same. This is because the root canal-treated teeth better and more consistently deliver the pathogen/toxin load into the blood and lymphatic fluids than cavitations. Also, root canal-treated teeth can continually seed other areas of the body with pathogens while the sparser pathogen presence in cavitations does not typically end up seeding another infection remotely.

However large and interconnected cavitations can end up being a very large source of toxin exposure and a cause of significant chronic disease, just less predictably so. Studies show that a lesser number of teeth (which will always be associated with more cavitation-related disease) is related to a greater risk of all-cause mortality, including cardiovascular mortality. [11,12] Consistent with this greater tooth loss was found to be related to a greater incidence of metabolic syndrome and laboratory markers of inflammation, both of which are strongly related to and most likely causative of increased coronary artery disease. [13]

Repair of Cavitations and Removal of Root Canal-Treated Teeth

The toxin profiles of root canal-treated teeth and cavitations are essentially the same. Variable degrees of cavitation will also be routinely found around the floor of the extraction site of a root canal-treated tooth, usually nearest the root tips. The toxins and microbes associated with the root canal-treated tooth will always induce some degree of necrosis in the adjacent or surrounding bone in much the same fashion as they do in a cavitation.

For this reason a dentist or oral surgeon — one who has experience in the surgical repair of cavitations and the removal of periodontal ligaments — should perform the proper extraction of a root canal-treated tooth. Extracting a root canal-treated tooth correctly in order to have the least short-term and long-term negative impact on the health of the patient is substantially more involved than a routine dental extraction and continues to be done only very rarely by dentists or oral surgeons today.

The Problems with Dental Implants

A dental implant involves the insertion of a dental material at the site of a missing tooth. This material is typically an alloy of titanium and it is used for the purpose of later anchoring a prosthetic tooth, a bridge, or either a partial or complete denture. When technically successful a dental implant is mechanically a stable and strong option for the restoration of a missing tooth.

Physiologically, however, a dental implant is often another source of substantial toxicity and infection. The implant procedure is usually initiated shortly after the tooth extraction takes place. As such, the implant is typically being placed directly in and through an evolving cavitation. As noted above, a cavitation is characterized by the accumulation of necrotic material with the associated toxic metabolic byproducts of the microorganisms that get trapped there after the extraction takes place.

Even when the implant heals in sufficiently to result in a mechanically sound anchoring device the infection and toxins associated with the evolving cavitation are routinely inserted deeply into the jawbone. As a result previously healthy bone gets exposed to toxins and microbes that would not normally have reached it as the implant is physically screwed or tapped into the bone beyond the developing cavitation. Because of this, the implant placement can facilitate the formation of an associated cavitation.

An additional downside to the dental implant is that the immune system will typically mount some degree of immune reaction or rejection whenever a foreign material is placed inside any tissue, including bone. Over time a substantial number of patients will develop chronic autoimmune problems. An autoimmune process presents an additional significant stressor on the immune system and an additional antioxidant-depleting effect to the body beyond just the toxic and infectious stress of the commonly associated cavitations at the tips of the implants.

As a practical point dental implants will not consistently have the same enormous negative impact on the health of the patient as the root canal-treated teeth or the larger cavitations. However dental implants will consistently have some negative impact on the general health. Just as with the root canal-treated teeth and cavitations, the older, more immunocompromised patients will suffer the greatest harm from dental implants.

Even when an implant is placed through an area of completely healed and healthy bone some of the microbes from the mouth can be expected to find their way into the implant site. Such an implant can be expected to cause fewer problems early on but many of them will still evolve into significantly toxic and infected entities. Also the autoimmune challenge presented by the implant will be initiated as soon as the implant is placed regardless of the health of the bone at the implant site.

Most Dental Materials: Highly Toxic

Amalgam Dental Fillings Are Astonishingly Toxic

Mercury amalgam fillings continue to be placed regularly and frequently inside the mouths of trusting patients. The so-called "silver" fillings that you may have in your mouth and that you see in the mouths of so many others are more than 50% mercury. Only a very small amount of the filling is actually silver. Furthermore, mercury is not only the most toxic heavy metal known to science; it is also the most toxic non-radioactive element in existence. Mercury amalgam fillings have been placed in greater numbers than any other type of filling for over a century now. And although public health awareness groups are gradually bringing one of dentistry's oldest dirty little secrets into the light of day, these fillings continue to be placed at an alarmingly high rate by dentists who refuse to change, much less scientifically examine the overwhelming body of evidence indicating how toxic these fillings are for so many people. [14]

While the debate continues to rage over how dangerous a mouthful of mercury amalgam fillings can be it remains undeniable that these fillings continuously release mercury vapor over time. This vapor is virtually completely inhaled and/or absorbed immediately by the mucous membranes or saliva in the mouth. Furthermore toxins like mercury are characterized by steady accumulation in the tissues with very little spontaneous excretion and no significant metabolic breakdown. No toxin that is not readily eliminated from the body and/or metabolized into non-toxic byproducts should be ignored in the pursuit of good health, much less one as toxic and difficult to eliminate as mercury.

Roughly another 30% of the mercury amalgam filling is composed of copper. This was not always the case. Until the 1970s most amalgam fillings had a much lower amount of copper. Then the high-copper amalgam was introduced and the toxicity of the fillings skyrocketed. Not only was the copper highly toxic and pro-oxidant in nature by itself, the increased percentage of the copper in the filling caused a much larger release of mercury vapor. Copper is also strongly carcinogenic (cancer-causing).

Toxic Reconstruction Materials Used in Implants, Bridges, and Crowns

Nickel is another highly toxic, yet commonly used, dental material. Nickel is used extensively in the metal alloys used in dental restorations because it is very durable, resistant to corrosion, and cheap. However it is also one of the most carcinogenic metals known to medicine. Once again it seems that modern dentistry only really concerns itself with the mechanical properties and cost of a dental substance, leaving the physiological consequences of such a substance virtually unaddressed. Ironically, many dentists do realize that nickel is carcinogenic. Yet they do not seem to realize how much of it is present in the stainless steel and other common metal alloys that they utilize. Years ago orthopedic surgeons used nickel-containing metals in their procedures. This was largely discontinued when the carcinogenic nature of nickel was fully realized. Dentistry, however, has never followed suit. Nickel remains a very commonly used metal in dental procedures and appliances.

Literally thousands of different dental materials are used today in dentistry. Aside from the toxic metals noted above, a wide variety of different chemicals, many toxic as well, are used in the production of these materials. Because of this a very large number of these chemical-based dental materials are noxious and toxic to some degree after placement in the mouth.

Biocompatibility Testing Provides Helpful Guidance

Serum biocompatibility testing can provide some degree of guidance or help in selecting the least toxic and immunoreactive materials for use in a given patient. Years of testing dental materials for this immune reactivity have revealed many of them to be consistently toxic with many others consistently non-toxic or only minimally toxic. Specific testing for an individual is always best to minimize the chances of having problems after dental work is performed, although selecting a consistently non-toxic material without specific testing will improve the chances of a good outcome. What should not be done is just to allow your dentist to use the materials that he or she likes the most, which is very often the case.

Periodontal (Gum) Disease Is Hazardous to Health, Too

The presence of infected and inflamed gums (periodontal disease or periodontitis) has now been established to be an independent risk factor or marker for coronary heart disease.[15-20] Angiographic studies have also clearly established that patients with periodontal disease are at an increased risk for developing coronary artery narrowings greater than 50%.[21]

This should come as no surprise since the same microorganisms that seed themselves in root canal-treated teeth and cavitations will also seed themselves in the spaces between the gums and the teeth when the gums are not healthy. Once such microbes get deep enough into these gum-teeth (crevicular) spaces, a relatively anaerobic (oxygen-starved) environment will exist, and the bacteria trapped there can be expected to produce many of the same potent toxins seen with root canal-treated teeth and cavitations. Heavily diseased gums, due to the overall quantity of infection, can compromise general health just as much as having several root canal-treated teeth. Periodontal disease has also been linked to an increased incidence of stroke [22] as well as to more generalized vascular disease. [23]

Conclusion

Today very many adults in the United States are dealing with illnesses that have resulted from any of a number of dental interventions. Root canal-treated teeth are such infected and highly toxic entities that a majority of cancers and heart attacks today are caused by them. Additionally cavitations, dental implants, toxic dental materials, and periodontal disease all contribute significantly to the depletion of the antioxidant defenses of the patient. While many different things can be done to improve the antioxidant status of someone, many of these interventions are largely without a great deal of effect in the pursuit of optimal health if the major sources of dental toxicity remain unaddressed. As Dr. Hal Huggins, the champion of toxin-free denistry once said, "You can't dry off while you're still in the shower."

SECTION FIVE:

Now What?

CHAPTER 15

Getting Good Care in a Sea of Bad Medicine

Work with a Physician Who Will Work with You

It is difficult for a patient to be his own doctor and receive the best of care. Whenever possible seek out a competent healthcare practitioner to help you protect or regain your health. This book has shed light on the widespread travesty of tradition-based medical practices that reject, ignore, or are unaware of the large volume of science that repudiates those traditions. This new light, however, should not be construed as a recommendation to reject one's physician and go it alone.

In spite of the arrogant "know-it-all" superiority that often accompanies the earning of a medical degree, some physicians are open and teachable. If your physician is willing to consider new information, share your perspectives, concerns, and even this book with him or her. You will help yourself and very likely you'll benefit many other patients that follow you. If you are scorned or barely tolerated don't try to walk through a brick wall. Find someone else to help you. Your doctor should be a compassionate, ever-learning partner, not a dictator.

Although membership in a particular organization is not a guarantee of any individual's personal position or integrity, there are three groups that can provide a good starting place should you need to find a new physician:

> 1) **American College for Advancement in Medicine** (ACAM). A listing of these doctors is on the website www.acam.org.
>
> 2) **American Academy of Anti-Aging Medicine** (A4M). A directory of these physicians is on the www.worldhealth.net website.
>
> 3) A third group of recommended doctors can be found at www.orthomolecular.org.

Once you have a doctor with whom you are comfortable you need to disclose everything you are doing and taking with him or her. Your clinical status, along with periodic laboratory testing, must be part of how you and your doctor decide whether to add, drop, or modify a given part of whatever protocol you are following.

It is also very important to realize that there is often more than one approach or protocol that can make you well and protect you from future disease. Many different therapies can produce good results. Ultimately, any approach, therapy, or protocol that decreases the oxidative stress inside your body will make you better and there is certainly more than one way to accomplish this goal.

For any reader who wants to contact me directly my email address is televymd@yahoo.com. I answer all my emails personally. However, I cannot directly advise anyone on how to proceed with treatment for their conditions and I cannot address too many emails from one individual. If your physician wants to pose questions regarding my antioxidant-centered approaches to medical care to me I am always available by email. But I cannot give that same advice directly to a patient. I can only offer my help to the doc who is helping you. Further information is also available on my website, www.peakenergy.com.

CHAPTER 16

Reversing Bone Damage

Suggested Osteoporosis Protection / Reversal Protocol

The effective treatment of osteoporosis and any other chronic degenerative disease must incorporate the following goals in order to maximize the potential of clinical improvement that is possible:

1) Minimize new toxin exposure.
2) Eradicate acute and chronic infections.
3) Eliminate accumulated toxins.
4) Improve or normalize critical regulatory hormones (sex, thyroid).
5) Optimize antioxidant and nutrient levels, especially vitamin C, throughout the body.
6) Selectively and appropriately use prescription medications.

1) Minimize New Toxin Exposure

Calcium: The primary two toxin exposures of greatest clinical significance in osteoporosis patients come from excess calcium ingestion and from ongoing toxin exposure from dental sources. Both exposures also play a great role in the appearance and worsening of all other chronic degenerative diseases. Pure calcium supplements should never be taken and all multi-ingredient supplements containing calcium are also best completely avoided. As well, calcium-containing antacid formulations should never be taken. When taken regularly for the control of an upset or acid stomach these preparations can be an exceptionally large source of calcium, virtually assuring a state of advanced calcium excess throughout the body.

While vitamin D uncombined with anything else needs to be supplemented on a regular basis it is best to avoid any calcium-rich foods that have had vitamin D added to them. Dairy intake should be minimized but need not be completely avoided. Milk, however, is best never ingested as a beverage as such a practice will also reliably induce a state of calcium excess in the body.

Additional supplements or supplement components that need to be strictly avoided are copper and iron. Copper should simply never be supplemented and iron should only be supplemented when there exists a documented iron deficiency anemia. Furthermore, iron supplementation for such an anemia should not be continued after the anemia has been resolved. When such an iron deficiency anemia exists the reason for the anemia must be diagnosed and treated appropriately. Most commonly in older patients with osteoporosis, such an anemia comes from blood loss in the gastrointestinal tract. Such blood loss will usually end up coming from a bleeding ulcer, benign or malignant, or a bleeding lower bowel cancer.

In summary, you should:

- Discontinue **all** calcium-containing supplements.
- Discontinue **all** calcium-containing antacids.
- Avoid **all** calcium-rich foods with vitamin D added.
- Avoid milk as a beverage.
- Avoid copper-containing supplements.
- Avoid iron-containing supplements (unless there is a documented iron-deficiency anemia).

Dental Toxins/Infections: For the individual wanting to give their body its best chance to restore healthy antioxidant levels throughout the organs and tissues a Total Dental Revision (TDR) is advisable. This involves addressing as many different sources of dental toxicity and infection as possible. A TDR includes the following:

- Extraction of root canal-treated teeth with complete removal of the periodontal ligament and surrounding infected bone; also, similar extraction of any acutely or chronically infected/abscessed teeth.
- Proper gum care to prevent or at least minimize chronic infection.
- Surgical evacuation and complete cleaning of cavitations.
- Proper removal of mercury amalgams with restorations using optimally biocompatible materials.
- Replacement of any other dental restorations (crowns, bridges, plates) with optimally biocompatible materials.
- Proper removal of infected dental implants.

While a complete TDR is optimal in minimizing dental sources of toxicity and infection, most individuals can get a enormous boost to their immune systems and body-wide antioxidant levels by addressing only the root canals and other infected teeth, along with proper gum care. Any infection and inflammation in the gums is usually quite effectively addressed by daily water irrigation (as with a Waterpik) with a large cupful of warm water, one to two tablespoons of 3% hydrogen peroxide, and a splash of preferred mouthwash for taste. Individuals with limited financial resources and/or significant apprehension regarding a TDR need to realize that removal of root canal-treated teeth and proper gum care are the most important and will almost always eliminate a majority of their dental toxin exposure.

It is also vital to understand that ignoring the dental aspects of the protocol does not completely prevent the protocol from significantly helping the patient. However, much of the time it will only slow osteoporosis progression rather than cause any actual improvement in the quality of the diseased bone. As well, the slowing of the disease process will nearly always be accompanied by lessened symptomatology and an improved quality of life.

Dietary/Digestive: What is eaten and how well it is digested are very important factors in any protocol attempting to minimize new daily toxin exposure. Of the two factors the quality of daily digestion is actually far more important than the quality of the food. This subject is covered more thoroughly in Chapter 13. A summary of important considerations discussed there is as follows:
- Chew all food thoroughly.
- Combine foods properly.

- Minimize beverages with meals including water.
- Eliminate milk as a beverage. Increase vegetable intake.
- Decrease/minimize (but not eliminate) meat intake.
- Minimize foods with a high glycemic index and eliminate refined sugar as much as possible.
- Minimize/eliminate highly toxic seafoods.

2) Eradicate Old Infections

While there is some overlap between this and the goal of minimizing new toxins discussed above, there are other sources of infections besides the mouth. Many individuals develop secondary locations of infection after having had the presence of dental infections for a long enough period of time.

Generally if the patient responds to the rest of the protocol very well both clinically and with substantial normalization of previously abnormal laboratory tests it is not really necessary to undergo further testing looking for additional sources of infection and toxicity. A lack of response to the protocol, however, suggests that secondary sources are at work. Individuals with rheumatoid arthritis, for example, often have low-grade infections seeded in their joints stemming from dental sites or infected tonsils.

One source of infection that is often overlooked lurks in seemingly healthy, yet chronically infected tonsils. This is particularly true when root canals have been present in the mouth for a long enough period of time, or when other dental sources of infection have been chronically present and the tonsils have had to chronically filter blood and lymph for dental pathogens.

Even when tonsils have a normal external appearance upon examination the possibility of chronically infected tonsils should be high on the list of suspects when the rest of the protocol produces no substantial improvement. When the tonsils are obviously infected and have sustained recurrences of tonsillitis, they should always be removed promptly rather than as a last resort, in order to minimize the inevitable damage inflicted on the immune system.

3) Eliminate Old Toxins

Some toxins, like mercury for example, are not readily eliminated from the body but rather deposit in tissues throughout the body. As long as these toxins remain in the body they continue to cause damage.

For some individuals, elimination or excretion of these accumulated toxins can be of major consequence; in others this is of minor or little importance. As such, the treating clinician must make his own best determination as to how vigorously this aspect of the protocol should be approached.

Much experience has been accumulated on the different chemical ways to chelate (bind) and excrete various toxins from the body. No attempt will be made here to advise of a "best way" to chemically chelate toxins as the choice of chelator will vary depending on the:

- Nature of the toxin accumulated
- Tissues in which the toxins have accumulated
- Severity of the patient's condition
- Perception of the treating clinician as to how big a role toxin accumulation is playing in the diseases of the patient

Commonly utilized chelators include dimercaptosuccinic acid (DMSA), dimercaptopropane sulfonate (DMPS), dimercaprol (BAL), ethylenediaminetetraacetic acid (EDTA), penicillamine, deferoxamine, and deferasirox. Significant nutrient chelators include alpha lipoic acid (ALA) and inositol hexaphosphate (IP6).

In addition, substantial natural chelation takes place inside the body via glutathione and glutathione-related detoxification enzymes. Because of this, any supplementation known to help restore normal glutathione levels inside the cells of the body can work to bind and excrete toxins via this mechanism. Such supplements would include whey protein, N-acetylcysteine, and liposome-encapsulated glutathione.

4) Correct Critical Hormone Deficiencies

As patients age deficiencies in critical regulatory hormone levels in the body become increasingly common. Testosterone, estrogen, and thyroid hormone deficiencies are actually more the rule than the exception when the patient population is old enough. It is very important to identify these deficiencies as early as possible in the management of patients with chronic degenerative diseases to optimally impact their morbidity and mortality. Sex hormone and thyroid hormone deficiencies have a negative impact on virtually every cell in the body. And just as importantly, these deficiencies must be corrected, or at least improved, in a very slow and deliberate fashion, as highly-dosed and inappropriately-administered replacement hormone therapy can definitely do more harm than good.

5) Optimize Antioxidant Levels

For the osteoporosis patient, antioxidant levels, particularly vitamin C, are extremely low in the bones themselves and they are always significantly depressed throughout the body as well. Optimizing the levels of vitamin C and other critical antioxidants and nutrients throughout the body is the overriding goal of the protocol. It is essential to realize, however, that this goal is unattainable as long as the toxins, infections, and hormone deficiencies remain unaddressed. This portion of the protocol cannot be adopted and followed by itself with the expectation that dramatic clinical and laboratory results will occur. However, this regimen of supplementation can still be expected to be of clear benefit in helping to control the evolution and symptomatology of chronic diseases such as osteoporosis even if no other aspects of the treatment protocol are followed.

After toxin exposures, chronic infections, and critical hormone deficiencies have been successfully addressed, much greater success can be realized in restoring important antioxidant and nutrient levels in the body. For osteoporosis, a good regimen of supplementation should include the items in the table on the next page in roughly a descending order of importance.

The lysine and proline supplementation is included in the regimen since the typical osteoporosis patient already has some underlying atherosclerosis and coronary artery disease. While higher amounts of lysine and proline would be appropriate in the treatment of established atherosclerosis, these lesser recommended amounts are appropriate for slowing the progression, or even reversing, any undiagnosed coronary artery disease at the time of supplementation initiation.

6) Appropriate Prescription Medication Use

Prescription medications for osteoporosis should be considered only when application of the protocol discussed fails to produce a satisfactory response as determined clinically and in follow-up blood testing. When significant portions of the suggested protocol are not followed there

Supplement	Daily Oral Dose	Special Instructions
Vitamin C as sodium ascorbate or ascorbic acid	6,000 to 15,000 mg	Depending upon bowel tolerance, in two to four divided doses throughout the day
Vitamin C in liposome-encapsulated form	1,000 to 2,000 mg	
Vitamin C in a fat-soluble form as ascorbyl palmitate	1,000 to 2,000 mg	Divided into two doses
Lysine	2,500 mg	
Proline	500 mg	
Vitamin D3	5,000 units (Starting Dose!)	Adjust by blood testing to stay as close to a 50 ng/cc blood level as possible over time
Vitamin K2 (menaquinone-4, or menatetrenone)	3 to 6 mg	
Magnesium glycinate	400 mg	Divided into two doses
Omega-3 fish oil (EPA and DHA content)	1 to 2 grams	Divided into two doses
Mixed tocopherols (vitamin E source)	800 IU	Divided into two doses
Beta carotene (vitamin A source)	25,000 to 50,000 IU	
Complete B vitamin complex (as from Life Extension Foundation)	1 to 2 Capsules	Divided into two doses if taking 2 capsules
Specifically AVOID any supplementation with copper, calcium, or iron; iron should only be taken for laboratory-documented iron deficiency anemia		

will be a greater likelihood that the osteoporotic bone will not strengthen or even stabilize. In this case attention to the missed portions of the protocol should be followed prior to prescription drug interventions that are likely to be recommended by your physician.

If and only if the protocol fails to produce satisfactory results, prescription medications can be useful tools. Frequently these medications come with significant side effects. However, the strong antioxidant support offered by the protocol should substantially lessen and sometimes eliminate such side effects in individuals requiring such medicine. The decision to treat with prescription medicines should rest on clinical and laboratory grounds, with the goal that bone strengthening or stabilization must not be accompanied with further increases in the excess calcium status outside of the bones.

The decision to go with prescription therapy will also be strongly affected by how old the patient is and how advanced the osteoporosis is when treatment is initiated. A younger patient with less brittle bones should never require prescription intervention while a very old patient with an imminent risk of osteoporotic fracture may require more aggressive intervention in order to be stabilized, even following the institution of the full osteoporosis protocol presented here.

The main prescription medicines in question here are selective estrogen receptor modulators (SERMs), bisphosphonates, calcitonin, strontium ranelate, and different forms of parathyroid hormone. On the positive side, all of these prescription drugs have been shown to have some positive effects on bone mineral density accompanied by a decreased incidence of some fractures, which is the primary goal of antiosteoporosis therapy.

Side effect profiles for these prescription drugs include the following:

While the side effects noted below are substantial and potentially fatal consequences can result, these drugs

Drug	Possible Side Effects
SERMs (selective receptor modulators)	Increased incidence of venous thromboembolism
Bisphosphonates	Gastric upset/intolerance, erosive esophagitis, possible increased risk of esophageal cancer, renal failure, osteonecrosis of the jaw, and atypical femoral fracture
Calcitonin	Allergy and possible anaphylaxis, headache, dizziness, tremor, impaired glucose tolerance, and gastric upset/intolerance
Strontium ranelate	Increased incidence of venous thromboembolism, seizures, allergy with hives and swelling, potentially fatal skin reactions (Stevens-Johnson syndrome, toxic epidermal necrolysis), and gastric upset/intolerance
Parathyroid hormone	Possible increased risk of osteosarcoma, nausea, transient hypercalcemia

do have their place — especially in old and brittle osteoporosis patients that do not respond favorably to the rest of the suggested treatment protocol. The decision to utilize any of these pharmaceuticals must be a thoughtful, balanced one, carefully weighing potential benefits against potential side effects in any given patient. Also, while it is likely that the increase in the antioxidant capacity of the body resulting from the suggested protocol could mitigate and even block most or all of the side effects associated with the drugs mentioned, this cannot be completely relied upon to be the case. The clinician still needs to exert appropriate caution in the use of these drugs.

As very many osteoporosis patients have other medical problems and are often on multiple prescription drugs that are not specifically treating the osteoporosis, a calcium channel blocker drug should be utilized whenever possible. High blood pressure can be treated with many different drugs but including a calcium channel blocker in the treatment of this condition can have a wide array of other positive effects. These benefits include a decreased risk of all-cause mortality as well as symptomatic benefit in diseased tissues that have the most increased oxidative stress from increased intracellular calcium levels.

While high blood pressure would be the most common example, a calcium channel blocker should also be used for any other condition established to benefit from this class of drugs. And another important note, while most prescription drugs have significant side effect profiles the calcium channel blocker does not. All prescription calcium channel blockers are quite effective for the treatment of hypertension and they are all tolerated very well. For more information about calcium channel blockers please see Appendix A.

CHAPTER 17

Decalcifying Coronary Arteries

Suggested Heart Disease Protection / Reversal Protocol

The same six goals of the osteoporosis treatment protocol apply to the proper treatment of coronary artery disease, or atherosclerosis. A very brief summary of the recommendations from that protocol is included here. For a more complete understanding of those recommendations, refer to Chapter 16. Most of this chapter concentrates on the differences in how the common six goals are best achieved in atherosclerosis.

As a reminder, the six goals are to:

1) Minimize new toxin exposure.
2) Eradicate acute and chronic infections.
3) Eliminate accumulated toxins.
4) Improve or normalize critical regulatory hormones (sex, thyroid).
5) Optimize antioxidant and nutrient levels, especially vitamin C, throughout the body.
6) Selectively and appropriately use prescription medications.

1) Minimize New Toxin Exposure

Calcium, iron, and copper supplementation all need to be carefully avoided and calcium ingestion in general needs to be minimized. In heart disease patients iron excess and the need to mobilize and excrete it are usually of greater urgency than in the osteoporosis patient.

Bear in mind, however, that the commonest diseases following menopause are osteoporosis and atherosclerotic heart disease. As such the careful clinician will often find the best approach to osteoporosis and heart disease patients is a combination of the osteoporosis and coronary artery disease protocols. How the protocols are best combined will depend upon the likely or known predominance of one condition over the other in any given patient.

In summary, you should:

- Discontinue **all** calcium-containing supplements.
- Discontinue **all** calcium-containing antacids
- Avoid **all** calcium-rich foods with vitamin D added.
- Avoid milk as a beverage.
- Avoid iron-containing supplements (unless there is a documented iron-deficiency anemia).
- Avoid copper-containing supplements.

Addressing dental toxins and infections is of paramount importance in treating any patient known to have coronary artery atherosclerosis. It is, in fact, the coronary arteries that are the first parts of the arterial system to be exposed to dental toxicity. As such, the continual release of pathogens and toxins from root canal-treated teeth into the venous drainage makes this toxin/infection source especially important for the heart disease patient. Due to their proximity to the outflow tract in the left ventricle of the heart the blood pressure in the coronary arteries is quite forceful. This makes them much more prone to seeding by any pathogens and toxins in the blood and this is why the low-pressure venous system does not get similarly seeded.

Therefore it is essential that the heart patient and treating physician realize that:

> **The presence of one or more root canal-treated teeth is the single greatest cause of significant coronary heart disease.**

As with osteoporosis, it is also highly advisable that any other teeth identified to be infected get properly extracted and that the gums be given warm water/hydrogen peroxide irrigations on a daily basis, such as with a Waterpik. The rest of the total dental revision (TDR) is important but addressing root canals, other infected teeth, and proper gum care will make the most difference and should not be neglected if there is any realistic hope for lessening the degree of narrowings in the coronary arteries.

A summary of the TDR priorities includes the following:

- Extraction of root canal-treated teeth, with complete removal of the periodontal ligament and surrounding infected bone; also, similar extraction of any acutely or chronically infected/abscessed teeth.
- Proper gum care to prevent or at least minimize chronic infection.
- Surgical evacuation and complete cleaning of cavitations.
- Proper removal of mercury amalgams, with restorations using optimally biocompatible materials.

- Replacement of any other dental restorations (crowns, bridges, plates) with optimally biocompatible materials.
- Proper removal of infected dental implants.

The same guidelines for minimizing poor diet/digestion-related pathogens and toxins as discussed in the osteoporosis treatment protocol apply equally to the coronary artery disease protocol. Those are:

- Chew all food thoroughly.
- Combine foods properly.
- Minimize beverages with meals including water.
- Eliminate milk as a beverage. Increase vegetable intake.
- Decrease/minimize (but not eliminate) meat intake.
- Minimize foods with a high glycemic index and eliminate refined sugar as much as possible.
- Minimize/eliminate highly toxic seafoods.

2) Eradicate Old Infections

This part of the protocol is much the same as the second part of the osteoporosis treatment protocol. However, just as mentioned in the preceding section, pathogens and toxins from the head and neck that drain into the venous system are especially important since they often selectively find their way into the inner lining of the coronary arteries. Because of this greater attention needs to be paid to making sure that occult infections, such as might be found in normal-appearing tonsils, are identified and eradicated, as they can single-handedly block most of the positive effects that could be accomplished with the rest of the protocol.

Obviously-infected tonsils must always be removed promptly but strong consideration needs to be given to tonsil removal when there is only a history of root canals, even though they might have been long since extracted. This option becomes particularly important when laboratory tests such as the C-reactive protein remain significantly elevated even after all infections are felt to have been identified and eradicated. While tonsils are designed to be a protective barrier against the dissemination of pathogens and toxins from the mouth they are often transformed from chronic protectors to chronic infectors when they have been subjected long enough to the chronic toxins and pathogens coming from root canal-treated teeth. As well, a history of frequent bouts of tonsillitis can also indicate likely "burned-out" tonsils that are more likely ongoing infection sources than barricades against infections.

3) Eliminate Old Toxins

Accelerating the elimination of old toxins is another part of the protocol that is largely the same for osteoporosis and coronary artery disease.

One big difference is how vigorously iron should be eliminated from the system, as a ferritin level greater than only 50 ng/cc ("normal" range for one prominent laboratory is 30 to 400 ng/cc) is clearly associated with a negative impact on the coronary arteries. If a cardiac patient is known to have significant, but not critical stenoses, and that patient is clinically stable, iron chelation need not be initiated. Instead, periodic phlebotomy can lower the ferritin to a safe level that does not further aggravate or accelerate the coronary atherosclerosis.

An additional means of reducing ferritin levels can be accomplished with inositol hexaphosphate (IP6). It can be taken orally (1 to 3 grams) when the stomach is empty and upon absorption iron is one of the substances that will naturally be bound and excreted. Far infrared sauna therapy is also exceptionally effective at eliminating iron from the body in addition to a wide variety of other heavy metals and toxins. If the heat can be tolerated, taking a 20 to 30 minute sauna several times a week can be enormously beneficial to the health in general, as well as in lowering iron levels. The sauna is also a good idea for the osteoporosis patients as sauna sweats will also eliminate calcium, but many of these patients are older and do not tolerate the heat well. It is never a good idea to risk having a patient pass out while taking a sauna regardless of the potential health benefits.

When ferritin levels are 400 ng/cc or more or the patient is very symptomatic and considered marginally stable with lesser elevations of ferritin (200 to 400 ng/cc), strong consideration should be given to prescription iron chelation. Probably the best choice here would be deferasirox, 125 mg or more orally before the evening meal, three times weekly. When ferritin levels drop below 100 ng/cc the chelation therapy can usually be terminated. The ultimate target ferritin level for long-term maintenance should be between 12 and 25 ng/cc as long as no evidence of iron deficiency anemia appears. As long as the oral deferasirox can do the job the injectable iron chelator, deferoxamine, is not recommended because of its significant side effects.

4) Correct Critical Hormone Deficiencies

This should be addressed in the same manner as for osteoporosis, as both testosterone and thyroid deficiencies can play significant roles in hastening the evolution of both osteoporosis and heart disease. However, testosterone, estrogen, and thyroid hormone deficiencies have all separately been shown to be associated with an increased risk of metabolic syndrome, a condition featuring multiple significant coronary artery disease risk factors. Therefore, for known coronary artery disease patients there is a greater urgency to address these deficiencies than even in the osteoporosis patient.

The greater urgency to treat, however, should not be confused with aggressive, highly-dosed replacement therapy. Either the sex or the thyroid hormone deficiencies must be corrected slowly, with low doses, and with bioidentical hormone replacement if available.

Furthermore, especially in older patients, a full-restoration of hormones will not typically be the goal. The initial goal should be to reach low to mid-range normal hormone values on follow-up laboratory testing. If the patient appears to be responding well with no evidence of any therapy-induced laboratory abnormalities the ultimate goal of therapy can be pushed a bit further to mid-range normal or slightly higher. Under no circumstances should the goal ever be to push the laboratory results into the high-normal range.

Many individuals on sex and thyroid hormone replacement therapy will start to mobilize fat stores with a resulting release of toxins and other pro-oxidant products such as cytokines. As such, this release will often be reflected in an increase in inflammatory biomarkers such as the C-reactive protein (CRP).

A significant enough increase in the evidence of inflammation needs to be countered with a still lower and slower approach to the hormone replacement therapy. Also, if the laboratory values are only minimally abnormal then a more vigorous approach to the antioxidant supplementation might be all that is needed. The ultimate desired goal of the hormone replacement therapy is the elimination of, or at least the dramatic lessening of, abnormalities in the major cardiac risk factors, including a complete normalization of any previously elevated inflammatory biomarkers like CRP.

5) Optimize Antioxidant Levels

The only significant difference in supplementation for established coronary artery disease versus osteoporosis is the need for larger amounts of lysine and proline. Lysine and proline are vital in optimizing the chances of lessening or even eliminating atherosclerotic narrowings in the coronary arteries. When the rest of the protocol has been carefully followed a reversal of arterial narrowings is actually the rule and not the exception. The atherosclerosis patient should take at least 2,500 mg of lysine twice daily orally along with 500 mg of proline twice daily. More can be taken if desired and with the monitoring of your healthcare practitioner.

It is also reasonable to administer a series of highly-dosed vitamin C infusions after the rest of the protocol has been initiated and especially after toxins and infections have been addressed as thoroughly as possible. The intravenous dosing of the vitamin C under these circumstances acts as a loading dose in the hopes of getting a good initial penetration in and around the endothelial cells of the coronary arteries. Following this series of infusions the rest of the protocol supplements can then work to maintain a strong antioxidant presence in the coronary arteries. Just as deeply-seated infections require a large loading dose of antibiotics followed by extended dosing at lower levels, the same pharmacokinetic principles apply to loading the vitamin C into the coronary arteries with initial high dosing.

In order to achieve the loading dose effect a high enough intravenous dose of vitamin C needs to be administered. A good rule of thumb to follow is to base the amount on body weight, at least roughly. Most individuals

Decalcifying Coronary Arteries

Supplement	Daily Oral Dose	Special Instructions
Vitamin C as sodium ascorbate or ascorbic acid	6,000 to 15,000 mg	Depending upon bowel tolerance, in two to four divided doses throughout the day
Vitamin C in liposome-encapsulated form	1,000 to 2,000 mg	
Vitamin C in a fat-soluble form as ascorbyl palmitate	1,000 to 2,000 mg	Divided into two doses
Lysine	5,000 mg	Divided into two doses
Proline	1,000 mg	Divided into two doses
Vitamin D3	5,000 units (Starting Dose!)	Adjust by blood testing to stay as close to a 50 ng/cc blood level as possible over time
Vitamin K2 (menaquinone-4, or menatetrenone)	3 to 6 mg	
Magnesium glycinate	400 mg	Divided into two doses
Omega-3 fish oil (EPA and DHA content)	1 to 2 grams	Divided into two doses
Mixed tocopherols (vitamin E source)	800 IU	Divided into two doses
Beta carotene (vitamin A source)	25,000 to 50,000 IU	
Complete B vitamin complex (as from Life Extension Foundation)	1 to 2 Capsules	Divided into two doses if taking 2 capsules
Specifically AVOID any supplementation with copper, calcium, or iron; iron should only be taken for laboratory-documented iron deficiency anemia		

should do very well with 1.0 to 1.5 grams of vitamin C per kilogram body weight per infusion. As a practical point, this works out to a range of 50 to 150 grams for body sizes ranging from a small woman to a large man.

Since a loading dose effect is the goal of these infusions the IV rate should be as rapid as possible, with the entire amount infusing over 30 to 60 minutes. This can cause a reflex release of insulin from the pancreas as it interprets the vitamin C load as a load of the closely-related molecule, glucose. Because of this hypoglycemic symptoms might be encountered, but the patient should be coached to try to tolerate the feeling since the insulin surge is helping deliver more vitamin C into the cells and it would be best not to give glucose or sugar to relieve symptoms as it would blunt the delivery effect.

There is no one precise number of intravenous infusions that could be considered optimal to begin the process of increasing vitamin C levels in the arterial walls but at least six infusions over a two-week period would probably suffice for most individuals. To optimize the acute effects of these infusions an additional 3,000 to 4,000 mg of oral liposome-encapsulated vitamin C should be taken to further bolster the goal of endothelial penetration of the vitamin C at the beginning of each infusion. In the event that the patient feels poorly during or immediately after a vitamin C infusion a "mop-up" vitamin C infusion can be given. This is discussed at greater length in section 5 of the cancer treatment protocol, where such negative effects of a vitamin C infusion can occur more frequently.

6. Appropriate Prescription Medication Use

As was mentioned in the protocol for the treatment of osteoporosis, calcium channel blocker drugs should be used as the first option when medically reasonable. Many coronary artery disease patients also have high blood pressure and at least occasional symptoms of angina pectoris. Both of these conditions benefit nicely from calcium channel blockers and the long-term evolution of those conditions as well as any other chronic degenerative diseases will benefit as well. In fact a strong case can be made for taking a calcium channel blocker solely for the benefits of limiting the calcium uptake by the cells throughout the body, although many docs might not be comfortable with prescribing such a drug without a more clear-cut "condition."

Statin drugs should be avoided in general, as much of the lipid abnormalities for which the statins are prescribed will resolve or at least substantially improve under the full protocol. Also, statins often have substantial side effects that are best avoided if possible. However patients who do not undergo any parts of the total dental revision, root canal extraction(s) in particular, will often have persistent and substantial cholesterol and lipid abnormalities and most physicians will strongly push their patients to take statins.

CHAPTER 18

Neutralizing the Mutagenic Effects of Calcium

Suggested Cancer Protection / Reversal Protocol

Cancer is a very diverse disease with many different cell types involved and many different clinical presentations. It must be understood that the treatment protocol for cancer is presented as a good baseline protocol from which many further adjustments and additions can be made for a given patient.

Most of this chapter concentrates on the differences in how the common six goals are best achieved in the cancer patient versus the other protocols offered.

As a reminder, the six goals are to:

1) Minimize new toxin exposure.

2) Eradicate acute and chronic infections.

3) Eliminate accumulated toxins.

4) Improve or normalize critical regulatory hormones (sex, thyroid).

5) Optimize antioxidant and nutrient levels, especially vitamin C, throughout the body.

6) Selectively and appropriately use prescription medications.

1) Minimize New Toxin Exposure

Although it is always desirable to minimize new toxin exposure to alleviate any chronic disease process, cancer, along with heart disease noted in Chapter 17, is especially severely impacted by excesses of calcium, iron, and copper.

In summary, you should:
- Discontinue **all** calcium-containing supplements.
- Discontinue **all** calcium-containing antacids.
- Avoid **all** calcium-rich foods with vitamin D added.
- Avoid milk as a beverage.
- Avoid iron-containing supplements (unless there is a documented iron-deficiency anemia).
- Avoid copper-containing supplements.

Infectious dental toxicity, particularly root canals and chronic gum disease, must be addressed as well. As with coronary artery disease, it also needs to be clearly stated that:

> **The presence of one or more root canal-treated teeth is the single greatest cause of cancers of the head, neck, and chest.**

Because of the enormous role played by root canals in head, neck, and chest cancers, it is very important to realize that leaving such teeth unextracted will greatly impair whatever recovery is anticipated with the remainder of the protocol. Very few people completely recover from cancer and maintain good health beyond the expected lifespan with root canals left in place. And even when one cancer appears to disappear with any of a number of chemotherapy and/or immune support protocols, the likelihood of the eventual recurrence of the old cancer or the appearance of a new cancer is very high when root canals stay and chronically impair immune function.

As with osteoporosis and heart disease it is very important to extract any other teeth found to be infected and to irrigate the gums with a warm water/hydrogen peroxide solution on a regular basis.

A summary of the Total Dental Revision (TDR) priorities includes the following:

- Extraction of root canal-treated teeth, with complete removal of the periodontal ligament and surrounding infected bone; also, similar extraction of any acutely or chronically infected/abscessed teeth.
- Proper gum care to prevent or at least minimize chronic infection.
- Surgical evacuation and complete cleaning of cavitations.
- Proper removal of mercury amalgams with restorations using optimally biocompatible materials.
- Replacement of any other dental restorations (crowns, bridges, plates) with optimally biocompatible materials.
- Proper removal of infected dental implants.

The same guidelines for minimizing poor diet/digestion-related pathogens and toxins as discussed in the osteoporosis treatment protocol apply equally to the cancer protocol. Those are:

- Chew all food thoroughly.

- Combine foods properly.
- Minimize beverages with meals including water.
- Eliminate milk as a beverage. Increase vegetable intake.
- Decrease/minimize (but not eliminate) meat intake.
- Minimize foods with a high glycemic index and eliminate refined sugar as much as possible.
- Minimize/eliminate highly toxic seafoods.

2) Eradicate Old Infections

Cancers of the head, neck, and chest are just as severely impacted by chronically-infected tonsils as is coronary artery disease. While it is important to eliminate any clearly identified sources of chronic infection to optimally support the immune system in the treatment of any chronic degenerative disease, it is especially important to do so for cancer and heart disease.

3) Eliminate Old Toxins

The elimination of old toxins is important to the long-term health of the cancer patient. However, it is very important that any form of chelation or toxin elimination does not get the job done too rapidly. It is critical to remember that:

Detoxification is also retoxification.

That is to say, no manner of toxin mobilization and elimination is completely free of causing increased oxidative stress in the blood and lymph. As toxins are freed from areas of storage, some degree of acute toxic, or pro-oxidant effect, results. If a chelator is used, the stronger the bond between toxin and chelator the less the acute pro-oxidant effect.

Far infrared sauna therapy also has at least some mild pro-oxidant effects as toxins are excreted and any patient using this therapy should start at lower temperatures for shortened periods of time. Time and temperature in the sauna can then gradually be increased as comfortably tolerated.

The main way to monitor this is simply by how good (or bad) one feels. If you are invigorated after the sauna, you are proceeding in a safe manner. However, if you feel completely wiped out and symptomatic in any manner (headache, muscle ache, malaise in general) you should either scale down the temperature and time or just stop it completely until your immune system strengthens sufficiently over time. As a practical point, younger cancer patients will generally tolerate the sauna better than older cancer patients. But if the sauna is well-tolerated at any age, it should be used regularly.

4) Correct Critical Hormone Deficiencies

Correcting critical hormone deficiencies is always an important goal in any patient. However, in the new cancer patient it is probably best to complete the initial phases of cancer treatment before addressing these deficiencies. This is important since any effective cancer therapy will kill cancer cells, releasing significant amounts of reactive iron and pro-oxidant debris into the blood and lymph, at least early in the course of the therapy.

Sex hormone and thyroid hormone replacement, especially together, will often initiate a phase of fat mobilization with some significant release of cytokines, toxins, and other pro-oxidants. It is best not to subject the immune system of the cancer patient to an avoidable excess of oxidative stress while trying to optimize the chances of a complete recovery.

5) Optimize Antioxidant Levels

The supplementation protocol as described in the treatment of the osteoporosis patient will largely suffice for the cancer patient. It is repeated here for your convenience. Especially important, however, is to give the cancer patient the opportunity to respond to a series of highly-dosed vitamin C infusions after the rest of the protocol has been initiated. The dose size in these IVs should be similar to the dose size of the IVs recommended for the coronary artery disease patient. Specifically, 1.0 to 1.5 grams of vitamin C per kilogram of body weight is a good dose, with anywhere from roughly 25 to 150 grams for body sizes ranging from a small child to a large man. For the especially small and the especially large persons, lower and higher amounts of vitamin C would be appropriate in the infusions.

Unlike the vitamin C IVs for the cardiac patient, however, the vitamin C should generally be infused more slowly in an attempt to bathe the affected cells for a longer period of time with increased vitamin C in the extracellular fluids. The more prolonged presence of increased levels of vitamin C is more desirable than a rapid rise and fall of the levels for the resolution of cancer. If a patient is hospitalized or in the position to receive intravenous infusions continually, a protocol that delivers 250 to 300 gram in a continuous fashion every 24 hours via infusion pump could offer optimal benefit. This is especially applicable for some cancer patients who might not otherwise respond well.

For the cancer patient not demonstrating an adequate response to highly-dosed vitamin C infusions along with rest of the protocol, strong consideration should be

Supplement	Daily Oral Dose	Special Instructions
Vitamin C as sodium ascorbate or ascorbic acid	6,000 to 15,000 mg	Depending upon bowel tolerance, in two to four divided doses throughout the day
Vitamin C in liposome-encapsulated form	1,000 to 2,000 mg	
Vitamin C in a fat-soluble form as ascorbyl palmitate	1,000 to 2,000 mg	Divided into two doses
Lysine	2,500 mg	
Proline	500 mg	
Vitamin D3	5,000 units (Starting Dose!)	Adjust by blood testing to stay as close to a 50 ng/cc blood level as possible over time
Vitamin K2 (menaquinone-4, or menatetrenone)	3 to 6 mg	
Magnesium glycinate	400 mg	Divided into two doses
Omega-3 fish oil (EPA and DHA content)	1 to 2 grams	Divided into two doses
Mixed tocopherols (vitamin E source)	800 IU	Divided into two doses
Beta carotene (vitamin A source)	25,000 to 50,000 IU	
Complete B vitamin complex (as from Life Extension Foundation)	1 to 2 Capsules	Divided into two doses if taking 2 capsules
Specifically AVOID any supplementation with copper, calcium, or iron; iron should only be taken for laboratory-documented iron deficiency anemia		

given to adding other agents to further upregulate the increased intracellular oxidative stress in the cancer cells. This can make the difference in whether the entire cancer cell population can reach the point of apoptosis (cell death) or outright cellular necrosis and rupture. Many different agents have this ability, but only two will be mentioned here:

> **Sulindac:** This is a nonsteroidal anti-inflammatory (NSAID) drug which is known to independently upregulate reactive oxygen species and free radicals inside the cells. It can be taken orally, 150 mg twice daily with food. Sulindac and anything else that can further increase intracellular oxidative stress, can be expected to enhance cancer cell-killing effects.
>
> **Iron:** Never to be given chronically, iron sucrose (100 mg in 5 cc) can be injected slowly over a 5-minute period after the vitamin C infusion has been started. This will transiently increase the levels of reactive iron inside the cancer cells and further allow the vitamin C, via the Fenton reaction to increase oxidative stress to the point of cell death.

Finally, the "mop-up" vitamin C infusion is crucial to the long-term success of highly-dosed vitamin C therapy, as a lack of patient compliance can greatly decrease or even effectively block the ultimate success of vitamin C-centered cancer therapy. It is generally desirable to push the amounts of vitamin C being administered by vein to the point that the patient actually does feel bad. This is a strong indicator that cancer cells are being effectively killed and disrupted, with significant reactive iron and pro-oxidant cellular debris being released into the blood and lymph and causing the symptomatology.

While some patients with a fairly small cancer mass in their bodies can recover without ever feeling poorly during a vitamin C IV, many cancer patients with larger cancer cell masses will feel poorly when enough cancer cells are killed during a treatment session. This is often referred to as a "Herxheimer" or "Herxheimer-like" reaction. This initially referred to the massive kill-off of syphilis spirochete organisms after the first dose of penicillin in a patient with a heavy pathogen load. It has "evolved," however, to typically refer to any patient who feels poorly after an infusion of any agent intended to kill a pathogen or a cancer cell. It has also been used to just refer to a patient who releases a significant amount of stored cellular toxins after a therapeutic infusion, which can occasionally occur in a "normal" patient who receives a large enough dose of vitamin C given relatively quickly.

The "mop-up" vitamin C infusion, then, employs the concept of "low and slow." Even though highly-dosed vitamin C can sometimes result in a flood of pro-oxidant debris in the treatment of the cancer patient, it is, ironically enough, vitamin C that will promptly remedy the situation it just caused.

If a cancer patient is receiving a 100-gram infusion of vitamin C over a 2-hour period and starts feeling poorly just before the IV infusion is complete, temporarily stop the vitamin C infusion and instead just infuse normal saline for 15 minutes. Following this restart the vitamin C infusion, but at only 25% of the rate of the initial infusion. So, if 90 grams was given in about a hour and 45 minutes give the remaining 10 grams of the vitamin C over the next 45 minutes to an hour. With only the rarest of exceptions the patient will be feeling very well by the time the rest of the vitamin C is given. It should be noted how much vitamin C over what period of time precipitated the symptoms. This will allow a slight scaling down of dose and rate for future infusions to maximize patient compliance and long-term positive outcome.

6. Appropriate Prescription Medication Use

For cancer as well as osteoporosis and coronary heart disease the use of a calcium channel blocker drug is always a good idea when medically reasonable. However, this is a drug that is probably best started or used only when a cancer has been successfully resolved. A calcium channel blocker has its effects by inhibiting calcium influx into cells, thereby decreasing the increased oxidative stress that is seen with excessive intracellular calcium.

At least theoretically, a calcium channel blocker could work counter to the treatment goal of increasing intracellular oxidative stress in cancer cells to the point of inducing cell death. And quite possibly a calcium channel blocker would have no discernible effect on how well vitamin C or chemotherapy does its task. Until a study directly addresses this issue, however, it would be best to use these agents when cancer is no longer present and then they can have their established positive effects in preventing future cancer and in reducing all-cause mortality.

Another issue that should be addressed is the ill-grounded fear that vitamin C, along with the other quality antioxidants and nutrient supplements, will decrease the effectiveness of traditional chemotherapy in killing cancer cells. Since many individuals will never feel comfortable completely avoiding the traditional drugs used to treat cancer it is important that they realize that the vitamin C is doing nothing but improving their chances of permanent cancer remission, even cure, as well as long-term improvement in day-to-day health and ultimately, longevity.

The only "interference" that the protocol being presented can have on the effect of standard chemotherapy drugs has to do with the timing of administration or ingestion of the nutrients and the drugs. All chemotherapy drugs that are used to kill cancer cells are pro-oxidant in nature and thereby toxic. When vitamin C and/or other potent antioxidants are circulating in the blood when the chemotherapy is given there will be a neutralization of the toxic drug in direct relation to the amount of vitamin C/antioxidants that are in the blood at that time. However, by taking the chemotherapy first and the vitamin C/antioxidants a few hours later there is no loss of effect of the cancer-killing effects of the chemotherapy. There is, however, a substantial repair of the normal cells that are damaged during each chemotherapy administration, resulting in otherwise "standard" side effects to the chemotherapy being greatly lessened and often eliminated.

CHAPTER 19

Tracking the Progress of a Treatment Protocol

◇◇

How Do You Know If It's Working?

◇◇

As long as the patient is not too old with diseases too advanced when the treatment protocol is initiated, both subjective and objective parameters should demonstrate that the underlying disease is stabilizing and is at least becoming more easily manageable. When the protocol interventions are initiated at a young enough age and when the disease is not overly advanced, these same parameters should very often demonstrate clear reversal of critical aspects of that disease.

This book has demonstrated the profoundly toxic nature of excess calcium and that critical health issues start with its deposition outside the bones. It only follows that any laboratory test that can demonstrate interval change in the calcium content of the body outside of the bones should be of particular utility in monitoring the progress of a patient.

Computed tomography of the coronary arteries produces a computer-generated coronary artery calcium (CAC) score. For both known coronary heart disease and any other chronic degenerative disease this CAC score is a very good way to determine whether the overall protocol of treatment being followed is having a clearly positive effect on the disease process. Quite simply, any detection of coronary artery calcium (CAC score greater than zero) is abnormal.

Follow-up testing, preferably on the same testing machine, will clearly indicate whether underlying disease is progressing rapidly, progressing slowly, showing no change, or actually reversing. And even though it is the calcium content in the coronary arteries that is being measured, the calcium content of these arteries correlates directly with abnormal calcium levels and calcium depositions throughout the body. If or when a detectable CAC score reverts to zero the patient has an excellent indication that disease reversal is taking place and the protocol being followed is optimal or near-optimal.

A zero calcium score, however, does not mean clinical normalcy by itself. It just means the individual being tested is definitely healthier with a zero measured level than with any detectable level of calcium. Other serial testing needs to be performed to properly monitor individuals whose first CAC score is zero.

Specific Tests for Tracking Progress of Atherosclerosis Protocols

Although significant coronary artery disease can develop in the absence of detectable coronary artery calcium it is the exception rather than the rule. As such, cardiac computed tomography with venous contrast injection as well as the much more invasive procedure of coronary angiography can establish the presence of coronary atherosclerotic plaques and narrowings. If availability permits, these additional tests can be used to confirm progress.

If arterial narrowings are detected, even with a CAC score of zero, follow-up cardiac computed tomography visualization of the coronary arteries over time will also give excellent guidance as to the overall clinical progress of the patient. If arterial narrowings lessen in degree or even disappear the protocol is excellent. As with the CAC score, the reversal of atherosclerosis is also about as good an indicator as there is to verify that any coexisting chronic disease process in the body is also improving.

Basically, as the heart goes, so goes the rest of the body. It would truly be extraordinary to see atherosclerosis clearly resolving while any coexisting chronic disease is clearly worsening. What makes a heart artery healthy again literally makes everything else in the body better as well.

Specific Tests for Tracking Progress of Cancer Protocols

In cancer patients an objective improvement in any of a number of tumor marker tests is clear evidence of an effective treatment protocol. Over 20 tumor markers have now been identified and have proven to be useful in a clinical setting. Some examples include:

1. Alpha-fetoprotein, for tracking liver cancer and germ cell tumors.
2. CA15-3 and CA27.29, cancer antigens for tracking breast cancer.
3. CA19-9, cancer antigen for tracking pancreatic, gallbladder, bile duct, and gastric cancer.
4. CEA, carcinoembryonic antigen, for tracking colorectal and breast cancer.
5. CA-125, cancer antigen, and HE4, human epididymal protein, for tracking ovarian cancer.

6. HER2, human epidermal growth factor receptor, for tracking breast, cancer, and esophageal cancer.
7. PSA, prostate-specific antigen, for tracking prostate cancer.
8. CD20, cluster of differentiation, for tracking lymphomas.
9. B2M, beta-2 microglobulin, for tracking multiple myeloma, lymphoma, and chronic lymphocytic leukemia.
10. Beta-hCG, beta-human chorionic gonadotropin, for tracking choriocarcinoma and testicular cancer.

General Chronic Degenerative Disease Protocol and Testing

The basic protocol for the treatment of any chronic degenerative disease is essentially the same as the protocol outlined for osteoporosis. The primary variations from that basic protocol would result when multiple chronic degenerative diseases are present. Certainly, many older individuals have some degree of osteoporosis, coronary heart disease, and even undiagnosed cancers. As a result, when more than one diagnosis is established, some minimal adjustments/additions can be made, as with giving more lysine and proline when coronary artery disease is definitely present. However the six basic principles apply regardless of the underlying disease.

In monitoring patients with any chronic degenerative disease a number of common blood tests can be very useful. These tests are especially helpful in monitoring progress. Are abnormal values normalizing or are normal values becoming abnormal? No single one of these tests should be over-interpreted as to their significance if there is no support from any of the other tests. However when a number of these blood tests collectively normalize or worsen, they are strong indicators that the treatment protocol is working well, fair, poorly, or not at all. Blood tests to follow regularly include the following:

1. CBC and biochemistry panel (especially glucose, uric acid, BUN, creatinine, calcium, phosphorus, albumin, SGPT, alkaline phosphatase, CPK, cholesterol [total, HDL, LDL], triglycerides, hemoglobin, WBC, MCV, and MCHC; also HbA1C
2. Lipoprotein (a)
3. ANA (antinuclear antibody)
4. RF (rheumatoid factor)
5. Ferritin (for tracking overall iron content in the body)
6. Parameters of chronic inflammation:
    a. CRP (C-reactive protein)
    b. Cytokines
    c. Interleukins
    d. Sedimentation rate

Certainly, this list of important laboratory tests is not exhaustive. However it will serve nearly anyone quite well who wants to see clear evidence that body metabolism is functionally normal or at least substantially improving. Improved laboratory tests, lessened clinical symptoms, and documentation of decreased calcium stores in the body together should always be seen in a patient whose osteoporosis and/or other chronic degenerative disease has stabilized or improved.

Recap

Osteoporosis, coronary heart disease, cancer, and all other chronic degenerative diseases have a lot in common. While their optimal treatment protocols vary a bit, they share strong common themes. Generally increased toxicity, lessened antioxidant stores, and deficient sex and/or thyroid hormone levels will cause or aggravate all known medical conditions. The medical condition of one patient will often differ from that of another patient depending upon genetic predispositions. Nevertheless, once any chronic diseases are established the protocols outlined are the best ways to stabilize, reverse, or even resolve them.

CHAPTER 20

"But I really like milk!"

How to Have Some Dairy and Good Health, Too

For the many individuals who cannot conceive of a life without dairy there is a little bit of good news, but only a little. It still involves a significant change in dietary habits, particularly with regard to frequency of dairy ingestion and serving sizes.

Let's start by re-emphasizing a point already made several times: There is no room in a healthy diet for milk as a beverage, including for children. It turns out to be less of a negative for kids and young adults than for the older folks, but that is only because skeletal growth is still utilizing increased amounts of calcium from the diet relative to later years. You do outgrow your need for milk, and it occurs when you stop weaning as an infant. And that's your need for human milk, not cow's milk with its four-fold greater content of calcium.[1] Cows have very large bones, and they need the increased calcium early in development much more than humans.

Except for its use in milk-derived foods, such as cheese and yogurt, there is no place for cow's milk in the diet of a health-seeking individual. The ways to be discussed in which you can minimize calcium intake will also lessen the negative impact of milk should you continue to ingest it as a beverage but they cannot be expected to protect you completely. The calcium content in a limited list of foods is noted in Chapter 12. Remember to look at food labels with a wary eye as you begin your process of minimizing calcium in your diet. Never assume something to be true if it cannot be validated.

Calcium Intake

Calcium intake is minimized when milk and dairy are avoided completely. However they represent comfort foods to very many people and when avoiding them completely is not an option, consider the following approach:

1. Avoid completely any dairy product, especially milk, that has had vitamin D added to it. Depending on where you live, you might have an option of obtaining dairy products derived from raw milk. If you must consume milk, raw milk has significantly less negative impact on your health than the pasteurized, processed milks with added vitamin D.
2. Make your dairy a special treat. Having your favorite cheese or yogurt once every week or two will minimize the negative impact of the extra calcium.
3. Make a deliberate effort to find new non-dairy foods that you might never have eaten before and make them your new snack foods. Any of a wide variety of nuts, seeds, and fresh fruits could be viable options. Ask your health-conscious friends what their favorite snacks are. Go to the Internet and do a little research there as well. You'll be

surprised at the many good tastes that exist outside of dairy.
4. When you do indulge in dairy take an extra 100 to 300 mg of magnesium glycinate beforehand. Magnesium, as noted earlier, is Nature's natural calcium antagonist. Less calcium from your snack is likely to accumulate or enter your cells with larger amounts of bioavailable magnesium available to compete with that calcium.
5. Read all labels. Many products, such as orange juice, can have large amounts of calcium added to them in a presumed attempt to promote good health and make the calcium-spiked products more nutritious.

Calcium Excretion

In addition to doing everything you can to limit calcium intake you can also try to increase the elimination of calcium from your body. While not generally realized, inducing a good sweat on a regular basis can eliminate a substantial amount of calcium from your body over time.[2] In fact individuals with a syndrome of excessive sweating (hyperhidrosis) have significantly lower plasma levels of calcium compared to control subjects.[3] Male endurance athletes, who sweat profoundly, often realize a sharp drop in their calcium blood levels.[4]

One of the best things you can do for your general health is to purchase and use a good far infrared sauna. In addition to sweating out much of your excess calcium you will also eliminate large amounts of a wide variety of toxins that you have taken in over the years, including toxic metals.[5,6] Sweating in a sauna is also probably the least toxic way to detoxify your body, as most chelators and other toxin mobilizers result in greater degrees of toxin redistribution and clinical retoxification.

Further evidence of the health-giving effects of repeated sauna therapy, completely consistent with the documented excretion of a wide variety of toxins, including excess calcium, is seen in the clinical benefits observed in the following studies:

1. Improved vascular health in the setting of coronary risk factors [7]
2. Effective therapy for anorexia nervosa [8]
3. Reduction of cardiac events in patients with congestive heart failure [9]
4. Reduced incidence of the common cold [10]
5. Improvement in pulmonary hypertension during exercise in chronic lung disease patients [11]
6. Effective therapy for chronic fatigue syndrome [12]
7. Effective for chronic pain [13]

Sweating is also a little-known but very reliable way to lower elevated iron levels in your body. Since, in addition to having too much calcium, most adults have an excess of iron contributing to increased oxidative stress, iron elimination is highly desirable. Studies on young athletes clearly show that many readily sweat themselves into a state of iron deficiency anemia. [14,15]

Probably the main downside to the use of a sauna on a regular basis is the overall time investment involved, which will usually average about an hour or so, considering sauna warm-up time and after-sauna showering and dressing. You should also clear this with your healthcare practitioner as some individuals might not tolerate it well and the stress of the heat and loss of fluid could acutely aggravate some of the more delicate underlying conditions. And until you clearly establish how well you tolerate sauna therapy you should have someone available to check on you. Passing out in a sauna is never good for your health.

If you do acquire a sauna and use it on a regular basis over months to years you can actually lower your iron levels to the point of becoming anemic. As such you should periodically monitor your ferritin levels and your complete blood count. When the ferritin level is below a level of 30 ng/cc and an early iron deficiency anemia appears (which is easily diagnosed), a limited course of oral iron therapy can rapidly correct this without raising the overall levels of iron throughout the body. And don't be concerned about reaching the point of being anemic for a while. Chronically elevated levels of iron in the body over the years are of vastly more negative consequence to health than a few weeks to a few months of an iron deficiency anemia.

Aside from any sweat-induced iron deficiency, any other sauna-induced mineral deficiencies are addressed with a balanced diet and the supplementation regimen outlined earlier. However you need not worry that you will sweat out too much calcium. That is simply not a realistic possibility. If you decide to include sauna sweats as a regular part of your calcium excess treatment protocol it is also probably best to add a supplemental source of zinc, such as a zinc glycinate chelate, 30 mg daily, to the rest of the supplements recommended earlier in the treatment protocols.

Recap

The most important points to take away from this final chapter are that you should never take a calcium supplement and you should never drink milk as a beverage – period. If you follow this advice, you will likely enjoy a longer and a significantly healthier life. Even if you cannot break the habits of consuming a large amount of dairy-related products on a regular basis do not feel that there is nothing to gain from just stopping the calcium supplementation and the milk. Furthermore, if you add the treatment protocol suggestions outlined earlier along with no milk or calcium pills you may well mobilize and excrete your excess calcium without having to overly restrict the rest of your dairy intake. Serial coronary artery calcium scores, initially at six-month intervals, will be your best way to know if you need to be more restrictive with your calcium intake over time.

APPENDIX A

More About Calcium Channel Blockers

Small portals are embedded in the membranes of the cells throughout the body. These portals, also called channels, allow the entrance and/or exit of certain substances from the cell. One type of such portals control the entrance of calcium into the cell; these portals are called calcium channels.

Normally the concentration of calcium outside the body's cells is about 10,000 times greater than the concentration inside. So when the calcium channel opens in response to specific stimuli, calcium floods in. In smooth muscle tissues, including those in the heart and coronary arteries, calcium functions as an electrolyte that conducts the electrical impulses that cause muscles to contract or constrict.

Calcium channel blockers comprise a group of drugs designed to prevent or restrict the opening of these calcium channels and therefore limit the influx/uptake of calcium into cells. High blood pressure [hypertension] is often the result of excessive constriction of arterial muscles. By limiting the calcium uptake in these muscles the vessels actually dilate. As a positive consequence the pressure required to pump blood through them is reduced. Initially developed as vasodilators, [1] calcium channel blocker drugs have been found to be exceptionally safe and effective and they have been used as frontline antihypertensive agents for several decades. [2-5]

The side effect profile of these drugs is primarily that of excessively limiting calcium entrance into cells, resulting in low blood pressure [frank hypotension] caused by a state of depleted intracellular calcium. Depending on the type of calcium channel blocker used, an overdose could adversely affect the heart rate (either abnormally high or abnormally low). However, even when calcium channel blockers have been unintentionally overdosed, fatality is very rare and the long-term outlook is good. [6]

Calcium channel blockers have been found to exert a positive effect in treating a host of maladies unrelated to high blood pressure, including cancer, angina pectoris, epilepsy, peripheral neuropathy, Alzheimer's disease, and Parkinson's disease. The effectiveness of these drugs in such divergent illnesses is further solid evidence that excessive intracellular calcium is an integral part of most chronic degenerative diseases.

When calcium channel blockers are used to treat conditions in patients who do not have high blood pressure, it would be expected that a frequent side effect would include low blood pressure if intracellular calcium levels were normal. Notably this is not the case.

This begs two questions:

1) How can non-hypertensive patients take calcium channel blockers for extended periods of time without having to deal with low blood pressure?
2) If the primary function of calcium channel blockers limits cellular uptake of calcium,

how can they exert such a positive effect on so many medical conditions and diseases?

The obvious answer to the first question is: Non-hypertensive patients who respond well to calcium channel blockers must have elevated intracellular calcium levels.

Morbidity (disease) and mortality (death) statistics related to atherosclerosis — a disease that is marked by arterial calcification — provide overwhelming evidence of this reality. In 2008, more than 30% of the deaths in the U.S. were from heart disease and stroke.[7] Many cancers are also characterized by calcifications. To deny the impact of excess calcium on health is to simply deny the existence of a very large body of data that does not lead to any other reasonable conclusion.

The second question requires more discussion. Certainly limiting cellular calcium intake produces a major, if not **the** major, health benefit realized from the use of calcium channel blockers. Increased calcium concentrations in selective intracellular components — the nucleus, mitochondria, and endoplasmic reticulum — and not just the gel-like substance that fills the cell and surrounds the other internal structures [cytoplasm] also signal increased pathology [development of disease] and even imminent cell death.

In an animal model of Parkinson's disease, calcium entry into the mitochondria contained inside the cells increases oxidative stress in those sites, promoting the evolution of that disease.[8] Another component inside the cells, the endoplasmic reticulum, appears to help mediate cancer cell death when their levels of calcium are sufficiently increased.[9] Clearly, everywhere calcium concentrations increase chronically, pathology develops and the chance of cell death escalates.[10]

But, there are apparently other properties that are at work as well. One such property is that calcium channel blockers have also been found to have antioxidant effects.[11-14] This antioxidant property of calcium channel blockers fits well with the observed clinical effects of these drugs, although it is clear that direct antioxidant effects are not the primary effects of this class of drugs.

Calcium channel blockers have also been observed to actually decrease atherosclerotic plaque burden and decrease fibrous plaque content,[15] an outcome that is not clearly due to calcium channel blocking effects. This could represent a clinical setting in which the antioxidant effect of the calcium channel blocker played a more prominent role in the anti-atherosclerosis effect than the calcium channel blocking effect.

In addition to the reduction of oxidative stress resulting from a decrease of intracellular calcium, these drugs seem to posses more direct antioxidant properties. Research shows that they have the ability to directly quench free radicals as well as to suppress their formation.[16-17]

Calcium channel blockers also appear to decrease the increased intracellular oxidative stress seen in cancer cells. Sustained elevations of intracellular calcium ultimately lead to increased cellular proliferation, as seen in cancer cells.[18,19] In studies on cancer cells, effective calcium channel blocker therapy can significantly reduce cancer proliferation and migration[20,21] and sometimes induce programmed cell death.[22] In fact studies looking for the cause of disease have indicated that calcium channel blocker use is inversely related to prostate cancer incidence.[23]

Virtually all chronic degenerative diseases feature increased intracellular oxidative stress and anything that can decrease this stress will nonspecifically promote clinical improvement and ultimately increase survival from all medical conditions.[24]

A significant part of the positive effects of calcium channel blockers on cancer also relates to the fact that some calcium channels appear to facilitate iron uptake by cells.[25] Cancer cells thrive on increased cytoplasmic iron levels and anything that would lessen the size of this iron pool would be detrimental to cancer growth and survival.

Currently the oral calcium channel blockers commonly used for hypertension include the following:

- Benzothiazepines, represented by diltiazem
- Dihydropyridines, represented by amlodipine, felodipine, isradipine, nicardipine, nifedipine, and nisoldipine
- Diphenylalkylamines, represented by verapamil

All of these prescription calcium channel blockers are quite effective for the treatment of hypertension and they are all tolerated very well. It should be noted, however, that the reduction of all-cause mortality due to the administration of dihydropyridine calcium channel blockers was seen with long-acting forms of nifedipine.

The bottom line is that there are actually few prescription drugs as safe as calcium channel blockers when administered in appropriate doses. Not only have the long-acting calcium channel blockers been demonstrated to be effective antihypertensive agents, they also have been demonstrated to reduce the incidence of hypertension-associated cardiac events, such as stroke, heart attack, angina, and heart failure.[26,27] They have also been found to have anti-atherosclerosis effects beyond their blood pressure-lowering effects.[28]

APPENDIX B

A Guide to the Optimal Administration of Vitamin C

The causal relationship between vitamin C deficiency and osteoporosis is clear. And in truth, vitamin C deficiencies have been implicated in the causation and/or worsening of most, if not all, chronic degenerative diseases.

Realizing that an individual with a chronic degenerative disease such as osteoporosis is substantially deficient in vitamin C and the other important components of the general antioxidant matrix in the body is straightforward. However, restoring the levels of vitamin C and other important antioxidants to normal or near-normal levels is not is as simple as one would hope. While popping a vitamin C pill of any size daily will help just about everyone, it falls far short of the goal of reaching the state of optimized health that a normal antioxidant balance will bring in the body.

Many conditions, especially acute infections and acute toxin exposures, can readily be addressed and resolved with an aggressive administration of multigram doses of vitamin C for several days.[1] However, optimizing vitamin C levels in the tissues of the body to minimize the impact and evolution of chronic diseases is a different story. This appendix will endeavor to outline the different ways in which vitamin C can be most effectively administered, along with important suggestions for both reaching and maintaining optimal tissue levels of vitamin C.

Important Factors in the Effective Administration of Vitamin C

1) Dose
2) Route
3) Rate
4) Frequency
5) Duration of treatment period
6) Type of vitamin C
7) Adjunct therapies
8) Safety
9) Quality of overall protocol

1) Dose: The Most Critical Factor for Effective Results

While all of the factors of vitamin C administration to be discussed are important, inadequate dosing is the single most important factor in preventing complete clinical success with the vitamin C treatment. If enough vitamin C is not given to deal with the amount of increased oxidative stress involved with an infection, poisoning, or with an ongoing medical condition, complete clinical success will never be realized. It is also important to emphasize that some success short of an optimal response will always be seen no matter how little vitamin C is given. In sick individuals vitamin C is always in short supply, and any amount will help some. More will help even more. Optimal success will be seen when all

A Guide to the Optimal Administration of Vitamin C

excess oxidative stress has been neutralized and continues to be neutralized as it recurs.

In the treatment of acute infections and acute poisonings optimal dosing is especially critical, since many such conditions can kill or cause long-term secondary organ damage if present in the body long enough before effective treatment. Determining the initial dose requires clinical evaluation. And even more importantly, follow-up clinical evaluation is needed after the initial dose has been given to determine whether future dosing needs to be higher, the same, or even a little lower. It is always optimal to work with a healthcare practitioner familiar with vitamin C to monitor clinical progress and make dosing changes as indicated.

While not an absolute rule, a reasonable guide for selecting the initial dose of vitamin C to be given intravenously would be roughly from 1 to 1.5 grams per kilogram of body weight. Practically speaking this would mean 25 grams for most children old enough to readily tolerate an IV line, 50 to 75 grams for a 100- to 150-pound person, and 75 to 150 grams for a 150- to 250-pound person. Larger children will

GENERAL VITMAMIN C DOSAGE GUIDE

Vitamin C Type	Typical Dose	Maximum Dose	Dose Frequency	Dose Monitoring/ Adjustments
Liposome-Encapsulated	1,000 to 5,000 mg daily	No absolute dosage	Not necessary to divide into multiple doses	Increase until symptomatic improvement no longer seen
Ascorbyl Palmitate (not liposome-encapsulated)	1,000 to 2,000 mg daily	5,000 mg	Best to divide doses throughout day	Increase until no symptomatic improvement no longer seen
Pill or Powder	5 to 15 grams	To bowel tolerance	Best to divide doses throughout day	Bowel tolerance and/or until symptomatic improvement no longer seen

benefit most by starting at 50 grams. Lower doses and higher doses can always be given as deemed clinically appropriate.

When determining long-term vitamin C dosing for general healthcare maintenance as well as chronic disease management, factors of convenience, symptom relief, and laboratory test results play significant roles in selecting both the type(s) and amounts of vitamin C to be taken orally daily. The General Vitamin C Dosage Guide on the previous page provides a basic starting reference.

> **Convenience:** Vitamin C, in pill or powder form is best given several times a day due to its rapid clearance through the kidneys. This is less of a concern with the liposome-encapsulated form of vitamin C, as the intracellular uptake of this form of vitamin C substantially slows its excretion. The optimal dosage of vitamin C is best determined over a few days by how much sodium ascorbate or ascorbic acid it takes to reach bowel tolerance (just before the onset of diarrhea). Most reasonably healthy individuals will end up with a bowel tolerance dose throughout the day between 5 and 15 grams of vitamin C. Some people have much more sensitive bowels and cannot take more than one or two grams. Such individuals should take more of the liposome-encapsulated vitamin C, as bowel tolerance is not an issue with that form of vitamin C. Other individuals have very high bowel tolerances of 20, 30, 40 grams or more of vitamin C and a handful of individuals cannot reliably reach a bowel tolerance level. Generally these individuals have significant toxin levels in their bodies, often secondary to dental infections, such as root canal-treated teeth.

Symptom relief: Very few individuals have completely symptom-free lives. As all symptoms are mediated by increased oxidative stress in some area of the body. At the very least vitamin C can always be expected to lessen a symptom when dosed correctly. Individuals who begin supplementing vitamin C quickly develop a sense for what amount of vitamin C makes them feel the best and this is a good way to help determine long-term dosing. Other individuals who have no discernible symptoms will nevertheless begin to develop an increased "health awareness" the longer they supplement vitamin C. Such individuals often begin to feel better without having realized they were not feeling optimally before. Also they quickly realize when they are having a toxic or infectious challenge, as their sense of wellness becomes slightly impaired. In these instances the vitamin C dose can be increased above maintenance levels for a few days to deal with that challenge and not permit outright sickness to develop.

Laboratory testing: Rarely do all the scores in a broad array of baseline laboratory tests fall within the normal range. As vitamin C is administered over time many abnormal tests will significantly improve or even normalize. An astute healthcare practitioner will be able to determine optimal doses over time through evaluation of routine laboratory testing. Laboratory testing is an especially elegant way to fine-tune vitamin C dosing, as some individuals may still feel well even while certain laboratory test scores are moving the wrong direction.

2) Route: What's the Best Avenue for Vitamin C Administration?

Vitamin C can be given intravenously, intramuscularly, by mouth, per rectum, by misting inhalers, topically on the eyes or in the ears, and both on the skin as well as through it (transdermally). Most commonly it is given orally and intravenously. The success of any vitamin C treatment, however, depends primarily on getting vitamin C molecules in direct contact with the pro-oxidant molecules in the site(s) of increased oxidative stress.

When using vitamin C in the treatment of delicate areas, such as the eyes or the respiratory tract, it is important to always use pH-neutral solutions of vitamin C (sodium ascorbate or properly buffered ascorbic acid). Intramuscular injections, discussed further below, are great for babies and small children. Rectal administrations can also be an option if oral or intravenous routes are not feasible or if a retention enema application is being used, as for a condition such as chronic ulcerative colitis. Conditions such as colitis do not require rectal administration however. Any inflammatory condition of the intestine or colon can also be very effectively treated by oral administration of sodium ascorbate powder in water or juice up to bowel tolerance.

3) Rate: How Fast Should Vitamin C Be Administered?

How fast a dose of vitamin C is given intravenously is a very important factor for maximizing the benefit of vitamin C therapy. Depending on the condition being treated and the effect that is desired, vitamin C can be given in seconds as an IV push or it can be infused rapidly, slowly, or even as a continuous infusion over 24 or more hours.

IV Push: When a patient is in imminent danger of death, such as might be seen after an acute exposure to life-threatening amounts of venom or toxin that are still largely circulating in the bloodstream, multigram doses of vitamin C (sodium ascorbate or well-buffered ascorbic acid) can be admnistered via IV push. The idea is to get as much vitamin C in direct contact with circulating toxins as rapidly as possible. The results can be dramatic. Dr. Klenner described how he treated a cyanotic patient who was acutely poisoned by the bite of a venomous Puss Caterpillar only 10 minutes earlier and complaining of severe chest pain, the inability to take a deep breath, and the feeling that he was dying:

> "Twelve grams of vitamin C was quickly pulled into a 50 c.c. syringe and with a 20 gauge needle was given intravenously as fast as the plunger could be pushed. Even before the injection was completed, he exclaimed, 'Thank God.' The poison had been neutralized that rapidly." [2]

Rapid Infusion: Rapid infusion generally means an infusion rate that is as rapid as a wide-open IV line will permit. Practically speaking, this translates to 500 to 700 cc of vitamin C solution being administered in a time frame between 40 and 60 minutes, typically containing between 50 and 100 grams of vitamin C.

When such an amount of vitamin C is infused this rapidly the pancreas perceives the vitamin C load as a glucose load because glucose and vitamin C molecules are extremely similar chemically. Consequently the pancreas secretes substantial insulin into the blood to deal with what it considers to be an acute excess of glucose. For most individuals the insulin release is significant enough that a pronounced hypoglycemia, sometimes as low as 20 to 25 mg/dL, ensues and is maintained until the IV is completed or some oral or IV forms of glucose are supplied to increase the glucose level. This type of vitamin C infusion, then, can be viewed as an endogenously-induced form of insulin potentiation therapy (IPT).

IPT, involving the deliberate induction of substantial hypoglycemia with insulin injections, has been documented to be a very effective way to increase the cellular uptake of most nutrients and/or medications given at the same time.[3] The endogenously-induced IPT will have the same effect, assuring a much larger uptake of vitamin C into the cells than would otherwise take place when it is infused at a slower rate and no significant release of insulin is stimulated. In cell studies insulin has been documented to stimulate vitamin C accumulation.[4-6] Such studies, along with known effects of IPT, reliably indicate that similar mechanisms are in play for insulin promoting vitamin C uptake in all the metabolically active cells in the body.

Slow Infusion: As noted, rapid infusions can acutely push much more vitamin C inside the cells. However a much greater portion of the vitamin C also ends up being excreted through the kidneys in the process. Many chronic degenerative disease patients, including heart patients and cancer patients, will benefit optimally when their infusion take place over two or more hours. Many such patients will benefit from both rapid and slow infusions during the course of their protocol administration. Vitamin C, like regular antibiotic therapy, can offer more benefit when given several times as a high-concentration, rapidly-infused "loading dose," to be followed over a more extended period of time with repeated slow infusions. This simply allows the underlying disease to be exposed to more vitamin C more of the time, often resulting in dramatic symptom lessening and even disease reversal.

Continuous Infusion: This is a form of administration that should be of great value but has not yet been done with any frequency. Dr. Klenner first made the suggestion with regard to the possible treatment of cancer:

> "This is the reason we believe a dose range of 100 grams to 300 grams daily by continuous intravenous drip for a period of several months might prove surprisingly profitable." [7]

Perhaps the only flaw in Dr. Klenner's assertion is that it would seem unlikely that most cancers would require months to resolve with such an approach. Of course the practical "flaw" is that as of the writing of this book no hospital in the United States will permit any infusion of vitamin C, much less a continuous infusion. Should circumstances ever permit this approach, however, it is likely that an enormous amount of good could be done not only with cancer, but also with any other chronic degenerative disease, including neurological conditions like multiple sclerosis and Alzheimer's disease.

4) Frequency: What's the Optimal Interval Between Vitamin C Administrations?

The appropriate frequency of vitamin C dosing in any of its forms is completely based on the clinical response to the previous administration(s) of vitamin C. When treating an acute infectious disease or an acute intoxication/poisoning, the improvement of vital signs and the reported relief of any associated acute symptomatology dictate how soon and how sizeable the next dose of vitamin C should be. When no significant improvement is seen more vitamin C should be given immediately and generally infused more rapidly. IV push should be reserved for those circumstances when death or coma appear imminent.

If an appropriately-sized dose of vitamin C is administered the first time a positive response should nearly always result, especially if intravenous administration is being utilized. The decision of when and how much the second dose of vitamin C should be will still be dictated by the clinical expertise of the treating healthcare practitioner. An oral vitamin C regimen can also be pushed in a vigorous fashion by a caregiver at home if no healthcare provider is involved. The lowering of elevated temperatures, rapid heart rates, and rapid breathing, along with normalization of elevated or depressed blood pressures and the overall increased comfort level of the patient are the most important parameters to follow in the early stage of treatment. It is also important to give sizeable doses of both regular vitamin C and liposome-encapsulated vitamin C orally regardless of whether the patient is also receiving any intravenous administrations.

5) Duration: How Long Should Vitamin C Administrations Be Continued?

Especially for significant acute infectious diseases, the duration of a vitamin C treatment regimen by whatever route of administration, is important. A patient can and usually does respond very dramatically to a large initial dose of vitamin C. However, even when clinical normalcy appears to have been restored it is very important to give sizeable doses of vitamin C for at least 48 hours after the patient "appears" completely cured. Many infections, especially viral ones, can rebound promptly when vitamin C therapy is not extended for this length of time. Giving a large amount of vitamin C orally, IV, and/or IM every 4 to 6 hours around the clock will reliably resolve an acute infectious syndrome much more rapidly than would be seen with a very large single dose with no follow-up dose for another 24 hours.

6) Type: What's the Best Chemical Form of Vitamin C to Use?

The essence of vitamin C is its ascorbate anion. The associated cations include the following:
- Hydrogen (ascorbic acid)
- Sodium (ascorbate)
- Calcium (ascorbate)
- Magnesium (ascorbate)
- Potassium (ascorbate)
- Manganese (ascorbate)
- Zinc (ascorbate)
- Molybdenum (ascorbate)
- Chromium (ascorbate)

Ascorbic acid: This is really the prototypical form of vitamin C. This is always a desirable form of

Vitamin C Type	Advantages	Disadvantages
Liposome-Encapsulated	• Highest bioavailability • No digestive upset or diarrhea • Slower excretion rate • Best intracellular delivery	• Most expensive
CAUTION: *Inexpensive brands are often just emulsions and not truly liposome-encapsulated.*		
Ascorbic Acid	• Most desirable regular form if no concern of stomach upset • Inexpensive	• Frequent dosing and potential of diarrhea can make less convenient • Most prone to stomach upset
Sodium Ascorbate	• Best tolerated of pill/powder forms if large doses are desired • Sodium content not a concern for those worried about fluid retention or high blood pressure • Inexpensive	• Frequent dosing and potential of diarrhea can make less convenient
Calcium Ascorbate	• Calcium acts as buffer, easier on stomach	• More expensive than other forms
CAUTION: *Added calcium is always undesirable.*		
Magnesium Ascorbate	• Brings magnesium and ascorbate into body	• More expensive than other forms
Potassium Ascorbate	• Brings potassium into the body	• More expensive than other forms • Limited to small doses • Requires a measure of regular monitoring
CAUTION: *Potassium can be toxic — too much can be fatal.*		
Other Forms of Ascorbate	• Brings other trace elements into the body	• More expensive than other common forms • Limited to small doses
CAUTION: *Not recommended. Potential of toxicity, especially with manganese, molybdenum, zinc, and chromium forms.*		
Ascorbyl Palmitate	• Fat-soluable, so it provides extra protection for fat-rich tissues • Less potential for digestive upset	• More expensive than other forms

vitamin C to take when there is no concern with stomach upset due to excess acid effect, or no concern of excess acidity causing pain at the catheter site when given intravenously.

Sodium ascorbate: This is probably the optimal form of regular vitamin C that has not been encapsulated with liposomes. This is because very large amounts can be given up to the point of inducing a diarrhea-like, vitamin C-flush effect when what is known as bowel tolerance is reached. If exceeding the bowel tolerance level is well-tolerated this is also a very desirable effect as it neutralizes and eliminates a large amount of gut-generated toxins before they get absorbed. The amount of sodium ascorbate needed to exceed the bowel tolerance point can also be useful as a rough guide to the degree of infection or toxicity that is present in the patient. Generally the greater the infectious and/or toxic challenge the more vitamin C gets absorbed from the gut and the less of it reaches the colon, with the bowel tolerance point not being reached as readily. [8,9]

It should also be noted that large amounts of sodium ascorbate can be taken by most individuals, including those with high blood pressure and heart disease, without causing fluid retention or an increase in blood pressure. This is because it is sodium chloride, not sodium associated with another anion like ascorbate, citrate, or bicarbonate, that reliably causes fluid retention and aggravates high blood pressure in individuals sensitive to volume overload. The term "sodium-dependent" hypertension should forever be replaced with the term "sodium chloride-dependent" or "table salt-dependent" hypertension.[10,11] In any event, large doses of sodium ascorbate should not be avoided for fear of provoking elevated blood pressure.

Calcium ascorbate: This form is typically marketed as Ester C or buffered vitamin C. This form just adds another unnecessary source of calcium to the supplementing individual. While it is true that it is easy on the stomach, sodium ascorbate is tolerated just as easily and does not aggravate the preexisting state of calcium excess already present in most older individuals.

Magnesium ascorbate: This is an excellent form of vitamin C since it brings both magnesium and ascorbate into the body. The only practical limit to dosage with this form of vitamin C would be the amount that starts to approach bowel tolerance and that results in diarrhea. Probably the main reason against supplementing magnesium ascorbate on a regular basis is that it adds significant cost to what are two exceptionally inexpensive supplements when taken separately.

Potassium ascorbate: This is also a good form of ascorbate for supplementation. The only problem is that it is relatively easy to overdose on potassium, which can cause fatal cardiac arrhythmias, especially if it is taken with the same abandon as so many other completely nontoxic supplements. Potassium should never really be taken on a regular basis unless advised or prescribed by a healthcare practitioner who has done appropriate clinical and laboratory testing beforehand. For people who are in need of potassium supplementation this can be a excellent supplement. It just needs some measure of regular monitoring.

The other forms of ascorbate: These are forms other than the specific forms mentioned above. They are not really good forms of vitamin C to ingest in large amounts on a regular basis. While ascorbate has no real toxicity concerns, most of the mineral ascorbates, especially manganese, molybdenum, zinc, and chromium, can very easily be overdone. Also, as mentioned above they are needlessly expensive and do not end up providing the amounts of vitamin C that most individuals should be taking on a regular basis. Better to take a quality supplement with a wide range of minerals along with multigram amounts of sodium ascorbate separately.

Ascorbyl Palmitate: Unlike all the other ascorbate forms listed above, this is a form of vitamin C that is fat-soluble. Including at least a gram or two of ascorbyl palmitate in a daily supplementation regimen can provide important additional antioxidant coverage in fat-rich tissues and areas not otherwise well-protected by the more common forms of vitamin C.[12-14] Ascorbyl palmitate has been demonstrated to protect the cell membrane of intact red blood cells[15] as well as to protect important anti-atherosclerotic lipoproteins in the body.[16] It has also been employed as an antioxidant to prevent skin aging.[17] Liposome delivery systems containing ascorbyl palmitate have been demonstrated to kill cancer cells *in vitro* as well as to slow tumor growth in mice more effectively than with free ascorbic acid.[18] All of these studies indicate the importance of including ascorbyl palmitate as part of an optimally effective vitamin C-centered protocol.

"Vitamin C Complex": There is also a vitamin C supplement being marketed as "Vitamin C Complex," with the basic assertion that vitamin C must be present in a "food form" with multiple associated substances, such as antioxidant bioflavonoids like rutin and quercetin, to be of any benefit. Many of the sellers of a product like this even make the incredibly outlandish assertion that pure vitamin C, as ascorbic acid or sodium ascorbate, is not of much benefit and will not even reverse scurvy by itself. In a nutshell, this is all marketing hyperbole by companies trying to carve out a piece of the vitamin C sales pie.

Just as has been asserted several times in this book, vitamin C does function optimally with as large a network of other antioxidants as can be assimilated. However it is completely wrong and frankly ridiculous to assert that it will not reverse scurvy by itself or that it is of very limited utility by itself. All the work of vitamin C pioneer, Frederick Klenner, M.D., with infectious diseases and toxins demonstrated unequivocally the incredible and typically curative value of vitamin C utilized by itself in high doses in these conditions. [19]

Just as crazy, some sellers of this product claim ascorbic acid is not vitamin C, which is as crazy as a statement can be. Presumably this assertion is made in order to convince vitamin consumers that their product is the only one that can deliver the many benefits of vitamin C ingestion. Not surprisingly this form of vitamin C supplementation is substantially more expensive that regular supplemental forms of vitamin C. Although this is a product that will certainly provide benefits more benefit is available for less money spent on just ascorbic acid or sodium ascorbate. Buyer beware!

7) Adjunct Therapies: Will Vitamin C Administration Compete with Other Treatments?

Unless another therapy is inherently pro-oxidant or toxic in nature, vitamin C will only add to the desired effects. For example, if an individual is receiving chemotherapy for cancer the vitamin C can neutralize the chemotherapy drug itself if both are circulating in the blood at the same time. The chemotherapy is a toxic, electron-seeking agent, and the vitamin C is an antioxidant, electron-donating agent. When any chemotherapy agent has received the electrons it is seeking it ceases to be toxic and can no longer kill or help to kill a cancer cell.

However this effect is easily avoided by staggering the dosing of any inherently toxic drug and any administered vitamin C by a few hours or so. It should also be noted that when vitamin C is given after a cancer chemotherapy agent it helps both to kill the cancer cell even more effectively while also repairing the damage that was done to normal cells by the chemotherapy. When the vitamin C is given before such chemotherapy a greater cancer-killing effect is also seen and many normal cells that would have been damaged are protected by the greater concentration of vitamin C present.

It is also important to note that vitamin C does not interfere with the antimicrobial effects of antibiotics. Quite the contrary, vitamin C enhances the effects of many antibiotics and one should never avoid indicated antibiotic therapy if there is the possibility to take it along with the vitamin C. Vitamin C has many different supportive effects on the immune system[20] including increasing the degree of antibody response to a pathogen. Even though vitamin C can often do the job on a bacterial infection by itself here is no reason to avoid its synergistic effect with an appropriate antibiotic in resolving the infection.

8) Safety: How Safe is Vitamin C?

An important factor in the administration of any therapy to treat a medical condition is how safe it is. Many traditional medical therapies can often have a desired clinical effect, but they can also have a significant side effect or toxicity much of the time. "First, do no harm" continues to be the appropriate standard by which any therapeutic intervention is measured regardless of how effective it might be some of the time.

Except in patients with significant chronic renal insufficiency or chronic renal failure, vitamin C has no definable toxicity. Of course nearly all drugs have to be administered with caution in patients with kidney failure, and vitamin C is no exception. It should also be noted that many patients with deteriorating kidney function can benefit greatly from well-monitored vitamin C therapy. This is because inflammation, which is only another way of describing increased oxidative stress, is at the root of evolving kidney failure.

Outside of the context of poor kidney function vitamin C is enormously safe given in the highest of doses over extended periods of time in even the sickest of patients.[21] Also, vitamin C has no relation to the development of kidney stones in spite of the continued efforts by the scientific media to convince doctors and the public otherwise. In fact vitamin C reliably **decreases** the chances of kidney stones and the persons with the highest blood levels of vitamin C have the lowest incidence of kidney stone disease.

One very rare side effect of vitamin C can occur in patients with G6PD deficiency, an X-linked recessive hereditary disease. G6PD (glucose-6-phosphate dehydrogenase) is an enzyme that is especially important in red blood cell metabolism. When is it severely deficient in the red blood cells, a hemolysis (rupture) of many of the red blood cells can be provoked by any of a number of agents, anemia being the result of an acute development.

The blood test measuring G6PD is readily available and it is appropriate to obtain this test before initiating vitamin C therapy if possible. However even when this deficiency is present it is still unlikely that the vitamin C will provoke any red blood cell hemolysis.

If a test is positive and the need for vitamin C is urgent treatment should proceed, but with closer clinical monitoring, slower infusion, lower doses, and a slower increasing of the vitamin C dose over time. It should also be noted that the initial doses of vitamin C will decrease the susceptibility of the red blood cells to subsequent hemolysis as well, since vitamin C helps to bolster intracellular glutathione levels, which strongly protects them from hemolysis.

When time permits, the administration of other agents that increase intracellular glutathione levels inside the red blood cells (N-acetyl cysteine, whey protein, liposome-encapsulated glutathione) can also stabilize the red blood cells and increase their resistance to hemolysis before the initiation of vitamin C therapy.

9) Overall Protocol of Administration

This factor is much more important in the treatment of chronic degenerative diseases than when treating acute infectious diseases or acute toxin exposures. Toxins and infections will generally respond favorably and rapidly to the aggressive administration of vitamin C as discussed above. However, how effective it is with a chronic condition depends on how effectively several other factors that use up the antioxidant capacity of the body are addressed. Discussed at greater length in Chapters 16, 17, and 18, these factors are:

- How effectively new toxins are being avoided.
- How completely chronic infections and occult acute infections have been eradicated.
- How effectively old toxins have been eliminated and how effectively they are continuing to be eliminated in the most minimally toxic manner possible.
- Whether deficient levels of critical regulatory hormones (testosterone, estrogen, and thyroid) have been restored to normal.
- Whether appropriate prescription medications have been utilized.

Multi-C Protocol

As the ultimate goal of an optimally effective vitamin C protocol is to get as much of the active (reduced) vitamin C into as many areas of the body in the highest concentrations possible, the Multi-C Protocol utilizes multiple forms of vitamin C for supplementation. The basic outline of this protocol is as follows:

1) One to five grams of liposome-encapsulated vitamin C taken orally daily.
2) Multigram doses of sodium ascorbate powder taken orally several times daily in juice or water up to or reaching bowel tolerance (the induction of watery diarrhea).
3) One to three grams daily of ascorbyl palmitate orally daily.
4) 25 to 150 grams of vitamin C intravenously up to several times weekly and occasionally daily depending on the condition and the need to get vitamin C blood levels at very high levels for longer periods of time.

The reasoning behind the Multi-C Protocol is as follows:

1) Liposome-Encapsulated Vitamin C

Liposomes utilize a very unique biodelivery system, achieving an intracellular delivery of a substantial percentage of their payload [22,23] without the expenditure of energy in the process. When that payload is vitamin C the result is cells containing more vitamin C leading to decreased intracellular oxidative stress without an accompanying depletion of the energy resources in the body in order to achieve that goal.

All other forms of regular unencapsulated vitamin C, administered either orally or intravenously, need to consume energy for cells to end up with an increased content of active reduced vitamin C. While oxidized vitamin C circulating in the blood can be taken into cells passively without the immediate consumption of energy, energy must still be spent inside the cells to reduce it back to its active antioxidant state. [24,25]

When choosing a liposome-encapsulated vitamin C...

An additional practical point is that it is very important to take a supplement with a high concentration of liposomes of an appropriately tiny size. Although advertised otherwise, many commercial formulations, as well as homemade formulations, are emulsions only and have zero liposome content.

An emulsion can contain two or more substances that do not normally go into solution, like fat and water, in what can be characterized as a smooth watery suspension containing small fat globules. However, these globules are as much larger than liposomes as a house is larger than a grain of sand. There are none of the unique intracellular biodelivery characteristics of incredibly tiny liposomes shared by large globules of fat. And these globules do not contain vitamin C, anyway.

An emulsified supplement containing vitamin C and lecithin-derived phosphatidylcholine can certainly provide some clinical benefit since both substances are individually quality supplements. Phosphatidylcholine has been demonstrated to have multiple positive effects. [27-31] However, an emulsion does not have the ability to put anything directly inside cells without the consumption of energy like liposomes of the appropriately tiny size.

Once again, buyer beware, as multiple manufacturers are trying to jump on the liposome bandwagon without going through the substantial expense and care involved in producing a consistently high-quality product. The benefits of vitamin C properly encapsulated in liposomes are literally exponentially better that the same amount of vitamin C delivered orally in an emulsion just containing phosphatidylcholine.

Reduced (unoxidized) vitamin C circulating in the blood, however, requires an active transport mechanism to get inside the cell, which means that energy must be consumed for the transport system to work.[26] Therefore, even when regular vitamin C is delivered straight into the blood, significant energy consumption must take place to increase the levels of active vitamin C inside the cells.

Liposome-encapsulated vitamin C, even though taken orally, does not deplete any of the energy stores in the body to deliver its payload inside the cells.

In addition to their energy-sparing system of delivery, liposomes have an exceptionally rapid and enhanced form of absorption in the gastrointestinal tract. Unlike regular forms of vitamin C, nearly all of the liposome-encapsulated vitamin C is absorbed.[27]

The payload encapsulation by lipids also prevents potential stomach upset by the liposome contents (in this case, vitamin C). It also prevents any premature breakdown or degradation of the liposome contents that might otherwise occur from enzyme and/or stomach acid exposure.

In the case of liposome-encapsulated vitamin C, there is no issue of bowel tolerance and diarrhea as is seen with regular forms of vitamin C, although a very large dose of liposomes could potentially result in oily, greasy stools in a few individuals.

For all these reasons the unique intracellular delivery of vitamin C encapsulated in liposomes makes it an essential part of any protocol that strives to optimize support of intracellular vitamin C and antioxidant levels.

2) Sodium Ascorbate Powder

The consumption of vitamin C on a regular (optimally daily) basis as sodium ascorbate powder facilitates the direct neutralization of toxins that are formed by the incomplete digestion, or putrefaction, of different foods. When the doses are pushed high enough and bowel tolerance is reached, further intake results in a watery diarrhea. This watery diarrhea, also known as a C-flush, further ensures that a substantial amount of toxins are directly eliminated without the need for neutralization. Inducing a C-flush at least once weekly is a great idea for general health support, as it allows for toxins to be eliminated, toxins to be neutralized and it helps keep the bowels regular even when the amounts of vitamin C being ingested are not up to bowel tolerance levels. If desired, inducing a C-flush even more frequently is fine.

Anything that induces bowel movements at least once a day, and preferably twice a day, will definitely promote good health. When ingested foodstuffs stay in the gut for more than 24 hours, significant putrefaction and anaerobic bacterial toxin formation will always result. Because of this, any degree of constipation is a substantial additional challenge to maintaining a healthy level of vitamin C and other antioxidants in the body, as many of the most potent toxins generated in a sluggish gut are equal in toxicity to those seen in chronic dental infections, like root canals and other chronically (or acutely) infected teeth.

The regular ingestion of sodium ascorbate also assures a regular uptake of vitamin C into the extracellular fluids and spaces of the body. Just as the liposome-encapsulated vitamin C targets the intracellular spaces the vitamin C powder continually supplies the extracellular areas while providing all of its other benefits in producing a healthy gut. Of course some of the extracellular vitamin C also eventually makes its way inside the cells as well, just not with the efficiency of oral liposome-encapsulated vitamin C.

3) Ascorbyl Palmitate

As discussed in greater detail above, ascorbyl palmitate is a unique form of vitamin C that is fat-soluble rather than water-soluble. As such, this allows the antioxidant effects of vitamin C to reach areas normally not as readily accessible to regular water-soluble vitamin C.

4) Intravenous Vitamin C (IVC)

IVC allows the administration of vastly higher doses of vitamin C than can be given by any other route. It results in very high concentrations in the blood and extracellular fluids. It also eventually increases intracellular vitamin C levels as well, even though energy consumption is required to achieve this (see above). Although all forms of vitamin C have been documented to have potent antitoxic and antimicrobial properties, a very large body of scientific evidence collected since the early 1940's has shown that properly dosed and administered IVC can result in a degree of toxin (poison) neutralization and infection resolution that simply has not been rivaled by any other agent. [32]

It is also important to emphasize that vitamin C need not be used instead of other traditional agents for combating toxins and infections, as it works well along with any other traditional measures used for these conditions. However, the evidence does clearly show that vitamin C works better as a monotherapy than any other single agent that modern medicine has to offer.

Another parenteral (non-oral) application of vitamin C that is little used today but that can be highly effective in certain situations is the intramuscular route. Frederick Klenner, MD, who singularly pioneered the field of the effective clinical applications of vitamin C, would often use intramuscular injections in young patients who were not optimal candidates for taking anything intravenously or for ingesting sufficient quantities of anything orally. Regarding the intramuscular injection of vitamin C, Dr. Klenner had the following to say:

> "In small patients, where veins are at a premium, ascorbic acid can easily be given intramuscularly in amounts up to two grams at one site. Several areas can be used with each dose given. Ice held to the gluteal muscles until red, almost eliminates the pain. We always reapply the ice for a few minutes after the injection. Ascorbic acid is also given, by mouth, as followup treatment. Every emergency room should be stocked with vitamin C ampoules of sufficient strength so that time will never be counted — as a factor in saving a life. The 4 gram, 20 c.c. ampoule and 10 gram 50 c.c. ampoule must be made available to the physician." [33]

It should also be noted that the typical injection used by Dr. Klenner was sodium ascorbate or ascorbic acid buffered with sodium bicarbonate, not just straight ascorbic acid. Additionally, great care needs to be taken to ensure that the entire injection is intramuscular, with none of it in the loose subcutaneous tissue. Whether by misguided intramuscular injection or by an infiltrated intravenous infusion of vitamin C, subcutaneous placement of any amount of vitamin C is enormously painful, often for up to an hour or so before resolving. While no damage is done by a subcutaneous infiltration, the pain is significant enough that the patient might not be so willing to permit future vitamin C infusions or injections.

A suggested formula for intramuscular injections would be:
- 2 cc of vitamin C (500 mg/cc)
- 1 cc of sterile water,
- 0.5 cc of 8.4% sodium bicarbonate
- 1 cc of 2% procaine

(Formula courtesy of Jason West, DC, NMD)

This makes a total volume of 4.5 cc, half injected into each buttock.

While Dr. Klenner gave 2 grams rather than 1 gram at each injection site, this protocol eliminates any significant pain resulting from these injections.

Practical IVC Considerations

In addition to how quickly vitamin C should be infused and how much should be given at a time, as discussed above, it is very important that the patient is completely comfortable and free of discomfort or pain in the process. Significant pain during the infusion of vitamin C, or anything else for that matter, will reliably lead to phlebitis, or inflammation of the vein, if not promptly addressed at the time of the infusion. No matter how good a vitamin C-centered protocol might be it will do no little or no good if the patient becomes severely noncompliant in returning for continued IV infusions. Since it is clear that most patients will get their best clinical results with optimally-dosed vitamin C versus other traditional therapies, it is important not to let the patient get to the point of refusing further IVC treatment.

It should first be emphasized that most patients have no problem with vitamin C infusions, tolerating them without any symptomatology of any kind. However, when significant discomfort appears during an IV infusion, the following factors should all be considered in making the infusion as comfortable as possible:

1) **Size of intravenous cannula, or infusion catheter.** A larger cannula inside a smaller vein can cause discomfort.
2) **Placement of cannula**. Even though a cannula might be completely inside the vein,

demonstrating venous backflow when tested, pain can ensue when the angle of the cannula abuts directly against the side of the vein or when a venous valve is at the tip of the cannula. Oftentimes nothing will stop the pain except cannula removal with reinsertion at another site in the vein, with greater care to insert the cannula in as coaxial an alignment as possible.

3) **Size of the vein.** While some individuals can tolerate IV infusions in the tiniest of veins, many cannot. The largest vein available should always be chosen except when it is already known that smaller, more distal veins tolerate the infusion well, as in a larger man with substantially-sized veins on the back of the hand. If the patient is a smaller woman, or even a child, consideration should be given to having a central line placed if there appears to be no other way to get the amount of vitamin C infused at the rate desired and repeated infusions are clearly warranted for the condition.

4) **Rate of flow.** Many individuals tolerate a slower infusion perfectly well, while always noticing increasing discomfort the more rapid the infusion becomes. If this sensitivity is severe, consideration should again be given to the placement of a central line if deemed appropriate. Some patients will complain of discomfort and get relief when the infusion rate is slowed and then later not feel any discomfort when the infusion rate is once again increased. Whatever the physiological reason is, it appears that the vein can show increased tolerance the longer it is exposed to the vitamin C infusion. Minimal discomfort can often be alleviated with cold (or even hot!) compresses gently applied and held over the infusion site.

5) **Concentration.** When a large enough vein cannot be found for infusion without significant discomfort a more dilute infusion of vitamin C is usually warranted.

6) **Temperature of the infusion solution.** Making sure the infusion solution is close to body temperature during the administration period can prevent a substantial amount of discomfort from ever developing in the first place. Many offices are quite cold and the IV solutions often tend to be room temperature, or less. One or more refrigerated vitamin C vials should be pre-warmed in a room temperature bag. To minimize any degradation (oxidation) of the vitamin C place the IV bag in hot water for 10 to 15 minutes before adding the vitamin C. The vitamin C vial can similarly be warmed immediately before being added to the IV bag.

7) **Presence of other solutes.** Generally, it is best to infuse vitamin C and nothing else. While other agents can be added, it is important not to blame the vitamin C for discomfort in the IV when something else is at fault.

8) **pH of the infusion.** The more acidic an infusion is the more likely it will hurt. A pH of 7.0 to 7.4 is ideal, and it is characteristically reached when sodium ascorbate powder is put into solution in sterile water. When ascorbic acid is used it must be buffered with sodium bicarbonate. Vials of ascorbic acid buffered with sodium bicarbonate are available but they are generally buffered only to be somewhere in the range of pH 5.5 to 7.0. For the exceptionally sensitive patient, pH test paper should be utilized to make sure pH is in the optimal range and more sodium bicarbonate should be added

to the infusion if necessary to get into that range.

9) **Nature of carrier solution.** Generally it is best to infuse vitamin C mixed in sterile water. While D5W, normal saline, or lactated Ringer's solution can be used, it is best to stick with vitamin C in sterile water, buffered as close to a pH of 7.0 to 7.4 as possible. D5W should really never be used, since it puts more glucose into the blood at the same time as the vitamin C and it prevents the maximal amount of vitamin C from getting into the cells, since glucose and vitamin C use the same mechanism for entering the cells.

10) **Presence of persistent or severe pain.** Any extravasation, or leakage, of vitamin C outside of the vein and into the subcutaneous tissue is severely painful, usually persisting for an hour or more before dissipation is complete. Sometimes the cannula can move back out of the vein transiently and a little leakage will take place. When the cannula comes completely out of the vein it will be obvious to the experienced practitioner.

11) **Vitamin C-induced hypoglycemia.** Rarely, some individuals are so sensitive to the infusion of multigram amounts of vitamin C that they will demonstrate some hypoglycemia secondary to increased insulin release from the pancreas at infusion rates well below what most other patients tolerate easily. When any unexplained agitation, sweating, minimal disorientation, or increase in blood pressure occurs, be prepared to give some fruit juice orally or some glucose intravenously. Also, while very rare, an occasional individual, typically cachetic and poorly nourished in general, can have a delayed

hypoglycemia reaction hours later at home. All patients should be encouraged to promptly eat after an infusion session is complete.

12) **Allergy-like reactions**. Technically the ascorbate anion should never cause an allergic reaction in anyone as it is a natural antioxidant molecule vital to health, as well as a substance that can be used to *treat* an allergic reaction. Nevertheless individuals may sometimes (rarely) demonstrate a rash and feel poorly. When this occurs shortly after the IV is started an allergy-like reaction is likely and the IV should be stopped. Consideration should then be given to obtaining vitamin C from a different source. Corn is commonly a source, but beet and casaba are also sources. When the reaction occurs late in the IV or shortly after its conclusion a detoxification from the cells is more likely. This type of reaction and how to deal with it is addressed below in the "Mop-Up Vitamin C" section. If different types of vitamin C, mixed in different carrier solutions, continue to produce the same effect, premedication with an injection of 100 to 250 mg of hydrocortisone will usually blunt or prevent the reaction. This is a one-time dose and further steroids should not be given following the infusion.

13) **No local anesthetics**. While used by some practitioners, I am not in favor of giving any types of anesthetic agents that would prevent the perception of pain in the vein. If pain is reported by the patient and pain relief through anesthesia is obtained, the pain-causing inflammation in the vein can still result in enough of a reaction that vein thrombosis and subsequent sclerosis can occur. Relieving infusion pain with anesthesia is not a good idea for the long-term health of the veins. However,

this does not refer to the use of a small amount of lidocaine in the subcutaneous tissue to lessen or block the pain of the initial needle stick for placement of the intravenous cannula if felt indicated.

Mop-Up IVC

Many individuals, especially sicker ones with acute and chronic infections as well as substantial toxin accumulations in their bodies, will feel anywhere from minimally to substantially ill late during an infusion of vitamin C or directly following it. These exacerbations of illness have been called Herxheimer, or Herxheimer-like reactions. The first described Herxheimer reaction occurred when syphilis patients with a high pathogen load took their first injection of penicillin. The kill-off of the pathogens was so extensive that massive amounts of pro-oxidant dead pathogen-related debris was released into the blood as a result. The clinical result was a much sicker patient, at least in the short term, while the body processed and eliminated the toxic debris. Following an infusion of vitamin C these Herxheimer-like reactions can occur because of one or more of the following reasons:

1) **Whenever an acute or chronic infection responds dramatically enough to the antimicrobial effect of vitamin C.** This results in the release of toxic pathogen-related debris into the blood and lymphatics similar to the syphilis example above.
2) **Whenever a legitimate detoxification occurs.** When some individuals with longstanding and substantial accumulations of toxins inside the cells receive a high enough dose of vitamin C quickly enough, toxins are then mobilized out of the cells and flood the blood and lymphatics.

Generally, this occurs only when toxin levels are so high that many of the natural enzymatic chelators and toxin mobilizers are themselves in an oxidized and relatively nonfunctional state. The massive administration then causes a big intracellular rise in vitamin C, the enzymes are repaired by reduction (electron donation) from the vitamin C, and the toxins are released in large quantities. It is very important to realize that detoxification is also retoxification, and many newly mobilized toxins are just as free to be redeposited anew somewhere else in the body as to be excreted via the urine or feces. Detoxification should never be deliberately done vigorously without the ability to sufficiently promote neutralization and excretion of those toxins after they are released from the cells.

3) **Whenever a substantial quantity of cancer cells are rapidly killed via necrosis**: When dosed and administered correctly, many different cancers will begin to resolve, often to the point of complete resolution. When a patient has a relatively large physical mass of cancer cells in their body this type of reaction is more likely to occur than when the collective cancer mass is small. This reaction can be very dramatic in some patients and several days may be needed for the patient to properly process and excrete the pro-oxidant debris. Of note as well, both cancer cells and most infectious agents have very large concentrations of reactive iron inside and the rupture of cancer cells and pathogens via vitamin C-fed mechanisms can quite abruptly release large amounts of reactive iron into the blood and lymphatics. Iron is highly toxic (pro-oxidant)

when concentrated in its unbound, reactive form.

The Mop-Up vitamin C infusion, at first, might seem paradoxical. That is to say, the very same agent (vitamin C) that caused the flood of pro-oxidant debris into the blood and lymphatics is also the very same agent best suited to deal with that. The trick is in the amount of vitamin C infused and the rate at which it is infused.

All three of the types of pro-oxidant reactions noted above share one thing in common. Namely they needed large amounts of vitamin C given quickly to become manifest. However, at the termination of such an infusion a "Low & Slow" follow-up infusion of vitamin C at 25% or less of the initial amount given, infused over two hours or more, will readily "mop-up" much or all of the pro-oxidant debris released by the larger rapid infusion.

The mop-up infusion does not significantly worsen the pro-oxidant release because of its low concentration and slow rate of infusion. However, it does very effectively neutralize the toxins already released while they are circulating in the blood and lymphatics. While the figures are not precise, this would mean that someone who was feeling well at the outset of a 50 gram infusion of vitamin C but began feeling poorly after the completion of the infusion in about one hour, should then receive about 12.5 grams of vitamin C infused over another two hours.

While most pro-oxidant debris release scenarios occur when stimulated, as with a vitamin C infusion it's also important to appreciate what is going on in a patient with an extended, chronic detoxification process. For example, when an older patient has an exceptionally large amount of stored toxins in the body the stage is set for a chronic release of toxins when enough other things occur. The relatively abrupt initiation of a quality supplement regimen, especially when accompanied or preceded by a removal of ongoing sources of toxin exposure, as from dental infections like root canals, can result in enough of a reactivation of natural detoxification enzymes inside the cells that a chronic detoxification results. As such, the patient can begin to feel poorly a greater percentage of the time the less the antioxidant capacity of the body is supported.

Just as with the acute pro-oxidant debris release scenario, the chronic one is readily dealt with by the same "Low & Slow" vitamin C infusions, with a good clinical response typically realized. However, many chronic detoxifications can take months or sometimes years before the individual truly feels well, so experimentation must take place with finding the best amounts of vitamin C to take orally that will neutralize the pro-oxidant products of detoxification without significantly further stimulating their release from the cells.

Another especially important consideration about the Mop-Up vitamin C infusion is that is allows the healthcare practitioners to push vitamin C doses higher than might have been possible otherwise. As long as a patient feels good by the time they leave the office they will generally come back for more treatment, even if they were a bit symptomatic toward the end of the initial infusion. Mop-Up vitamin C, then, is a tool that allows a large group of patients that could otherwise only tolerate substantially lower doses of vitamin C to push their doses into a range that will produce even more positive clinical outcomes that were not otherwise attainable.

Recap

All infections, all toxin exposures, and all chronic degenerative diseases will benefit some and often greatly from properly dosed and administered vitamin C. The different forms of vitamin C and the various ways to give it offer a wide range of treatment possibilities, capable of being appropriately individualized for optimal clinical response. The new concept of Mop-Up vitamin C now allows the vitamin C practitioner to push the therapeutic envelope to previously unattainable levels. Utilized properly, vitamin C-centered protocols have already gone and will continue to go where no protocols have gone before.

APPENDIX C

The Cause of All Disease: A Unified Theory

Overview

As mentioned at the end of the Introduction, osteoporosis is really a chronic focal scurvy, or severe vitamin C deficiency, of the bones. And even though this book is primarily concerned with osteoporosis and the negative health consequences of excessive calcium ingestion, the explanation of what causes osteoporosis falls quite nicely under a more general explanation of what causes all disease. Understanding these common denominators to all diseases allows for the reasoned, optimal choice of treatment for any given patient.

The clinical goal for all diseases is the same: Lessened oxidative stress in a given organ or target tissue. Clinically speaking all diseases will respond very positively to the practical suggestions offered in Chapters 16 through 18 unless secondary organ and/or tissue damage has advanced beyond the point of allowing a reasonable measure of reversal. Minor protocol modifications are usually necessary in the treatment of different diseases, however. An optimal protocol for one disease may differ slightly from the protocol for another disease in how the clinical goal is achieved. For example, the specific strategy for lessening the increased oxidative stress in the coronary arteries of heart disease patients will never be exactly the same as the method used to decrease the increased oxidative stress in different types of cancer or in other chronic degenerative diseases such as osteoporosis. Nevertheless, clinical improvements in all diseases can always be anticipated when a given patient is able to:

1) Lessen new toxin exposure,
2) Eliminate old stored toxins,
3) Normalize critical regulatory, "master" hormones (testosterone, estrogen, thyroid, and cortisol), and
4) Optimize antioxidant levels throughout the body.

An accurate model that can explain the nature of life, disease, and ultimately death can go a long way toward finding the most appropriate treatments available to deal with a given disease or medical condition.

The best model will consistently predict the best therapies and the best ways to maintain whatever clinical improvements are achieved with those therapies. Certainly there is a scientific reason for everything that happens in any given disease, even if that reason remains unknown to the clinician. Biological molecules do not behave in a random, illogical fashion, even if it sometimes appears that way. Whenever it seems that a biological process is behaving in a seemingly illogical manner the logical conclusion is that such a process is yet to be properly understood. While the science of biochemistry does not currently explain all of the potential interactions among molecules it has established some sound starting points.

What biochemistry has been able to clearly establish is that efficient and prolific electron transport, transfer, and sharing are at the heart of the state of life itself. A high level of electron flow among the biomolecules of the body literally defines good health. A decline of this flow defines both aging and disease, depending on where and to what degree the flow is compromised. Finally, the cessation or near-cessation of electron flow occurs when the organism dies.

While the science of physics maintains that the total sum of energy in the universe remains unchanged since energy is neither created nor destroyed, energy is constantly being transferred or transformed. In biological systems the flow of energy is achieved by electron transport in and among biological molecules. Electron flow, quite literally, is the fuel of life. A car will not function without gasoline combusting in the engine and a cell will not function without electron flow among its molecules. Electrons must continue to move through, between, and among biological molecules for life to exist and to flourish.

Oxidation in the body occurs when electrons are lost from biomolecules. When such oxidized biomolecules predominate in any given microenvironment, the amount of electron flow and transfer is decreased and that area is no longer capable of functioning optimally. The initiation of a disease state then commences and it progresses the longer this state of decreased electron flow is left uncorrected. Such a microenvironment with increased numbers of oxidized biomolecules is defined as an area of ***increased oxidative stress.***

All established diseases can be characterized as having decreased electron flow and increased oxidative stress at the molecular level in the affected tissues. Conversely, when reduced, electron-rich molecules (antioxidants and non-oxidized biomolecules) predominate in a biological microenvironment that area will have increased electron flow along with minimized, or physiological, amounts of oxidative stress and it will function in a clinically healthy fashion.

> It is the *effects of vitamin C* in diseased, infected, and toxic states that allow the understanding of why tissues become diseased in the first place, as well as how they are best treated. The *biochemistry of vitamin C is the major key* in understanding both the physiology of health and the pathophysiology of disease in man and animals.

Toxins, Vitamin C, and Electrons

Currently modern medicine has a straightforward yet only minimally effective approach to patients who present with pictures of acute and life-threatening poisoning from any of a wide variety of toxins.

The competent emergency room physician immediately makes sure an airway is maintained and respiratory support is provided if necessary. Depending upon the toxin ingested, attempts might be made to neutralize it in the stomach (activated charcoal as a nonspecific antidote) or to physically remove any of it remaining in the gut (emesis, gastric emptying, whole bowel irrigation). Then, if available, a specific antidote may be administered. Subsequently, depending on the patient's clinical response, techniques to enhance the elimination of the poison assimilated by the body may be undertaken, including additional doses of activated charcoal, urinary alkalinization, and extracorporeal procedures.

The ability of vitamin C to effectively neutralize the toxicity of a wide range of different toxins has been very clearly established in the scientific literature, [1,2] even if that ability remains to be appreciated, understood, and appropriately utilized by most physicians. As long as emergency room physicians continue to consult poison control centers and the treatment algorithms provided in the medical textbook rather than immediately administer intravenous vitamin C when a poisoned or toxic patient arrives, needless suffering and death will continue to occur.

In spite of an enormous body of clinical and laboratory evidence indicating vitamin C is the treatment of choice for virtually all cases of known or even suspected toxin ingestion, there is probably not a single emergency room in the United States that routinely infuses vitamin C in such patients.

All of the traditional interventions for the acutely poisoned patient noted above are useful and occasionally life-saving, but the intravenous vitamin C can and should be started as soon as intravenous access is obtained for all critically poisoned patients. Otherwise the best chance at saving the patient's life and avoiding tissue damage from the poisoning will been missed, as vitamin C is simply the best antidote available. Regardless of the poisoning, recovery is much more the rule rather than the exception with rapid administration of high doses of vitamin C. Vitamin C should also be as vigorously-dosed as possible orally before and along with the intravenous infusion if the condition of the patient allows.

Unlike the administration of vitamin C, antidotes or antiserums known to have significant toxicity and side effects should never be given "just in case." Prompt administration of vitamin C will always save precious time in poisoned patients where just a little time can make all the difference not only in just surviving, but also in avoiding long-term tissue and organ damage. A prime example of this is the acetaminophen-poisoned patient who barely survives the acute poisoning but ends up with enough liver damage to require liver transplantation to ensure a more prolonged survival.

Other interventions can be useful in acutely poisoned patients but they should never be utilized in the absence of vitamin C administration. In fact, antidotes to poisons, venoms, and toxic chemicals are really unnecessary when the patient receives enough vitamin C. Also, many antidotes, such as some antivenoms for snakebites, reliably inflict significant toxicities of their own. And even though it might never be known if such antivenoms were necessary for survival, the vitamin C can make the patient much more comfortable as it neutralizes the nearly inevitable and substantial toxic antivenom side effects. No patient should suffer antiserum toxicity by the ill-advised avoidance of vitamin C therapy. The point is even more significant when it later turns out the biting snake was not poisonous but the antiserum was given in order to "cover all the bases."

Sufficient oral doses of vitamin C, particularly when encapsulated in sufficiently tiny liposomes, can also be effective in many cases of clinical poisoning, especially when a substantial percentage of the acute toxicity is taking place inside the cells of the body (intracellular) rather than in the extracellular fluid or the bloodstream. When available, large multigram doses of intravenous vitamin C, oral liposome-encapsulated vitamin C, and even regular vitamin C as ascorbic acid or sodium ascorbate should be promptly administered, as both the intracellular and extracellular areas of the body are better covered by such an approach.

These consistently positive clinical responses of chemically diverse toxins to only vitamin C beg a very important question:

How can one simple and small molecule (vitamin C) block, reverse, and/or negate

the acute toxicity of virtually all toxins regardless of the chemical composition or nature of the toxin?

The answer to this question immediately cuts to the innermost layer of the proverbial onion. Understanding this answer explains not only why a state of disease is present, it also simultaneously makes clear what is necessary to ameliorate, reverse, or even cure such a disease. Two important definitions must first be stated:

> **Oxidation**: the chemical reaction resulting in the *loss* of electrons
>
> **Reduction:** the chemical reaction resulting in the *gain* of electrons

What causes all disease is as simple as it is elegant. All toxins oxidize, or cause to be oxidized, important biomolecules in the body. As toxin presence persists or increases, increased oxidative stress persists or further increases. It is this increased oxidative stress that is responsible, directly and indirectly, for the genesis of all diseases. Furthermore this increased oxidative stress is also directly responsible for causing all of the symptoms associated with those diseases. This increased oxidative stress will always be present when:

> **1) Toxin (prooxidant) levels are high, when**
> **2) Antioxidant levels are low, or when**
> **3) Both factors coexist**.

Many other factors determine the great variety of diseases seen in patients, but the underlying condition of increased oxidative stress secondary to these specific modulating factors is always present. There is really no other way for vitamin C (and other antioxidants) to block toxicity in general, while nonspecifically reducing the evolution and expression of chronic disease except by this mechanism.

Infections and Toxins

Localized infections as well as more systemic infectious diseases are also powerful promoters of increased oxidative stress in the body. Infections all have their own oxidized metabolic waste products which exert greater toxic effects the longer they are not mobilized and properly excreted.

An abscess is a perfect example of such waste products accumulating rather than being mobilized. The presence of one or more abscesses anywhere in the body is typically associated with enormous clinical toxicity, depletion of electrons, and progressive loss of antioxidant stores.

Furthermore different bacteria can produce potent endotoxins or exotoxins. Endotoxins result from the breakdown of the outer membrane of certain gram-negative bacteria. As such bacteria are disrupted, the released components of these membranes demonstrate a potent toxicity.

Many clinicians consider the Herxheimer reaction to be a classical example of endotoxin release. When such a reaction occurs the patient can demonstrate fever, chills, and a general, although temporary, worsening of the nonspecific symptoms of any disease process. This reaction was first described as resulting from the initially large kill-off of syphilis pathogens (spirochetes) following the first doses of antibiotics, typically penicillin, in infected patients.

Many other infections with a significant collective physical mass in the body can also demonstrate variations of this Herxheimer reaction. This happens as pro-oxidant microbial debris is suddenly produced when the offending pathogens are killed and/or otherwise disrupted. Similarly a cancer patient with an acute kill-off of enough cancer cells can demonstrate this type of reaction after the initial doses of an effective therapy.

Exotoxins, on the other hand, are toxic proteins produced by a variety of different bacteria, including such well-known genera as *Clostridium, Escherichia, Pseudomonas, Salmonella, Shigella, Staphylococcus,* and *Streptococcus*. Unlike endotoxins, exotoxins are not associated with bacterial breakdown but instead expressed as the pathogens proliferate. Exotoxins, one of which is the enormously potent botulinum toxin, are collectively the most clinically poisonous substances known.

All infectious diseases are associated with multiple mechanisms for depleting electron supply and inhibiting electron flow in the body. The deadliest infections produce the most potent toxins but all infections, even without clearly associated endotoxins or exotoxins, will interfere with normal cellular metabolism and produce varying degrees of increased oxidative stress. This can be due not only to the toxic nature of accumulating metabolic byproducts, but also because of the physical displacement of normal biomolecules that would otherwise continue to support normal physiological function.

Reduction-Oxidation [Redox] Chemistry

Redox chemistry refers to the effective transfer, or "flow", of electrons in and through a pool of molecules having a significant antioxidant and oxidized antioxidant content. Antioxidant molecules donate, or give up, their electrons, causing reduction in the molecules receiving the electrons. Pro-oxidant molecules (toxins) take away electrons from surrounding molecules, causing oxidation in those molecules losing the electrons. Furthermore, any oxidized antioxidant molecule immediately becomes an electron-seeking pro-oxidant after it has lost its electrons, allowing the electron "flow" that is characteristic of ongoing redox reactions.

There is a big difference between pro-oxidant molecules that are known toxins and oxidized antioxidant molecules, even though both species of molecules seek to take electrons from other molecules. Specifically, the oxidized antioxidant reverts to an electron-donating antioxidant once its electrons are restored. Pro-oxidant toxins, on the other hand, do not transform into electron-donating "antioxidants" after they have taken electrons from other antioxidants or other vital biomolecules. Instead toxins immediately stop the electron transfer or flow of the redox chemical reactions in the tissues by just holding onto the electrons they have acquired as they are further metabolized, stored, or excreted.

The assimilation of electrons by the typical pro-oxidant toxin, then, represents a practical blockage or impediment in the ongoing exchange of electrons or electron flow, while electrons that get restored to pro-oxidants like oxidized antioxidants are rapidly passed along once again to molecules seeking electrons, supporting electron flow.

Outside of the oxidized antioxidants present, it is really only the previously oxidized biomolecule or the newly-appearing toxin that is seeking new electrons. Because of this a high toxin influx prevents oxidized biomolecules from having their electron status normalized and cellular/tissue malfunction will result. When toxin levels are very low, however, newly ingested antioxidants on a daily basis will serve to prevent biomolecules from being oxidized in the first place or they will simply donate their electrons to previously oxidized biomolecules, restoring their normal electrically reduced status.

With regard to electron flow, then, the true antioxidant continues an ongoing cycle of taking and giving electrons, permitting and facilitating electron flow and transfer in the tissues. The true toxin, however, only takes electrons and never re-donates them to any other molecules, which stops or impedes electron flow to the extent that the toxin is present and concentrated. This is the primary difference between an oxidized antioxidant that is restored to a reduced antioxidant by electron donation from a toxin that procures electrons from surrounding molecules. The reduced, electron-endowed toxin does not re-donate its stolen electrons like the recharged, reduced antioxidants do. Rather, it holds onto them and only serves to block electron flow.

Early on, toxins just promote impaired metabolism locally. When toxicity is chronic and substantial, involving more tissues and/or organs, disease will become manifest. When toxins accumulate sufficiently or concentrate in vital areas impaired electron flow will become sufficiently pronounced so that the markedly increased oxidative stress will cause local cell and tissue death (apoptosis and necrosis) with death to the entire organism eventually occurring if the continued toxin accumulation goes unchecked.

Reactive Oxygen Species (ROS)

Reactive oxygen species (ROS) are a group of molecules that are strongly pro-oxidant and thereby toxins by definition, seeking to take electrons away from other molecules. Many ROS are free radicals which are highly unstable molecules that can only achieve chemical stability when additional electrons have been acquired. However, like any other toxin or pro-oxidant molecule, a free radical does not participate in the give-and-take of electrons in redox chemistry as described above. Free radicals, seeking to remain stable, do not re-donate their newly acquired electrons to additional molecules, unlike the oxidized antioxidant described above.

An antioxidant and an oxidized antioxidant are molecules of similar chemical stability such that electron "flow" can proceed readily in either direction in the right microenvironment. Toxins and ROS, however, are much more chemically stable once they have received electrons. They cannot naturally proceed to a more chemically unstable form by giving up the electrons they initially received in order to reach a more stable state. The primary difference between an antioxidant and a toxin that has acquired electrons by oxidizing a biomolecule is that the toxin will not naturally seek the less stable chemical configuration associated with giving up the electrons again. This all follows the basic tenet of biochemistry that molecules are always seeking their most stable chemical configurations.

Toxin Properties and Variables

If the common denominator among toxins is the oxidation of biomolecules and the impairment of electron flow in affected cells, what makes one toxin enormously potent and rapidly fatal to the organism, another toxin the cause of a chronic degenerative disease, and still another toxin only the cause of minimally increased oxidative stress and few or no clinical symptoms? The factors that dictate how toxic a toxin is include the following:

1) **Solubility properties.** Is a toxin fat-soluble, water-soluble, or some degree of combination of the two? These properties largely determine where (what tissue, what organ, intracellular, extracellular, cell membrane, etc.) a toxin will concentrate.
2) **Molecular size.** A smaller molecule will have greater physical access to multiple sites in cells and tissues than a larger molecule. Relatively small or tiny toxin molecules might penetrate target cells by

simple diffusion or passage through cell wall pores that larger toxin molecules could not achieve.

3) **Ionic charge or electrical neutrality.** Like molecular size, this property will play a big role on where a toxin molecule is permitted to penetrate or migrate.

4) **Unique molecular structure.** This property is the defining physical configuration of a given toxin molecule. This configuration combined with the first three properties just mentioned confers the three-dimensional character of a toxin molecule. It is this unique physical structure that determines what biomolecule optimally receives or "fits" a given toxin molecule, which means that biomolecule will be the one that gets "targeted" by the toxin.

5) **Binding with other molecules.** This also affects where the toxin can go and what gets targeted. [3]

6) **Chemical ease with which oxidation occurs.** No two substances that chemically react with each other will do so with equal ease. One given toxin may react very vigorously with a given chemical type of biomolecule, while much less so with another. Other toxins may require a certain optimal "microenvironment," such as a specific pH range within the cell to have their most pronounced oxidative effects. Said another way, due to the unique chemical nature of the substances themselves, electrons do not spontaneously flow from different biomolecules to different toxins with identical ease. This characteristic results in

one toxin affecting certain biomolecules to a greater or lesser degree than another toxin.

7) **Tendency to generate ROS that produce oxidative chain reactions.** When a toxin has the appropriate molecular structure, location, and concentration in the right area of the cell oxidative chain reactions can be triggered that further massively upregulate the amounts of oxidative stress generated. This property makes the given toxin a much more potent poison.

8) **Tendency to specifically oxidize important enzymes, amino acids, antioxidants, and antioxidant enzymes.** When a given toxin can uniquely access and oxidize critical molecules in the cell the increased oxidative stress generated can be further escalated when the normal role of those molecules before they were oxidized would have been to help control the generation of oxidative stress. For example, oxidizing the enzyme superoxide dismutase not only alters the structure of that molecule, it also stops or impairs its function of preventing further oxidative damage via the mopping up of highly reactive superoxide free radicals.

9) **Specific targeting of sodium and/or potassium cellular ion channels.** A toxin with this property can affect intracellular and extracellular electrolyte balance and biochemical stability. [4,5]

10) **Tendency to specifically accumulate where critical biomolecules need to interact.** When a toxin has acquired the electrons that it seeks it physically needs to reside somewhere if is it not promptly

mobilized and excreted. The more pronounced this physical accumulation is the more normal cellular biomolecules and antioxidants are blocked from directly interacting chemically with each other, impairing their normal biochemical functions.

11) **Toxin similarity to structural biomolecules.** Certain toxins will strongly resemble structural biomolecules in the cell and they can end up incorporated into cell structures in the place of normally functioning biomolecules. Additionally, such a toxin can be more difficult to mobilize and excrete versus one that is just in solution in the cytoplasm or the extracellular fluid.

12) **Mimicry of hormonal function.** Some toxins can cause the biological functions of estrogens. [6]

13) **Access to excretion by chelation.** The unique molecular structure of a toxin will also determine whether it has ready access and/or a natural proclivity to readily bind to endogenous (natural) and exogenous (administered) chelators. Toxins easily reached, bound, and ultimately excreted by such chelators will be less clinically toxic than those toxins that cannot be readily reached or bound by these chelators.

14) **Access to excretion without chelation.** Smaller, less chemically complex toxins will generally be less clinically toxic if they can be readily excreted without the assistance of endogenous and/or exogenous chelators. Does the toxin appear spontaneously in feces, urine, breath, or sweat?

15) **Access to excretion by sweating.** How readily a given toxin can be mobilized by the sweating mechanism relates directly to how readily it accumulates. Toxins that naturally reach the innermost tissues and intracellular compartments of the cells of the body will effectively be more toxic over time if they can avoid being readily flushed out of the body via the sweating mechanism. The avoidance of circumstances that promote sweating naturally increases toxin retention as well.

16) **Genetic susceptibilities of the patient.** This facilitates the oxidative potential of a toxin in affected tissues or organs when certain enzymes or other important biomolecules are lacking or deficient.

17) **Does the toxin stimulate an immune response?** Under these circumstances, chronic immunological reactions can sometimes become an additional disease process if the toxin exposure is chronic.

18) **How is the toxin encountered and/or assimilated?** Is it inhaled or ingested? [7] Is it in its final form when ingested? [8] Is it produced by a pathogen? Was it administered parenterally?

19) **Are there specific receptors for the toxin?** For example, specific receptors that mediate toxicity exist for anthrax. [9,10]

20) **Are the toxins endotoxins, exotoxins, or toxic metabolites of pathogens or other infectious agents?** [11] Clinical resolution depends on infection eradication as well as on toxin neutralization and elimination.

Any of a number of combinations of the factors itemized above can play a role in determining the unique clinical profile of a given toxin or poison. For example, when a toxin accumulates in brain or nervous tissue the clinical syndrome produced will be very different from one produced by a toxin that accumulates in the kidneys or liver. And when the toxin can reach and oxidize one or more critical enzymes needed for the respiratory production of energy a small amount can rapidly result in death of the organism even when the bulk of the organism is largely unaffected. This is the case with a toxin such as cyanide, which can result in death within seconds to minutes when inhaled as hydrogen cyanide.

Levels of Intracellular Oxidative Stress

All chronic degenerative diseases have increased oxidative stress to some degree in both the intracellular and extracellular spaces. While a chronic disease with primarily increased extracellular oxidative stress is typified by coronary artery atherosclerosis (basement membrane area surrounding the endothelial cells), cancer features primarily increased intracellular oxidative stress. Although many cancers also have some degree of increased *extracellular* oxidative stress, it is the increased *intracellular* oxidative stress that is a feature present in all cancers. It is the degree to which this oxidative stress is increased that determines how aggressive and primitive, or anaplastic, a given cancer might be. And it is the highest elevations of intracellular calcium that ultimately result in cell death.[12,13] The degrees of oxidative stress present inside various normal, diseased but non-malignant, and malignant cells can be categorized into at least eight stages:

1) **None, or not readily detectable**: This is seen in dormant and non-replicating cells.

2) **Minimal**: This can be considered the baseline physiological level of oxidative stress consistent with the metabolic activity seen in viable non-replicating cells of less metabolically active organs.

3) **Minimal to moderate**: This is the range of normal oxidative stress seen in viable non-replicating cells present in organs with a high level of physiological activity, like heart, kidneys, or liver. In less active organs and tissues this level of oxidative stress can still be physiological in degree but only transiently, as in multiple redox signaling functions resulting in the upregulation and downregulation of various metabolic reactions via selective and reversible oxidation of key biomolecules. [14,15]

4) **Moderate**: This can be a normal or abnormal level of intracellular oxidative stress, depending on whether the level appears transiently in order to support cell replication or in a redox signaling capacity centrally involved in any of a number of stress-related and/or homeostatic mechanisms. However, when present most or all of the time, this level heralds the arrival or imminent arrival of malignant transformation.

Also essential to the malignant state is that this chronic level of increased intracellular oxidative stress be accompanied by elevated intracellular levels of calcium and reactive iron with decreased to absent levels of catalase. When normal levels of intracellular catalase and reactive iron are present, however, this increased oxidative stress level is characteristic of the cells in many of the non-malignant chronic degenerative diseases.

5) **Moderate to elevated**: This degree of oxidative stress is characteristic of established and replicating cancer cells. It is never chronically present in non-malignant cells unless the cell is progressing to apoptosis (programmed cell death), in which case very elevated intracellular oxidative stress will be transiently present before completion of the apoptotic process. [16,17]

6) **Elevated**: This is seen in the most metabolically active of cancer cells such as those that are highly invasive and actively metastasizing. [18] This can also be transiently present in normal cells proceeding to apoptosis, as noted above.

7) **Greatly elevated**: This is present in cancer cells with markedly upregulated Fenton chemistry activity in the cytoplasm, such as when primed by a pro-oxidative chemotherapy agent. Depending on the duration and degree of upregulation of this oxidative stress this level can either return back to the chronically moderate to elevated stages or proceed to apoptosis or frank cell necrosis.

8) **Maximal**: This is the highest level of oxidative stress that can exist in a still technically live cancer cell. When these levels are present remaining cell life is fleeting and the degree of the oxidative stress will generally take the cell directly to frank cell necrosis and rupture, as the apoptosis form of cell death is associated

with less massive rises in intracellular oxidative stress.

Summary

The cause of all disease is excess oxidative stress in the extracellular space as well as inside the cells. Excess oxidative stress is invariably caused by the increased presence of toxins (pro-oxidants) and/or a decreased presence of antioxidants. The effects of properly-dosed vitamin C on all forms of toxin exposure lend the strongest credence to this unified theory of disease. As a practical point, most chronic degenerative diseases can be approached as variable presentations of chronic focal scurvy. This is certainly the case for osteoporosis, which has been shown to be a chronic focal scurvy of the bones.

References

CHAPTER 1 CITATIONS

1. **Demer L (1995)** A skeleton in the atherosclerosis closet. *Circulation* 92:2029-2032. PMID: 7554176
2. **Kruger M, Horrobin D (1997)** Calcium metabolism, osteoporosis and essential fatty acids: a review. *Progress in Lipid Research* 36:131-151. PMID: 9624425
3. **Danilevicius C, Lopes J, Pereira R (2007)** Bone metabolism and vascular calcification. *Brazilian Journal of Medical and Biological Research* 40:435-442. PMID: 17401486
4. **Bolland M, A. Avenell, J. Baron, et al. (2010)** Effect of calcium supplements on risk of myocardial infarction and cardiovascular events: meta-analysis. *BMJ* 341:c3691. PMID: 20671013
5. **Bolland M, Grey A, Avenell A, et al. (2011)** Calcium supplements with or without vitamin D and risk of cardiovascular events: reanalysis of the Women's Health Initiative limited access dataset and meta-analysis. *BMJ* 342:d2040. PMID: 21505219
6. **Reid I, Bolland M, Avenell A, Grey A (2011)** Cardiovascular effects of calcium supplementation. *Osteoporosis International* 22:1649-1658. PMID: 21409434
7. **Michaelsson K, Melhus H, Lemming E, et al. (2013)** Long term calcium intake and rates of all cause and cardiovascular mortality: community based prospective longitudinal cohort study. *BMJ* 346:f228. PMID: 23403980
8. **Li K, Kaaks R, Linseisen J, Rohrmann S (2012)** Associations of dietary calcium intake and calcium supplementation with myocardial infarction and stroke risk and overall cardiovascular mortality in the Heidelberg cohort of the European Prospective Investigation into Cancer and Nutrition study (EPIC-Heidelberg). *Heart* 98:920-925. PMID: 22626900
9. **Bolland M, Barber P, Doughty R, et al. (2008)** Vascular events in healthy older women receiving calcium supplementation: randomised controlled trial. *BMJ* 336:262-266. PMID: 18198394
10. **Reid I, Bolland M (2008)** Calcium supplementation and vascular disease. *Climacteric* 11:280-286. PMID: 18645693
11. **Guzman R (2007)** Clinical, cellular, and molecular aspects of arterial calcification. *Journal of Vascular Surgery* 45:A57-A63. PMID: 17544025

12. **Taylor A, Bindeman J, Feuerstein I, et al.** (2005) Coronary calcium independently predicts incident premature coronary heart disease over measured cardiovascular risk factors: mean three-year outcomes in the Prospective Army Coronary Calcium (PACC) project. *Journal of the American College of Cardiology* 46:807-814. PMID: 16139129
13. **Yamamoto H, Ohashi N, Ishibashi K, et al.** (2011) Coronary calcium score as a predictor for coronary artery disease and cardiac events in Japanese high-risk patients. *Circulation Journal* 75:2424-2431. PMID: 21778594
14. **Fleckenstein A, Frey M, Thimm F, Fleckenstein-Grun G (1990)** Excessive mural calcium overload--a predominant causal factor in the development of stenosing coronary plaques in humans. *Cardiovascular Drugs and Therapy* 4:1005-1013. PMID: 2076386
15. **Ruiz-Garcia J, Lerman A, Weisz G, et al.**, (2012) Age- and gender-related changes in plaque composition in patients with acute coronary syndrome: the PROSPECT study. *EuroIntervention* 8:929-938. PMID: 23253546
16. **Kelly J, Thickman D, Abramson S, et al.** (2008) Coronary CT angiography findings in patients without coronary calcification. *American Journal of Roentgenology* 191:50-55. PMID: 18562724
17. **Chen C, Kuo Y, Liu C, et al.** (2012) Frequency and risk factors associated with atherosclerotic plaques in patients with a zero coronary artery calcium score. *Journal of the Chinese Medical Association* 75:10-15. PMID: 22240530
18. **Buyukterzi M, Turkvatan A, Buyukterzi Z (2013)** Frequency and extent of coronary atherosclerotic plaques in patients with a coronary artery calcium score of zero: assessment with CT angiography. *Diagnostic and Interventional Radiology* (Ankara, Turkey) 19:111-118. PMID: 23271579
19. **Gungor B, Polat A, Polat C, et al.** (2012) Do the calcifications in the thyroid gland predict malignancy? *Bratislavske Lekarske Listy* 113:552-555. PMID: 22979912
20. **Bai Y, Wang M, Han Y, et al.** (2013) Susceptibility weighted imaging: a new tool in the diagnosis of prostate cancer and detection of prostatic calcification. *PLoS One* 8:e53237. PMID: 23308170
21. **Gudermann T, Roelle S (2006)** Calcium-dependent growth regulation of small cell lung cancer cells by neuropeptides. *Endocrine-Related Cancer* 13:1069-1084. PMID: 17158754
22. **Zhang J, Liu G, Meng Y, et al.** (2009) MAG-2 promotes invasion, mobility and adherence capability of lung cancer cells by MMP-2, CD44 and intracellular calcium in vitro. *Oncology Reports* 21:697-706. PMID: 19212629
23. **Kaufmann R, Hollenberg M (2012)** Proteinase-activated receptors (PARs) and calcium signaling in cancer. *Advances in Experimental Medicine and Cancer* 740:979-1000. PMID: 22453980
24. **Ryu S, McDonnell K, Choi H, et al.** (2013) Suppression of miRNA-708 by polycomb group promotes metastases by calcium-induced migration. *Cancer Cell* 23:63-76. PMID: 23328481
25. **O'Brien K, Caballero B (1997)** High bone mass as a marker for breast cancer risk. *Nutrition Reviews* 55:284-286. PMID: 9279067

26. **Zhang Y, Kiel D, Kreger B, et al. (1997)** Bone mass and the risk of breast cancer among postmenopausal women. *The New England Journal of Medicine* 336:611-617. PMID: 9032046
27. **VandeVord P, Wooley P, Darga L, et al. (2006)** Genetic determinants of bone mass do not relate with breast cancer risk in US white and African-American women. *Breast Cancer Research and Treatment* 100:103-107. PMID: 16791482
28. **Hadji P, Gottschalk M, Ziller V, et al. (2007)** Bone mass and the risk of breast cancer: the influence of cumulative exposure to oestrogen and reproductive correlates. Results of the Marburg breast cancer and osteoporosis trial (MABOT). *Maturitas* 56:312-321. PMID: 17049767
29. **Gumus H, Gumus M, Devalia H, et al. (2012)** Causes of failure in removing calcium in microcalcification-only lesions using 11-gauge stereotactic vacuum-assisted breast biopsy. *Diagnostic and Interventional Radiology* (Ankara, Turkey) 18:354-359. PMID: 22477646
30. **Holmberg L, Wong Y, Tabar L, et al. (2013)** Mammography casting-type calcification and risk of local recurrence in DCIS: analyses from a randomised study. *British Journal of Cancer* 108:812-819. PMID: 23370209
31. **Lee A, Villena N, Hodi Z, et al. (2012)** The value of examination of multiple levels of mammary needle core biopsy specimens taken for investigation of lesions other than calcification. *Journal of Clinical Pathology* 65:1097-1099. PMID: 22918889
32. **Ling H, Liu Z, Xu L, et al. (2012)** Malignant calcification is an important unfavorable prognostic factor in primary invasive breast cancer. *Asia-Pacific Journal of Clinical Oncology* Jul 9 [Epub ahead of print]. PMID: 22897789
33. **Parkash J, Asotra K (2010)** Calcium wave signaling in cancer cells. *Life Sciences* 87:587-595. PMID: 20875431
34. **Alessandro R, Masiero L, Liotta L, Kohn E (1996)** The role of calcium in the regulation of invasion and angiogenesis. *In Vivo* 10:153-160. PMID: 8744794
35. **Lin Q, Balasubramanian K, Fan D, et al. (2010)** Reactive astrocytes protect melanoma cells from chemotherapy by sequestering intracellular calcium through gap junction communication channels. *Neoplasia* 12:748-754. PMID: 20824051
36. **Kass G, Orrenius S (1999)** Calcium signaling and cytotoxicity. *Environmental Health Perspectives* 107:25-35. PMID: 10229704
37. **Chi Y, Zhang X, Cai J, et al. (2012)** Formaldehyde increases intracellular calcium concentration in primary cultured hippocampal neurons partly through NMDA receptors and T-type calcium channels. *Neuroscience Bulletin* 28:715-722. PMID: 23160928
38. **Marty M, Atchison W (1998)** Elevations of intracellular Ca2+ as a probable contributor to decreased viability in cerebellar granule cells following acute exposure to methylmercury. *Toxicology and Applied Pharmacology* 150:98-105. PMID: 9630458
39. **Roos D, Seeger R, Puntel R, Barbosa N (2012)** Role of calcium and mitochondria in MeHg-mediated cytotoxicity. *Journal of Biomedicine and Biotechnology* 2012:248764. PMID: 22927718

40. **Saris N, Mervaala E, Karppanen H, et al. (2000)** Magnesium. An update on physiological, clinical and analytical aspects. *Clinica Chimica Acta* 294:1-26. PMID: 10727669
41. **Li J, Wang P, Yu S, et al. (2012)** Calcium entry mediates hyperglycemia-induced apoptosis through Ca(2+)/calmodulin-dependent kinase II in retinal capillary endothelial cells. *Molecular Vision* 18:2371-2379. PMID: 23049237
42. **Embi A, Scherlag B, Embi P, et al. (2012)** Targeted cellular ionic calcium chelation by oxalates: implications for the treatment of tumor cells. *Cancer Cell International* 12:51. PMID: 23216811
43. **Sakamoto M, Ikegami N, Nakano A (1996)** Protective effects of Ca2+ channel blockers against methyl mercury toxicity. *Pharmacology and Toxicology* 78:193-199. PMID: 8882354
44. **Li M, Inoue K, Si H, Xiong Z (2011)** Calcium-permeable ion channels involved in glutamate receptor-independent ischemic brain injury. *Acta Pharmacologica Sinica* 32:734-740. PMID: 21552295
45. **Kass G, Wright J, Nicotera P, Orrenius S (1988)** The mechanism of 1-methyl-4-phenyl-1,2,3,6-tetrahydropyridine toxicity: role of intracellular calcium. *Archives of Biochemistry and Biophysics* 260:789-797. PMID: 2963592
46. **Orrenius S, Burkitt M, Kass G, et al. (1992)** Calcium ions and oxidative cell injury. *Annals of Neurology* 32:S33-S42. PMID: 1510379
47. **Trump B, Berezesky I (1996)** The role of altered [Ca2+]i regulation in apoptosis, oncosis, and necrosis. *Biochimica et Biophysica Acta* 1313:173-178. PMID: 8898851
48. **Prasad A, Bloom M, Carpenter D (2010)** Role of calcium and ROS in cell death induced by polyunsaturated fatty acids in murine thymocytes. *Journal of Cellular Physiology* 225:829-836. PMID: 20589836
49. **Kawamata H, Manfredi G (2010)** Mitochondrial dysfunction and intracellular calcium dysregulation in ALS. *Mechanisms of Ageing and Development* 131:517-526. PMID: 20493207
50. **Surmeier D, Guzman J, Sanchez-Padilla J, Schumacker P (2011)** The role of calcium and mitochondrial oxidant stress in the loss of substantia nigra pars compacta dopaminergic neurons in Parkinson's disease. *Neuroscience* 198:221-231. PMID: 21884755
51. **Corona C, Pensalfini A, Frazzini V, Sensi S (2011)** New therapeutic targets in Alzheimer's disease: brain deregulation of calcium and zinc. *Cell Death & Disease* 2:e176. PMID: 21697951
52. **Jacobs P, Gondrie M, van der Graaf Y, et al. (2012)** Coronary artery calcium can predict all-cause mortality and cardiovascular events on low-dose CT screening for lung cancer. *American Journal of Roentgenology* 198:505-511. PMID: 22357989
53. **Kiramijyan S, Ahmadi N, Isma'eel H, et al. (2013)** Impact of coronary artery calcium progression and statin therapy on clinical outcome in subjects with and without diabetes mellitus. *The American Journal of Cardiology* 111:356-361. PMID: 23206921
54. **Graham G, Blaha M, Budoff M, et al. (2012)** Impact of coronary artery calcification on all-cause mortality in individuals with and without hypertension. *Atherosclerosis* 225:432-437. PMID: 23078882

55. **Grandi N, Brenner H, Hahmann H, et al.** (2012) Calcium, phosphate and the risk of cardiovascular events and all-cause mortality in a population with stable coronary heart disease. *Heart* 98:926-933. PMID: 22301505
56. **Nasir K, Rubin J, Blaha M, et al.** (2012) Interplay of coronary artery calcification and traditional risk factors for the prediction of all-cause mortality in asymptomatic individuals. *Circulation. Cardiovascular Imaging* 5:467-473. PMID: 22718782
57. **Rossi A, Targher G, Zoppini G, et al.** (2012) Aortic and mitral annular calcifications are predictive of all-cause and cardiovascular mortality in patients with type 2 diabetes. *Diabetes Care* 35:1781-1786. PMID: 22699285
58. **Bajraktari G, Nicoll R, Ibrahimi P, et al.** (2012) Coronary calcium score correlates with estimate of total plaque burden. *International Journal of Cardiology* Nov 21 [Epub ahead of print]. PMID: 23176773
59. **Pilz S, Tomaschitz A, Drechsler C, et al.** (2010) Parathyroid hormone level is associated with mortality and cardiovascular events in patients undergoing coronary angiography. *European Heart Journal* 31:1591-1598. PMID: 20439261
60. **Yu N, Donnan P, Flynn R, et al.** (2010) Increased mortality and morbidity in mild primary hyperparathyroid patients. The Parathyroid Epidemiology and Audit Research Study (PEARS). *Clinical Endocrinology* 73:30-34. PMID: 20039887
61. **Grandi N, Breitling L, Hahmann H, et al.** (2011) Serum parathyroid hormone and risk of adverse outcomes in patients with stable coronary artery disease. *Heart* 97:1215-1221. PMID: 21586795
62. **Schierbeck L, Jensen T, Bang U, et al.** (2011) Parathyroid hormone and vitamin D--markers for cardiovascular and all cause mortality in heart failure. *European Journal of Heart Failure* 13:626-632. PMID: 21415099
63. **Kritchevsky S, Tooze J, Neiberg R, et al.** (2012) 25-hydroxyvitamin D, parathyroid hormone, and mortality in black and white older adults: the health ABC study. *The Journal of Clinical Endocrinology and Metabolism* 97:4156-4165. PMID: 22942386
64. **van Ballegooijen A, Reinders I, Visser M, et al.** (2013) Serum parathyroid hormone in relation to all-cause and cardiovascular mortality: The Hoorn Study. *The Journal of Clinical Endocrinology and Metabolism* Feb 13. [Epub ahead of print]. PMID: 23408568
65. **Michaelsson K, Melhus H, Lemming E, et al.** (2013) Long term calcium intake and rates of all cause and cardiovascular mortality: community based prospective longitudinal cohort study. *BMJ* 346:f228. PMID: 23403980 PMID: 23403980
66. **Cooke A (1932)** Alkalosis occurring in the alkaline treatment of peptic ulcers. *The Quarterly Journal of Medicine* 25:527.
67. **Abreo K, Adlakha A, Kilpatrick S, et al.** (1993) The milk-alkali syndrome. A reversible form of acute renal failure. *Archives of Internal Medicine* 153:1005-1010. PMID: 8481062
68. **Beall D, Scofield R (1995)** Milk-alkali syndrome associated with calcium carbonate consumption. Report of 7 patients with parathyroid hormone levels and an estimate of prevalence among patients hospitalized with hypercalcemia. *Medicine* 74:89-96. PMID: 7891547

69. **Beall D, Henslee H, Webb H, Scofield R (2006)** Milk-alkali syndrome: a historical review and description of the modern version of the syndrome. *The American Journal of the Medical Sciences* 331:233-242. PMID: 16702792
70. **Picolos M, Lavis V, Orlander P (2005)** Milk-alkali syndrome is a major cause of hypercalcaemia among non-end-stage renal disease (non-ESRD) inpatients. *Clinical Endocrinology* 63:566-576. PMID: 16268810
71. **Caruso J, Patel R, Julka K, Parish D (2007)** Health-behavior induced disease: return of the milk-alkali syndrome. *Journal of General Internal Medicine* 22:1053-1055. PMID: 17483976
72. **Medarov B (2009)** Milk-Alkali syndrome. *Mayo Clinic Proceedings. Mayo Clinic* 84:261-267. PMID: 19252114
73. **Muldowney W, Mazbar S (1996)** Rolaids-yogurt syndrome: a 1990s version of milk-alkali syndrome. *American Journal of Kidney Diseases* 27:270-272. PMID: 8659505
74. **Watson, S., B. Dellinger, K. Jennings, and L. Scott (2012)** Antacids, altered mental status, and milk-alkali syndrome. *Case Reports in Emergency Medicine* 2012:942452. PMID: 23431478

CHAPTER 2 CITATIONS

1. **Yanez M, Gil-Longo J, Campos-Toimil M (2012)** Calcium binding proteins. *Advances in Experimental Medicine and Biology* 740:461-482. PMID: 22453954
2. **Galva C, Artigas P, Gatto C (2012)** Nuclear Na+/K+-ATPase plays an active role in nucleoplasmic Ca2+ homeostasis. *Journal of Cell Science* 125:6137-6147. PMID: 23077175
3. **Zwadlo C, Borlak J (2006)** Nifedipine represses ion channels, transporters and Ca(2+)-binding proteins in the hearts of spontaneously hypertensive rats. *Toxicology and Applied Pharmacology* 213:224-234. PMID: 16343576
4. **Gonzalez J, Suki W (1995)** Cell calcium and arterial blood pressure. *Seminars in Nephrology* 15:564-568. PMID: 8588116
5. **Kurnellas M, Donahue K, Elkabes S (2007)** Mechanisms of neuronal damage in multiple sclerosis and its animal models: role of calcium pumps and exhangers. *Biochemical Society Transactions* 35:923-926. PMID: 17956247
6. **Bangalore S, Parkar S, Messerli F (2009)** Long-acting calcium antagonists in patients with coronary artery disease: a meta-analysis. *The American Journal of Medicine* 122:356-365. PMID: 19332231
7. **Mason R (2012)** Pleiotropic effects of calcium channel blockers. *Current Hypertension Reports* 14:293-303. PMID: 22610475
8. **Ishii N, Matsumura T, Shimoda S, Araki E (2012)** Anti-atherosclerotic potential of dihydropyridine calcium channel blockers. *Journal of Atherosclerosis and Thrombosis* 19:693-704. PMID: 22653165
9. **Conde-Agudelo A, Romero R, Kusanovic J (2011)** Nifedipine in the management of preterm labor: a systemic review and metaanalysis. *American Journal of Obstetrics and Gynecology* 204:134. PMID: 21284967
10. **Kusama Y, Kodani E, Nakagomi E, et al. (2011)** Variant angina and coronary artery spasm: the clinical spectrum, pathophysiology, and management. *Journal of Nippon Medical School* 78:4-12. PMID: 21389642
11. **Siama K, Tousoulis D, Papageorgiou N, et al. (2013)** Stable angina pectoris: current medical treatment. *Current Pharmaceutical Design* 19:1569-1580. PMID: 23016717
12. **Montani D, Savale L, Natali D, et al. (2010)** Long-term response to calcium-channel blockers in non-idiopathic pulmonary artery hypertension. *European Heart Journal* 31:1898-1907. PMID: 20543192
13. **Huisstede B, Hoogvliet P, Paulis W, et al. (2011)** Effectiveness of interventions for secondary Raynaud's phenomenon: a systemic review. *Archives of Physical Medicine and Rehabilitation* 92:1166-1180. PMID: 21704799
14. **Aslan A, Gurelik M, Cemek M, et al. (2012)** Nimodipine can diminish oxidative stress in patients with severe head trauma. *Journal of Neurosurgical Sciences* 56:247-253. PMID: 22854593

15. **Iannetti P, Spalice A, Parisi P (2005)** Calcium-channel blocker verapamil administration in prolonged and refractory status epilepticus. *Epilepsia* 46:967-969. PMID: 15946342
16. **Iannetti P, Parisi P, Spalice A, et al. (2009)** Addition of verapamil in the treatment of severe myoclonic epilepsy in infancy. *Epilepsy Research* 85:89-95. PMID: 19303743
17. **Tatsushima Y, Egashira N, Narishige Y, et al. (2013)** Calcium channel blockers reduce oxaliplatin-induced acute neuropathy: a retrospective study of 69 male patients receiving modified FOLFOX6 therapy. *Biomedicine & Pharmacotherapy* 67:39-42. PMID: 23206755
18. **Anekonda T, Quinn J (2011)** Calcium channel blocking as a therapeutic strategy for Alzheimer's disease: the case for isradipine. *Biochimica et Biophysica Acta* 1812:1584-1590. PMID: 21925266
19. **Pasternak B, Svanstrom H, Nielsen N, et al. (2012)** Use of calcium channel blockers and Parkinson's disease. American *Journal of Epidemiology* 175:627-635. PMID: 22387374
20. **Shimizu H, Nakagami H, Yasumasa N, et al. (2012)** Cilnidipine, but not amlodipine, ameliorates osteoporosis in ovariectomized hypertensive rats through inhibition of the N-type calcium channel. *Hypertension Research* 35:77-81. PMID: 21881574
21. **Barabas P, Cutler Peck C, Krizaj D (2010)** Do calcium channel blockers rescue dying photoreceptors in the Pde6b (rd1) mouse? *Advances in Experimental Medicine and Biology* 664:491-499. PMID: 20238051
22. **Gillman M, Ross-Degnan D, McLaughlin T, et al. (1999)** Effects of long-acting versus short-acting calcium channel blockers among older survivors of acute myocardial infarction. Journal of the *American Geriatrics Society* 47:512-517. PMID: 10323641
23. **Gibson R, Hansen J, Messerli F, et al. (2000)** Long-term effects of diltiazem and verapamil on mortality and cardiac events in a non-Q-wave acute myocardial infarction without pulmonary congestion: post hoc subset analysis of the multicenter diltiazem postinfarction trial and the second Danish verapamil infarction trial studies. The *American Journal of Cardiology* 86:275-279. PMID: 10922432
24. **Lubsen J, Wagener G, Kirwan B, et al. (2005)** Effect of long-acting nifedipine on mortality and cardiovascular morbidity in patients with symptomatic stable angina and hypertension: the ACTION trial. *Journal of Hypertension* 23:641-648. PMID: 15716708
25. **Costanzo P, Perrone-Filardi P, Petretta M, et al. (2009)** Calcium channel blockers and cardiovascular outcomes: a meta-analysis of 175,634 patients. *Journal of Hypertension* 27:1136-1151. PMID: 19451836

CHAPTER 3 CITATIONS

1. **Committee to Review Dietary Reference Intakes for Vitamin D and Calcium (2010)** Food and Nutrition Board, Institute of Medicine. *Dietary Reference Intakes for Calcium and Vitamin D.* Washington, DC: National Academy Press.
2. **Seeman E (2010)** Evidence that calcium supplements reduce fracture risk is lacking. *Clinical Journal of the American Society of Nephrology* 5:S3-S11. PMID: 20089500
3. **Kurabayashi M (2012)** [Is calcium supplement useful in aged persons? Calcium supplement doesn't reduce the fracture and vascular risk in aged persons]. [Article in Japanese]. *Clinical Calcium* 22:736-739. PMID: 22549199
4. **Chung M, Lee J, Terasawa T, et al. (2011)** Vitamin D with or without calcium supplementation for prevention of cancer and fractures: an updated meta-analysis for the U.S. Preventive Services Task Force. *Archives of Internal Medicine* 155:827-838. PMID: 22184690
5. **Chapuy M, Arlot M, Duboeuf F, et al. (1992)** Vitamin D3 and calcium to prevent hip fractures in the elderly women. *The New England Journal of Medicine* 327:1636-1642. PMID: 1331788
6. **Jackson R, LaCroix A, Gass M, et al. (2006)** Calcium plus vitamin D supplementation and the risk of fractures. *The New England Journal of Medicine* 354:669-683. PMID: 16481635
7. **Bischoff-Ferrari H, Willett W, Wong J, et al. (2005)** Fracture prevention with vitamin D supplementation: a meta-analysis of randomized controlled trials. *The Journal of the American Medical Association* 293:2257-2264. PMID: 15886381
8. **Trivedi D, Doll R, Khaw K (2003)** Effect of four monthly oral vitamin D3 (cholecalciferol) supplementation on fractures and mortality in men and women living in the community: randomised double blind controlled trial. *BMJ* 326:469. PMID: 12609940
9. **Bischoff-Ferrari H, Willett W, Orav E, et al. (2012)** A pooled analysis of vitamin D dose requirements for fracture prevention. *The New England Journal of Medicine* 367:40-49. PMID: 22762317
10. **Rizzoli R, Boonen S, Brandi M, et al. (2013)** Vitamin D supplementation in elderly or postmenopausal women: a 2013 update of the 2008 recommendations from the European Society for Clinical and Economic Aspects of Osteoporosis and Osteoarthritis (ESCEO). *Current Medical Research and Opinion* Feb 7 [Epub ahead of print]. PMID: 23320612
11. **Sonneville K, Gordon C, Kocher M, et al. (2012)** Vitamin D, calcium, and dairy intakes and stress fractures among female adolescents. *Archives of Pediatrics & Adolescent Medicine* 166:595-600. PMID: 22393172
12. **Fardellone P, Cotte F, RouxC, et al. (2010)** Calcium intake and the risk of osteoporosis and fractures in French women. *Joint, Bone, Spine* 77:154-158. PMID: 20185352
13. **Warensjo E, Byberg L, Melhus H, et al., (2011)** Dietary calcium intake and risk of fracture and osteoporosis: prospective longitudinal cohort study. *BMJ* 342:d1473. PMID: 21610048

14. **Grant A, Avenell A, Campbell M, et al. (2005)** Oral vitamin D3 and calcium for secondary prevention of low-trauma fractures in elderly people (Randomised Evaluation of Calcium Or vitamin D, RECORD): a randomised placebo-controlled trial. *Lancet* 365:1621-1628. PMID: 15885294
15. **Bischoff-Ferrari H, Dawson-Hughes B, Baron J, et al. (2011)** Milk intake and risk of hip fracture in men and women: a meta-analysis of prospective cohort studies. *Journal of Bone and Mineral Research* 26:833-839. PMID: 20949604
16. **Dawson-Hughes B, Harris S, Krall E, Dallal G (1997)** Effect of calcium and vitamin D supplementation on bone density in men and women 65 years of age or older. *The New England Journal of Medicine* 337:670-676. PMID: 9278463
17. **Seeman E (2010)** Evidence that calcium supplements reduce fracture risk is lacking. *Clinical Journal of the American Society of Nephrology* 5:S3-S11. PMID: 20089500
18. **Bischoff-Ferrari H, Kiel D, Dawson-Hughes B, et al. (2009)** Dietary calcium and serum 25-hydroxyvitamin D status in relation to BMD among U.S. adults. *Journal of Bone and Mineral Research* 24:935-942. PMID: 19113911
19. **Browner W, Seeley D, Vogt T, Cummings S (1991)** Non-trauma mortality in elderly women with low bone mineral density. Study of Osteoporotic Fractures Research Group. *Lancet* 338:355-358. PMID: 1677708
20. **Stojanovic O, Lazovic M, Lazovic M, Vuceljic M (2011)** Association between atherosclerosis and osteoporosis, the role of vitamin D. *Archives of Medical Science* 7:179-188. PMID: 22291755
21. **Browner W, Pressman A, Nevitt M, et al. (1993)** Association between low bone density and stroke in elderly women. The study of osteoporotic fractures. *Stroke* 24:940-946. PMID: 8322393
22. **Hmamouchi I, Allali F, Khazzani H, et al. (2009)** Low bone mineral density is related to atherosclerosis in postmenopausal Moroccan women. *BMC* Public Health 9:388. PMID: 19828021
23. **Bezerra M, Calomeni G, Caparbo V, et al. (2005)** Low bone density and low serum levels of soluble RANK ligand are associated with severe arterial calcification in patients with Takayasu arteritis. *Rheumatology* 44:1503-1506. PMID: 16219645
24. **Demer L (1995)** A skeleton in the atherosclerosis closet. *Circulation* 92:2029-2032. PMID: 7554176
25. **Kruger M, Horrobin D (1997)** Calcium metabolism, osteoporosis and essential fatty acids: a review. *Progress in Lipid Research* 36:131-151. PMID: 9624425
26. **Danilevicius C, Lopes J, Pereira R (2007)** Bone metabolism and vascular calcification. *Brazilian Journal of Medical and Biological Research* 40:435-442. PMID: 17401486
27. **Fisher A, Srikusalanukul W, Davis M, Smith P (2013)** Cardiovascular diseases in older patients with osteoporotic hip fracture: prevalence, disturbances in mineral and bone metabolism, and bidirectional links. *Clinical Interventions in Aging* 8:239-256. PMID: 23460043

References

28. **Mussolino M, Madans J, Gillum R (2003)** Bone mineral density and mortality in women and men: the NHANES I epidemiologic follow-up study. *Annals of Epidemiology* 13:692-697. PMID: 14599733
29. **Chen J, Hogan C, Lyubomirsky G, Sambrook P (2011)** Women with cardiovascular disease have increased risk of osteoporotic fracture. *Calcified Tissue International* 88:9-15. PMID: 21046091
30. **Rennenberg R, Kessels A, Schurgers L, et al. (2009)** Vascular calcifications as a marker of increased cardiovascular risk: a meta-analysis. *Vascular Health and Risk Management* 5:185-197. PMID: 19436645
31. **Eisman J, Martin T, MacIntyre I (1980)** Presence of 1,25-dihydroxy vitamin D receptor in normal and abnormal breast tissue. *Progress in Biochemical Pharmacology* 17:143-150. PMID: 6259652
32. **Feldman D, Chen T, Hirst M, et al. (1980)** Demonstration of 1,25-dihydroxyvitamin D3 receptors in human skin biopsies. *The Journal of Clinical Endocrinology and Metabolism* 51:1463-1465. PMID: 6255007
33. **Haussler M, Manolagas S, Deftos L (1980)** Evidence for a 1,25-dihydroxyvitamin D3 receptor-like macromolecule in rat pituitary. *The Journal of Biological Chemistry* 255:5007-5010. PMID: 6246092
34. **Reinhardt T, Conrad H (1980)** Specific binding protein for 1,25-dihydroxyvitamin D3 in bovine mammary gland. *Archives of Biochemistry and Biophysics* 203:108-116. PMID: 6250480
35. **Wecksler W, Ross F, Mason R, et al. (1980)** Biochemical properties of the 1 alpha, 25-dihydroxyvitamin D3 cytoplasmic receptors from human and chick parathyroid glands. *Archives of Biochemistry and Biophysics* 201:95-103. PMID: 6893115
36. **Christakos S, Norman A (1981)** Studies on the mode of action of calciferol. XXIX. Biochemical characterization of 1,25-dihydroxyvitamin D3 receptors in chick pancreas and kidney cytosol. *Endocrinology* 108:140-149. PMID: 6257481
37. **Nagpal S, Na S, Rathnachalam R (2005)** Noncalcemic actions of vitamin D receptor ligands. *Endocrine Reviews* 26:662-687. PMID: 15798098
38. **Holick M (2007)** Vitamin D deficiency. *The New England Journal of Medicine* 357:266-281. PMID: 17634462
39. **Wacker M, Holick M (2013)** Vitamin D--effects on skeletal and extraskeletal health and the need for supplementation. *Nutrients* 5:111-148. PMID: 23306192
40. **Malm O (1975)** Calcium and magnesium. *Progress in Food and Nutrition Science* 1:173-182. PMID: 788034
41. **Morris H, O'Loughlin P, Anderson P (2010)** Experimental evidence for the effects of calcium and vitamin D on bone: a review. *Nutrients* 2:1026-1035. PMID: 22254071
42. **Sachan A, Gupta R, Das V, et al. (2005)** High prevalence of vitamin D deficiency among pregnant women and their newborns in northern India. *The American Journal of Clinical Nutrition* 81:1060-1064. PMID: 15883429
43. **Al-Mogbel E (2012)** Vitamin D status among adult Saudi females visiting primary health care clinics. *International Journal of Health Sciences* 6:116-126. PMID: 23580892

44. **Nesby-O'Dell S, Scanlon K, Cogswell M, et al. (2002)** Hypovitaminosis D prevalence and determinants among African American and white women of reproductive age: third National Health and Nutrition Examination Survey, 1988-1994. *The American Journal of Clinical Nutrition* 76:187-192. PMID: 12081833

References

CHAPTER 4 CITATIONS

1. **Gabbay KH, et al. (2020)** Ascorbate synthesis pathway: dual role of ascorbate in bone homeostasis" *J Biol Chem* Jun 18 285(25):19510-20. PMID: 20410296
2. **Yalin S, et al. (2005)** Is there a role of free oxygen radicals in primary male osteoporosis? *Clin Exp Rheumatol* Sep-Oct 23(5):689-92. PMID: 16173248
3. **Park JB (2010)** The Effects of Dexamethasone, Ascorbic Acid, and β-Glycerophosphate on Osteoblastic Differentiation by Regulating Estrogen Receptor and Osteopontin Expression" *J Surg Res* Oct 8. PMID: 21035140
4. **Hie M, Tsukamoto I (2011)** Vitamin C-deficiency stimulates osteoclastogenesis with an increase in RANK expression" *J Nutr Biochem* 2011 Feb 22(2):164-71. PMID: 20444587
5. **Gabbay, K., K. Bohren, R. Morello, et al. (2010)** Ascorbate synthesis pathway: dual role of ascorbate in bone homeostasis. The *Journal of Biological Chemistry* 285:19510-19520. PMID: 20410296
6. **Cervellati, C., G. Bonaccorsi, E. Cremonini, et al. (2013)** Bone mass density selectively correlates with serum markers of oxidative damage in post-menopausal women. *Clinical Chemistry and Laboratory Medicine* 51:333-338. PMID: 23089610
7. **Sheweita SA, Khoshhal KI (2007)** Calcium metabolism and oxidative stress in bone fractures: role of antioxidants, *Curr Drug Metab* Jun 8(5):519-25. PMID: 17584023
8. **Saito M (2009)** Nutrition and bone health. Roles of vitamin C and vitamin B as regulators of bone mass and quality, *Clin Calcium* Aug 19(8):1192-9. PMID: 19638704
9. **Maehata Y, et al. (2007)** Type III collagen is essential for growth acceleration of human osteoblastic cells by ascorbic acid 2-phosphate, a long-acting vitamin C derivative, *Matrix Biol* Jun 26(5):371-81. PMID: 17306970
10. **Hie M, Tsukamoto I (2011)** Vitamin C-deficiency stimulates osteoclastogenesis with an increase in RANK expression, *J Nutr Biochem* Feb 22(2):164-71. PMID: 20444587
11. **Bourne G (1942)** Vitamin C and repair of injured tissues, *Lancet* 2:661-664.
12. **Zhu L, Cao J, Sun M, et al. (2012)** Vitamin C prevents hypogonadal bone loss. *PLoS One* 7:e47058. PMID: 23056580
13. **Morton D, Barrett-Connor E, Schneide D (2001)** Vitamin C supplement use and bone mineral density in postmenopausal women, *Journal of Bone and Mineral Research* 16(1):135-140. PMID: 11149477
14. **Leveille S, et al. (1997)** Dietary vitamin C and bone mineral density in postmenopausal women in Washington State, USA, *Journal of Epidemiology and Community Health* 51(5):479-485. PMID: 9425455
15. **Chuin A, et al. (2009)** Effect of antioxidants combined to resistance training on BMD in elderly women: a pilot study, *Osteoporos Int* Jul 20(7):1253-8. PMID: 19020919

16. **Sahni S, et al. (2008)** High vitamin C intake is associated with lower 4-year bone loss in elderly men, *J Nutr* Oct 138(10):1931-8. PMID: 18806103
17. **Pasco JA, et al. (2006)** Antioxidant vitamin supplements and markers of bone turnover in a community sample of nonsmoking women, *J Womens Health* (Larchmt) Apr 15(3):295-300. PMID: 16620188
18. **Sugiura M, et al. (2011)** Dietary patterns of antioxidant vitamin and carotenoid intake associated with bone mineral density: findings from post-menopausal Japanese female subjects, *Osteoporos Int* Jan 22(1):143-52. PMID: 20480147
19. **Ruiz-Ramos M, et al. (2010)** Supplementation of ascorbic acid and alpha-tocopherol is useful to preventing bone loss linked to oxidative stress in elderly, *J Nutr Health Aging* Jun 14(6):467-72. PMID: 20617290
20. **Zinnuroglu M, et al. (2012)** Prospective evaluation of free radicals and antioxidant activity following 6-month risedronate treatment in patients with postmenopausal osteoporosis, *Rheumatol Int* Apr 32(4):875-880. PMID: 21221594
21. **Sahni S, et al. (2009)** Protective effect of total and supplemental vitamin C intake on the risk of hip fracture — a 17-year follow-up from the Framingham Osteoporosis Study, *Osteoporos Int* Nov 20(11):1853-61. PMID: 19347239
22. **Falch JA, Mowé M, Bøhmer T (1998)** Low levels of serum ascorbic acid in elderly patients with hip fracture, *Scand J Clin Lab Invest* May 58(3):225-8. PMID: 9670346
23. **Sahni S, Hannan M, Gagnon D, et al. (2009)** Protective effect of total and supplemental vitamin C intake on the risk of hip fracture--a 17-year follow-up from the Framingham Osteoporosis Study, *Osteoporosis International* 20:1853-1861. PMID: 19347239
24. **Martinez-Ramirez M, Perez S, Delgado-Martinez A, et al. (2007)** Vitamin C, vitamin B12, folate and the risk of osteoporotic fractures. A case-control study, *International Journal for Vitamin and Nutrition Research* 77:359-368. PMID: 18622945
25. **Falch J, Mowe M, Bohmer T (1998)** Low levels of serum ascorbic acid in elderly patients with hip fracture, *Scandinavian Journal of Clinical and Laboratory Investigation* 58:225-228. PMID: 9670346
26. **Park J, Lee E, Kim A, et al. (2012)** Vitamin C deficiency accelerates bone loss inducing an increase in PPAR-γ expression in SMP30 knockout mice, *International Journal of Experimental Pathology* 93:332-340. PMID: 22974214
27. **Maggio D, Barabani M, Pierandrei M, et al. (2003)** Marked decrease in plasma antioxidants in aged osteoporotic women: results of a cross-sectional study, *The Journal of Clinical Endocrinology and Metabolism* 88:1523-1527. PMID: 12679433
28. **Melhus H, Michaelsson K, Holmberg L, et al. (1999)** Smoking, antioxidant vitamins, and the risk of hip fracture, *Journal of Bone and Mineral Research* 14:129-135. PMID: 9893075
29. **Guzman R. (2007)** Clinical, cellular, and molecular aspects of arterial calcification. *Journal of Vascular Surgery* 45:A57-A63. PMID: 17544025

References

30. **Taylor A, Bindeman J, Feuerstein I, et al.** (2005) Coronary calcium independently predicts incident premature coronary heart disease over measured cardiovascular risk factors: mean three-year outcomes in the Prospective Army Coronary Calcium (PACC) project, *Journal of the American College of Cardiology* 46:807-814. PMID: 16139129
31. **Yamamoto H, Ohashi N, Ishibashi K, et al.** (2011) Coronary calcium score as a predictor for coronary artery disease and cardiac events in Japanese high-risk patients, *Circulation Journal* 75:2424-2431. PMID: 21778594

CHAPTER 5 CITATIONS

1. **Burge R, Dawson-Hughes B, et al. (2007)** Incidence and economic burden of osteoporosis fractures in the United States, 2005-2025, *J Bone Miner Res* 22(3):465-475 PMID:17144789
2. **Melton LJ 3rd, Atkinson EJ, O'Connor MK, et al. (1998)** Bone density and fracture risk in men, *J Bone Miner Res* 13:1915.
3. **Melton LJ 3rd, Chrischilles EA, Cooper C, et al. (1992)** Perspective. How many women have osteoporosis?, *J Bone Miner Res* 7:1005. PMID: 1414493
4. **Kanis JA, Johnell O, Oden A, et al. (2000)** Long-term risk of osteoporotic fracture in Malmo, *Osteoporos Int* 11:669.
5. **Carinci F, Pezzetti F, Spina A, et al. (2005)** Effect of vitamin C on pre-osteoblast gene expression, *Archives of Oral Biology* 50:481-496. PMID: 15777530
6. **Naito H, Dohi Y, Zimmermann W, et al. (2011)** The effect of mesenchymal stem cell osteoblastic differentiation on the mechanical properties of engineered bone-like tissue, *Tissue Engineering. Part A* 17:2321-2329. PMID: 21548844
7. **Choi K, Seo Y, Yoon H, et al. (2008)** Effect of ascorbic acid on bone marrow-derived mesenchymal stem cell proliferation and differentiation, *Journal of Bioscience and Bioengineering* 105:586-594. PMID: 18640597
8. **Maehata Y, Takamizawa S, Ozawa S, et al. (2007)** Type III collagen is essential for growth acceleration of human osteoblastic cells by ascorbic acid 2-phosphate, a long-acting vitamin C derivative, *Matrix Biology* 26:371-381. PMID: 17306970
9. **Gabbay K, Bohren K, Morello R, et al. (2010)** Ascorbate synthesis pathway: dual role of ascorbate in bone homeostasis, *The Journal of Biological Chemistry* 285:19510-19520. PMID: 20410296
10. **Hie M, Tsukamoto I (2011)** Vitamin C-deficiency stimulates osteoclastogenesis with an increase in RANK expression, *The Journal of Nutritional Biochemistry* 22:164-171. PMID: 20444587
11. **Park J, Lee E, Kim A, et al. (2012)** vitamin C deficiency accelerates bone loss inducing an increase in PPAR-γ expression in SMP30 knockout mice, *International Journal of Experimental Pathology* 93:332-340. PMID: 22974214
12. **Tsuchiya H, Bates C (1997)** Vitamin C and copper interactions in guinea-pigs and a study of collagen cross-links, *The British Journal of Nutrition* 77:315-325. PMID: 9135375
13. **Munday K, Fulford A, Bates C (2005)** Vitamin C status and collagen cross-link ratios in Gambian children, *The British Journal of Nutrition* 93:501-507. PMID: 15946412
14. **Nakamura K, Saito T, Kobayashi R, et al. (2011)** C-reactive protein predicts incident fracture in community-dwelling elderly Japanese women: the Muramatsu study, *Osteoporosis International* 22:2145-2150. PMID: 20936400
15. **Mikirova N, Casciari J, Rogers A, Taylor P (2012)** Effect of high-dose intravenous vitamin C on inflammation in cancer patients, *Journal of Translational Medicine* 10:189. PMID: 22963460

16. **Lacativa P, Farias M (2010)** Osteoporosis and inflammation, *Arquivo Brasileiros de Endocrinologia e Metabologia* 54:123-132. PMID: 20485900
17. **Hall S, Greendale G (1998)** The relation of dietary vitamin C intake to bone mineral density: results from the PEPI study, *Calcified Tissue International* 63:183-189. PMID: 9701620
18. **Morton D, Barrett-Connor E, Schneider D (2001)** Vitamin C supplement use and bone mineral density in postmenopausal women, *Journal of Bone and Mineral Research* 16:135-140. PMID: 11149477
19. **Zhu L, Cao J, Sun M, et al. (2012)** Vitamin C prevents hypogonadal bone loss, *PLoS One* 7:e47058. PMID: 23056580
20. **Leveille S, LaCroix A, Koepsell T, et al. (1997)** Dietary vitamin C and bone mineral density in postmenopausal women in Washington State, USA, *Journal of Epidemiology and Community Health* 51:479-485. PMID: 9425455
21. **Sahni S, Hannan M, Gagnon D, et al. (2009)** Protective effect of total and supplemental vitamin C intake on the risk of hip fracture—a 17-year follow-up from the Framingham Osteoporosis Study, *Osteoporosis International* 20:1853-1861. PMID: 19347239
22. **Martinez-Ramirez M, Palma S, Delgado-Martinez A, et al. (2007)** Vitamin C, vitamin B12, folate and the risk of osteoporotic fractures. A case-control study, *International Journal for Vitamin and Nutrition Research* 77:359-368. PMID: 18622945
23. **Maggio D, Barabani M, Pierandrei M, et al. (2003)** Marked decrease in plasma antioxidants in aged osteoporotic women: results of a cross-sectional study, *The Journal of Clinical Endocrinology and Metabolism* 88:1523-1527. PMID: 12679433
24. **Yilmaz C, Erdemli E, Selek H, et al. (2001)** The contribution of vitamin C to healing of experimental fractures, *Archives of Orthopaedic and Trauma Surgery* 121:426-428. PMID: 11510911
25. **Sarisozen B, Durak K, Dincer G, Bilgen O (2002)** The effects of vitamins E and C on fracture healing on rats, *The Journal of International Medical Research* 30:309-313. PMID: 12166348
26. **Alcantara-Martos T, Delgado-Martinez A, Vega M, et al. (2007)** Effect of vitamin C on fracture healing in elderly Osteogenic Disorder Shionogi rats. The Journal of Bone and Joint Surgery. British Volume. 89:402-407. PMID: 17356161
27. **Yilmaz C, Erdemli E, Selek H, et al. (2001)** The contribution of vitamin C to healing of experimental fractures, *Archives of Orthopaedic and Trauma Surgery* 121:426-428. PMID: 11510911
28. **Sarisozen B, Durak K, Dincer G, Bilgen O (2002)** The effects of vitamins E and C on fracture healing on rats, *The Journal of International Medical Research* 30:309-313. PMID: 12166348
29. **Alcantara-Martos T, Delgado-Martinez A, Vega M, et al. (2007)** Effect of vitamin C on fracture healing in elderly Osteogenic Disorder Shionogi rats, *The Journal of Bone and Joint Surgery*. British Volume. 89:402-407. PMID: 17356161
30. **Sugimoto M, Hirota S, Sato M, et al. (1998)** Impaired expression of noncollagenous bone matrix protein mRNAs during fracture healing in ascorbic acid-deficient rats, *Journal of Bone and Mineral Research* 13:271-278. PMID: 9495521

31. **Franceschi R (1992)** The role of ascorbic acid in mesenchymal differentiation, *Nutrition Reviews* 50:65-70. PMID: 1565288
32. **Sullivan T, Uschmann B, Hough R, Leboy P (1994)** Ascorbate modulation of chondrocyte gene expression is independent of its role in collagen secretion, *The Journal of Biological Chemistry* 269:22500-22506. PMID: 8077198
33. **Bourne G (1942)** Vitamin C and repair of injured tissues, *Lancet* 2:661-664.
34. **Ruskin S (1938)** Studies on the parallel action of vitamin C and calcium, *American Journal of Digestive Diseases* 5:408-411.
35. **Ruskin S, Jonnard R (1938)** Studies in calcium metabolism: II. Further contributions to the comparative studies of the physicochemical properties of the gluconate and cevitamate of calcium and of vitamin C, *American Journal of Digestive Diseases* 5:676-680.
36. **Parsey R, Matteson D (1993)** Ascorbic acid modulation of calcium channels in pancreatic beta cells, *The Journal of General Physiology* 102:503-523. PMID: 8245821
37. **Takuma K, Matsuda T, Asano S, Baba A (1995)** Intracellular ascorbic acid inhibits the Na(+)-Ca2+ exchanger in cultured rat astrocytes, *Journal of Neurochemistry* 64:1536-1540. PMID: 7891080
38. **Salter W, Aub J (1931)** Studies of calcium and phosphorus metabolism. IX. Deposition of calcium in bone in healing scorbutus, *Archives of Pathology* 11:380-382.
39. **Poal-Manresa J, Little K, Trueta J (1970)** Some observations on the effects of vitamin C deficiency on bone, *British Journal of Experimental Pathology* 51:372-378. PMID: 5485760
40. **Simon J, Murtaugh M, Gross M, et al. (2004)** Relation of ascorbic acid to coronary artery calcium: the Coronary Artery Risk Development in Young Adults Study, *American Journal of Epidemiology* 15003962
41. **Maikranz P, Holley J, Parks J, et al. (1989)** Gestational hypercalciuria causes pathological urine calcium oxalate supersaturations, *Kidney International* 36:108-113. PMID: 2811052
42. **Grases F, Garcia-Ferragut L, Costa-Bauza A (1998)** Development of calcium oxalate crystals on urothelium: effect of free radicals, *Nephron* 78:296-301. 9546690
43. **Selvam R (2002)** Calcium oxalate stone disease: role of lipid peroxidation and antioxidants, *Urological Research* 30:35-47. PMID: 11942324
44. **Auer B, Auer D, Rodgers A (1998)** The effect of ascorbic acid ingestion on the biochemical and physicochemical risk factors associated with calcium oxalate kidney stone formation, *Clinical Chemistry and Laboratory Medicine* 36:143-147. PMID: 9589801
45. **Schwille P, Schmiedl A, Herrmann U, et al. (2000)** Ascorbic acid in idiopathic recurrent calcium urolithiasis in humans--does it have an abettor role in oxalate, and calcium oxalate crystallization? *Urological Research* 28:167-177. PMID: 10929425
46. **Curhan G, Willett W, Rimm E, Stampfer M (1996)** A prospective study of the intake of vitamins C and B6, and the risk of kidney stones in men, *The Journal of Urology* 155:1847-1851. PMID: 8618271

47. **Curhan G, Willett W, Speizer F, Stampfer M (1999)** Intake of vitamins B6 and C and the risk of kidney stones in women, *Journal of the American Society of Nephrology* 10:840-845. PMID: 10203369
48. **Gerster H (1997)** No contribution of ascorbic acid to renal calcium oxalate stones, *Annals of Nutrition & Metabolism* 41:269-282. PMID: 9429689
49. **Simon J, Hudes E (1999)** Relation of serum ascorbic acid to serum vitamin B12, serum ferritin, and kidney stones in US adults, *Archives of Internal Medicine* 159:619-624. PMID: 10090119
50. **Gaker L, Butcher N (1986)** Dissolution of staghorn calculus associated with amiloride-hydrochlorothiazide, sulfamethoxazole and trimethoprim, and ascorbic acid, *The Journal of Urology* 135:933-934. PMID: 3959252
51. **Belfield W, Zucker M (1993)** *How to Have a Healthier Dog.* San Jose, CA: Orthomolecular Specialties.
52. **Pandey D, Shekelle R, Selwyn B, et al. (1995)** Dietary vitamin C and beta-carotene and risk of death in middle-aged men. The Western Electric Study, *American Journal of Epidemiology* 142:1269-1278. PMID: 7503047
53. **Kromhout D, Bloemberg D, Feskens E, et al. (2000)** Saturated fat, vitamin C and smoking predict long-term population all-cause mortality rates in the Seven Countries Study, *International Journal of Epidemiology* 29:260-265. PMID: 10817122
54. **Loria C, Klag M, Caulfield L, Whelton P (2000)** Vitamin C status and mortality in US adults, *The American Journal of Clinical Nutrition* 72:139-145. PMID: 10871572
55. **Khah K, Bingham S, Welch A, et al. (2001)** Relation between plasma ascorbic acid and mortality in men and women in EPIC-Norfolk prospective study: a prospective population study. European Prospective Investigation into Cancer and Nutrition, *Lancet* 357:657-663. PMID: 11247548
56. **Simon J, Hudes E, Tice J (2001)** Relation of serum ascorbic acid to mortality among US adults, *Journal of the American College of Nutrition* 20:255-263. PMID: 11444422
57. **Boekholdt S, Meuwese M, Day N, et al. (2006)** Plasma concentrations of ascorbic acid and C-reactive protein, and risk of future coronary artery disease, in apparently healthy men and women: the EPIC-Norfolk prospective population study, *The British Journal of Nutrition* 96:516-522. PMID: 16925857
58. **Jia X, Aucott L, McNeill G (2007)** Nutritional status and subsequent all-cause mortality in men and women aged 75 years or over living in the community, *The British Journal of Nutrition* 98:593-599. PMID: 17442130
59. **Dashti-Khavidaki S, Talasaz A, Tabeefar H, et al. (2011)** Plasma vitamin C concentrations in patients on routine hemodialysis and its relationship to patients' morbidity and mortality, *International Journal for Vitamin and Nutrition Research* 81:197-203. PMID: 22237767
60. **Deicher R, Ziai F, Bieglmayer C, et al. (2005)** Low total vitamin C plasma level is a risk factor for cardiovascular morbidity and mortality in hemodialysis patients, *Journal of the American Society of Nephrology* 16:1811-1818. PMID: 15814831

61. **Dashti-Khavidaki S, Talasaz A, Tabeefar H, et al.** (2011) Plasma vitamin C concentrations in patients on routine hemodialysis and its relationship to patients' morbidity and mortality, *International Journal for Vitamin and Nutrition Research* 81:197-203. PMID: 22237767
62. **Padayatty S, Sun A, Chen Q, et al.** (2010) Vitamin C: intravenous use by complementary and alternative medicine practitioners and adverse effects, *PLoS One* 5:e11414. PMID: 20628650
63. **Go K (1997)** The normal and pathological physiology of brain water, *Advances and Technical Standards in Neurosurgery* 23:47-142. PMID: 9075471

CHAPTER 6 CITATIONS

1. **Iseri L, French J (1984)** Magnesium: nature's physiological calcium blocker, *American Heart Journal* 108:188-193. PMID: 6375330
2. **Altura B (1994)** Introduction: importance of Mg in physiology and medicine and the need for ion selective electrodes, *Scandinavian Journal of Clinical and Laboratory Investigation. Supplementum* 217:5-9. PMID: 7939385
3. **Fawcett W, Haxby E, Male D (1999)** Magnesium: physiology and pharmacology, *British Journal of Anaesthesia* 83:302-320. PMID: 10618948
4. **Saris N, Mervaala E, Karppanen H, et al. (2000)** Magnesium. An update on physiological, clinical and analytical aspects, *Clinica Chimica Acta* 294:1-26. PMID: 10727669
5. **Mazur A, Maier J, Rock E, et al. (2007)** Magnesium and the inflammatory response: potential physiopathological implications, *Archives of Biochemistry and Biophysics* 458:48-56. PMID: 16712775
6. **Lin C, Tsai P, Hung Y, Huang C (2010)** L-type calcium channel blockers are involved in mediating the anti-inflammatory effects of magnesium sulphate, *British Journal of Anaesthesia* 104:44-51. PMID: 19933511
7. **Akhtar M, Ullah H, Hamid M (2011)** Magnesium, a drug of diverse use, *JMPA: The Journal of the Pakistan Medical Association* 61:1220-1225. PMID: 22355971
8. **Anghileri L (2009)** Magnesium, calcium and cancer, *Magnesium Research* 22:247-255. PMID: 20228002
9. **Rude R, Singer F, Gruber H (2009)** Skeletal and hormonal effects of magnesium deficiency, *Journal of the American College of Nutrition* 28:131-141. PMID: 19828898
10. **Steidl L, Ditmar R (1990)** Soft tissue calcification treated with local and oral magnesium therapy, *Magnesium Research* 3:113-119. PMID: 2133625
11. **Stendig-Lindberg G, Tepper R, Leichter I (1993)** Trabecular bone density in a two year controlled trial of peroral magnesium in osteoporosis, *Magnesium Research* 6:155-163. PMID: 8274361
12. **Sojka J, Weaver C (1995)** Magnesium supplementation and osteoporosis, *Nutrition Reviews* 53:71-74. PMID: 7770187
13. **Ryder K, Shorr R, Bush A, et al. (2005)** Magnesium intake from food and supplements is associated with bone mineral density in healthy older white subjects, *Journal of the American Geriatrics Society* 53:1875-1880. PMID: 16274367
14. **Forbes R (1971)** Attempts to alter kidney calcification in the magnesium-deficient rat, *The Journal of Nutrition* 101:35-44. PMID: 5540524
15. **Rufenacht H, Fleisch H (1984)** Measurement of inhibitors of calcium phosphate precipitation in plasma ultrafiltrate, *The American Journal of Physiology* 246:F648-F655. PMID: 6720969
16. **Wutzen J, Lewicki Z (1985)** Histological and ultrastructural changes in femoral muscle of rat caused by low-magnesium diet, *Materia Medica Polona* 17:147-152. PMID: 3831618

17. **Ishimura E, Okuno S, Kitatani K, et al.** (2007) Significant association between the presence of peripheral vascular calcification and lower serum magnesium in hemodialysis patients, *Clinical Nephrology* 68:222-227. PMID: 17969489
18. **Rayssiguier Y (1984)** Role of magnesium and potassium in the pathogenesis of arteriosclerosis, *Magnesium* 3:226-238. PMID: 6399344
19. **Fox C, Ramsoomair D, Carter C (2001)** Magnesium: its proven and potential clinical significance, *Southern Medical Journal* 94:1195-1201. PMID: 11811859
20. **Sun Y, Selvaraj S, Varma A, et al.** (2013) Increase in serum Ca^{2+}/Mg^{2+} ratio promotes proliferation of prostate cancer cells by activating TRPM7 channels, *The Journal of Biological Chemistry* 288:255-263. PMID: 23168410
21. **Barbagallo M, Dominguez L (2007)** Magnesium metabolism in type 2 diabetes mellitus, metabolic syndrome and insulin resistance, *Archives of Biochemistry and Biophysics* 458:40-47. PMID: 16808892
22. **Belin R, He K (2007)** Magnesium physiology and pathogenic mechanisms that contribute to the development of the metabolic syndrome, *Magnesium Research* 20:107-129 PMID: 18062585
23. **Ito M, Sekine I, Kummerow F (1987)** Dietary magnesium effect on swine coronary atherosclerosis induced by hypervitaminosis D, *Acta Pathologica Japonica* 37:955-964. PMID: 2820185
24. **Dimai H, Porta S, Wirnsberger G, et al. (1998)** Daily oral magnesium supplementation suppresses bone turnover in young adult males, *The Journal of Clinical Endocrinology and Metabolism* 83:2742-2748. PMID: 9709941
25. **Aydin H, Deyneli O, Yavuz D, et al. (2010)** Short-term oral magnesium supplementation suppresses bone turnover in postmenopausal osteoporotic women, *Biological Trace Element Research* 133:136-143. PMID: 19488681
26. **Landfield P, Morgan G (1984)** Chronically elevating plasma Mg^{2+} improves hippocampal frequency potentiation and reversal learning in aged and young rats, *Brain Research* 322:167-171. PMID: 6097334
27. **Rude R (1993)** Magnesium metabolism and deficiency, *Endocrinology and Metabolism Clinics of North America* 22:377-395. PMID: 8325293
28. **Rock E, Astier C, Lab C, et al. (1995)** Dietary magnesium deficiency in rats enhances free radical production in skeletal muscle, The *Journal of Nutrition* 125:1205-1210. PMID: 7738680
29. **Malpeuch-Brugere C, Nowacki W, Daveau M, et al. (2000)** Inflammatory response following acute magnesium deficiency in the rat, *Biochimica et Biophysica Acta* 1501:91-98. PMID: 10838183
30. **Nielsen F (2010)** Magnesium, inflammation, and obesity in chronic disease, *Nutrition Reviews* 68:333-340. PMID: 20536778
31. **Weglicki W (2012)** Hypomagnesiumia and inflammation: clinical and basic aspects, *Annual Review of Nutrition* 32:55-71. PMID: 22404119
32. **Bussiere F, Gueux E, Rock E, et al. (2002)** Protective effect of calcium deficiency on the inflammatory response in magnesium-deficient rats, *European Journal of Nutrition* 41:197-202. PMID: 12395213

33. **Johnson S (2001)** The multifaceted and widespread pathology of magnesium deficiency, *Medical Hypotheses* 56:163-170. PMID: 11425281
34. **Maier J (2012)** Endothelial cells and magnesium: implications in atherosclerosis, *Clinical Science* (London, England:1979) 122:397-407. PMID: 22248353
35. **Rayssiguier Y, Durlach J, Gueux E, et al. (1993)** Magnesium and ageing. I. Experimental data: importance of oxidative damage, *Magnesium Research* 6:369-378. PMID: 8155489
36. **Leone N, Courbon D, Ducimetiere P, Zureik M (2006)** Zinc, copper, and magnesium and risks for all-cause, cancer, and cardiovascular mortality, *Epidemiology* (Cambridge, Mass.) 17:308-314. PMID: 16570028
37. **Haglin L, Tornkvist B, Backman L (2007)** Prediction of all-cause mortality in a patient population with hypertension and type 2 DM by using traditional risk factors and serum-phosphate, -calcium, and -magnesium, *Acta Diabetologica* 44:138-143. PMID: 17721752
38. **Ishimura E, Okuno S, Yamakawa T, et al. (2007)** Serum magnesium concentration is a significant predictor of mortality in maintenance hemodialysis patients, *Magnesium Research* 20:237-244. PMID: 18271493
39. **Adamopoulos C, Pitt B, Sui X, et al. (2009)** Low serum magnesium and cardiovascular mortality in chronic heart failure: a propensity-matched study, *International Journal of Cardiology* 136:270-277. PMID: 18672302
40. **Reffelmann T, Ittermann T, Dorr M, et al. (2011)** Low serum magnesium concentrations predict cardiovascular and all-cause mortality, *Atherosclerosis* 219:280-284. PMID: 21703623
41. **Markaki A, Kyriazis J, Stylianou K, et al. (2012)** The role of serum magnesium and calcium on the association between adiponectin levels and all-cause mortality in end-stage renal disease patients, *PLoS One* 7:e52350. PMID: 23285003
42. **Woods K, Fletcher S (1994)** Long-term outcome after intravenous magnesium sulphate in suspected acute myocardial infarction: the second Leicester Intravenous Magnesium Intervention Trial (LIMIT-2), *Lancet* 343:816-819. PMID: 7908076
43. **Shechter M, Hod H, Rabinowitz B, et al. (2003)** Long-term outcome of intravenous magnesium therapy in thrombolysis-ineligible acute myocardial infarction patients, *Cardiology* 99:205-210. PMID: 12845247
44. **Sahmoun A, Singh B (2010)** Does a higher ratio of serum calcium to magnesium increase the risk for postmenopausal breast cancer? *Medical Hypotheses* 75:315-318. PMID: 20371155
45. **Chen G, Pang Z, Liu Q (2012)** Magnesium intake and risk of colorectal cancer: a meta-analysis of prospective studies, *European Journal of Clinical Nutrition* 66:1182-1186. PMID: 23031849
46. **Cheng M, Chiu H, Tai S, et al. (2012)** Calcium and magnesium in drinking-water and risk of death from lung cancer in women, *Magnesium Research* 25:112-119. PMID: 23073359

47. **Qu X, Jin F, Hao Y, et al.** (2013) Nonlinear association between magnesium intake and the risk of colorectal cancer, *European Journal of Gastroenterology & Hepatology* 25:309-318. PMID: 23222473
48. **Malm O (1975)** Calcium and magnesium, *Progress in Food and Nutrition Science* 1:173-182. PMID: 788034
49. **Hung J, Tsai M, Yang B, Chen J (2005)** Maternal osteoporosis after prolonged magnesium sulfate tocolysis therapy: a case report, *Archives of Physical Medicine and Rehabilitation* 86:146-149. PMID: 15641005
50. **Sivas F, Gunesen O, Ozoran K, Alemdaroglu E (2007)** Osteomalacia from Mg-containing antacid; a case report of bilateral hip fracture, *Rheumatology International* 27:679-681. PMID: 17171347

CHAPTER 7 CITATIONS

1. **No authors listed (2009)** Vitamin K2. Monograph, *Alternative Medicine Review* 14:284-293. PMID: 19803553
2. **Tareen B, Summers J, Jamison J, et al. (2008)** A 12 week, open label, phase I/IIa study using apatone for the treatment of prostate cancer patients who have failed standard therapy, International *Journal of Medical Sciences* 5:62-67. PMID: 18392145
3. **McCarty M, Barroso-Aranda J, Contreras F (2010)** Oxidative stress therapy for solid tumors--a proposal, *Medical Hypotheses* 74:1052-1054. PMID: 20089364
4. **Kitano T, Yoda H, Tabata K, et al. (2012)** Vitamin K3 analogs induce selective tumor cytotoxicity in neuroblastoma, *Biological & Pharmaceutical Bulletin* 35:617-623. PMID: 22466570
5. **Tomasetti M, Nocchi L, Neuzil J, et al. (2012)** Alpha-tocopheryl succinate inhibits autophagic survival of prostate cancer cells induced by vitamin K3 and ascorbate to trigger cell death, *PLoS One* 7:e52263. PMID: 23272231
6. **Ferland G (2012)** The discovery of vitamin K and its clinical applications, *Annals of Nutrition & Metabolism* 61:213-218. PMID: 23183291
7. **Vermeer C (2012)** Vitamin K: the effect on health beyond coagulation – an overview, *Food & Nutrition Research* 56:5329. PMID: 22489224
8. **Adams J, Pepping J (2005)** Vitamin K in the treatment and prevention of osteoporosis and arterial calcification, *American Journal of Health-System Pharmacy* 62:1574-1581. PMID: 16030366
9. **Theuwissen E, Smit E, Vermeer C (2012)** The role of vitamin K in soft-tissue calcification, *Advances in Nutrition* 3:166-173. PMID: 22516724
10. **Price P, Faus S, Williamson M (1998)** Warfarin causes rapid calcification of the elastic lamellae in rat arteries and heart valves, *Arteriosclerosis, Thrombosis, and Vascular Biology* 18:1400-1407. PMID: 9743228
11. **Schurgers L, Joosen I, Laufer E, et al. (2012)** Vitamin K-antagonists accelerate atherosclerotic calcification and induce a vulnerable plaque phenotype, *PLoS One* 7:e43229. PMID: 22952653
12. **Schurgers L, Spronk H, Soute B, et al. (2007)** Regression of warfarin-induced medial elastocalcinosis by high intake of vitamin K in rats, *Blood* 109:2823-2831. PMID: 17138823
13. **Falcone T, Kim S, Cortazzo M (2011)** Vitamin K: fracture prevention and beyond, *PM & R: The Journal of Injury, Function, and Rehabilitation* 3:S82-S87. PMID: 21703586
14. **Schurgers L, Uitto J, Reutelingsperger C (2013)** Vitamin K-dependent carboxylation of matrix Gla-protein: a crucial switch to control ectopic mineralization, *Trends in Molecular Medicine* 19:217-226. PMID: 23375872
15. **Rennenberg R, de Leeuw P, Kessels A, et al. (2010)** Calcium scores and matrix Gla protein levels: association with vitamin K status, *European Journal of Clinical Investigation* 40:344-349. PMID: 20486996

16. **Cranenburg E, Vermeer C, Koos R, et al. (2008)** The circulating inactive form of matrix Gla protein (ucMGP) as a biomarker for cardiovascular calcification, *Journal of Vascular Research* 45:427-436. PMID: 18401181
17. **Gast G, de Roos N, Sluijs I, et al. (2009)** A high menaquinone intake reduces the incidence of coronary heart disease, *Nutrition, Metabolism, and Cardiovascular Diseases* 19:504-510. PMID: 19179058
18. **Beulens J, Bots M, Atsma F, et al. (2009)** High dietary menaquinone intake is associated with reduced coronary calcification, *Atherosclerosis* 203:489-493. PMID: 18722618
19. **Shea M, O'Donnell C, Hoffman U, et al. (2009)** Vitamin K supplementation and progression of coronary artery calcium in older men and women, *The American Journal of Clinical Nutrition* 89:1799-1807. PMID: 19386744
20. **Graham G, Blaha M, Budoff M, et al. (2012)** Impact of coronary artery calcification on all-cause mortality in individuals with and without hypertension, *Atherosclerosis* 225:432-437. PMID: 23078882
21. **Kramer C, Zinman B, Gross J, et al. (2013)** Coronary artery calcium score prediction of all cause mortality and cardiovascular events in people with type 2 diabetes: systemic review and meta-analysis, *BMJ* 346:f1654. PMID: 23529983
22. **Kalsch H, Lehmann N, Berg M, et al. (2013)** Coronary artery calcification outperforms thoracic aortic calcification for the prediction of myocardial infarction and all-cause mortality: The Heintz Nixdorf Recall Study, *European Journal of Preventive Cardiology* Mar 6. [Epub ahead of print]. PMID: 23467675
23. **Rennenberg R, Kessels A, Schurgers L, et al. (2009)** Vascular calcifications as a marker of increased cardiovascular risk: a meta-analysis, *Vascular Health and Risk Management* 5:185-197. PMID: 19436645
24. **Noordzij M, Cranenburg E, Engelsman L, et al. (2011)** Progression of aortic calcification is associated with disorders of mineral metabolism and mortality in chronic dialysis patients, *Nephrology, Dialysis, Transplantation* 26:1662-1669. PMID: 20880929
25. **Ueland T, Gullestad L, Dahl C, et al. (2010)** Undercarboxylated matrix Gla protein is associated with indices of heart failure and mortality in symptomatic aortic stenosis, *Journal of Internal Medicine* 268:483-492. PMID: 20804515
26. **Schlieper G, Westenfeld R, Kruger T, et al. (2011)** Circulating nonphosphorylated carboxylated matrix GLA protein predicts survival in ESRD, *Journal of the American Society of Nephrology* 22:387-395. PMID: 21289218
27. **Geleijnse J, Vermeer C, Grobbee D, et al. (2004)** Dietary intake of menaquinone is associated with a reduced risk of coronary heart disease: The Rotterdam Study, *The Journal of Nutrition* 134:3100-3105. PMID: 15514282
28. **Azuma K, Ouchi Y, Inoue S (2013)** Vitamin K: novel molecular mechanisms of action and its roles in osteoporosis, *Geriatrics & Gerontology International* Mar 26. [Epub ahead of print]. PMID: 23530597

29. **Habu D, Shiomi S, Tamori A, et al. (2004)** Role of vitamin K2 in the development of hepatocellular carcinoma in women with viral cirrhosis of the liver, *The Journal of the American Medical Association* 292:358-361. PMID: 15265851

30. **Mizuta T, Ozaki I, Eguchi Y, et al. (2006)** The effect of menatetrenone, a vitamin K2 analog, on disease recurrence and survival in patients with hepatocellular carcinoma after curative treatment: a pilot study, *Cancer* 106:867-872. PMID: 16400650

31. **Kakizaki S, Sohara N, Sato K, et al. (2007)** Preventive effects of vitamin K on recurrent disease in patients with hepatocellular carcinoma arising from hepatitis C viral infection, *Journal of Gastroenterology and Hepatology* 22:518-522. PMID: 17376044

32. **Azuma K, Urano T, Ouchi Y, Inoue S (2009)** Vitamin K2 suppresses proliferation and motility of hepatocellular carcinoma cells by activating steroid and xenobiotic receptor, *Endocrine Journal* 56:843-849. PMID: 19550077

33. **Sakai I, Hashimoto S, Yoda M, et al. (1994)** Novel role of vitamin K2: a potent inducer of differentiation of various human myeloid leukemia cell lines, *Biochemical and Biophysical Research Communications* 205:1305-1310. PMID: 7802663

34. **Tamori A, Habu D, Shiomi S, et al. (2007)** Potential role of vitamin K(2) as a chemopreventive agent against hepatocellular carcinoma. *Hepatology Research* 37:S303-S307. PMID: 17877500

35. **Takami A, Nakao S, Ontachi Y, et al. (1999)** Successful therapy of myelodysplastic syndrome with menatetrenone, a vitamin K2 analog, *International Journal of Hematology* 69:24-26. PMID: 10641439

36. **van Summeren M, Braam L, Lilien M, et al. (2009)** The effect of menaquinone-7 (vitamin K2) supplementation on osteocalcin carboxylation in healthy prepubertal children, *The British Journal of Nutrition* 102:1171-1178. PMID: 19450370

37. **Furusyo N, Ihara T, Hayaski T, et al. (2013)** The serum undercarboxylated osteocalcin level and the diet of a Japanese population: results from the Kyushu and Okinawa Population Study (KOPS), *Endocrine* 43:635-642. PMID: 23001602

38. **Cheung A, Tile L, Lee Y, et al. (2008)** Vitamin K supplementation in postmenopausal women with osteopenia (ECKO trial): a randomized controlled trial, *PLoS Medicine* 5:e196. PMID: 18922041

39. **No authors listed (2009)** Docosahexaenoic acid (DHA). Monograph, *Alternative Medicine Review* 14:391-399. PMID: 20030466

40. **Thijssen H, Vervoort L, Schurgers L, Shearer M (2006)** Menadione is a metabolite of oral vitamin K, *The British Journal of Nutrition* 95:260-266. PMID: 16469140

41. **Yamaguchi M, Taguchi H, Gao Y, et al. (1999)** Effect of vitamin K2 (menaquinone-7) in fermented soybean (natto) on bone loss in ovariectomized rats, *Journal of Bone and Mineral Metabolism* 17:23-29. PMID: 10084398

42. **Iwamoto J, Takeda T, Sato Y (2006)** Menatetrenone (vitamin K2) and bone quality in the treatment of postmenopausal osteoporosis. *Nutrition Reviews* 64:509-517. PMID: 17274493

43. **Yamaguchi M, Taguchi H, Gao Y, et al. (1999)** Effect of vitamin K2 (menaquinone-7) in fermented soybean (natto) on bone loss in ovariectomized rats, *Journal of Bone and Mineral Metabolism* 17:23-29. PMID: 10084398

44. **Tasci A, Bilgili H, Altunay H, et al. (2011)** Prospective evaluation of vitamin K2, raloxifene and their co-administration in osteoporotic rats, *European Journal of Pharmaceutical Sciences* 43:270-277. PMID: 21575717

45. **Tsukamoto Y (2004)** Studies on action of menaquinone-7 in regulation of bone metabolism and its preventive role of osteoporosis, *Biofactors* 22:5-19. PMID: 15630245

46. **Prabhoo R, Prabhoo T (2010)** Vitamin K2: a novel therapy for osteoporosis, *Journal of the Indian Medical Association* 108:253-254, 256-258. PMID: 21114195

47. **Vermeer C (2012)** Vitamin K: the effect on health beyond coagulation – an overview, *Food & Nutrition Research* 56:5329. PMID: 22489224

48. **Sogabe N, Maruyama R, Baba O, et al. (2011)** Effects of long-term vitamin K(1) (phylloquinone) or vitamin K(2) (menaquinone-4) supplementation on body composition and serum parameters in rats. *Bone* 48:1036-1042. PMID: 21295170

49. **Iwamoto J, Matsumoto H, Takeda T, et al. (2010)** Effects of vitamin K2 on cortical and cancellous bone mass, cortical osteocyte and lacunar system, and porosity in sciatic neurectomized rats, *Calcified Tissue International* 87:254-262. PMID: 20556371

50. **Fusaro M, Noale M, Viola V, et al. (2012)** Vitamin K, vertebral fractures, vascular calcifications, and mortality: Vitamin K Italian (VIKI) dialysis study, *Journal of Bone and Mineral Research* 27:2271-2278. PMID: 22692665

51. **Cockayne S, Adamson J, Lanham-New S, et al. (2006)** Vitamin K and the prevention of fractures: systematic review and meta-analysis of randomized controlled trials, *Archives of Internal Medicine* 166:1256-1261. PMID: 16801507

52. **Azuma K, Inoue S (2009)** [Vitamin K function mediated by activation of steroid and xenobiotic receptor]. [Article in Japanese], *Clinical Calcium* 19:1770-1778. PMID: 19949268

53. **Nakano T, Tsugawa N, Kuwabara A, et al. (2011)** High prevalence of hypovitaminosis D and K in patients with hip fracture, *Asia Pacific Journal of Clinical Nutrition* 20:56-61. PMID: 21393111

54. **Vermeer C, Theuwissen E (2011)** Vitamin K, osteoporosis and degenerative diseases of aging, *Menopause International* 17:19-23. PMID: 21427421

55. **Knapen M, Drummen N, Smit E, et al. (2013)** Three-year low-dose menaquinone-7 supplementation helps decrease bone loss in healthy postmenopausal women, *Osteoporosis International* Mar 23. [Epub ahead of print]. PMID: 23525894

56. **Forli L, Bollerslev J, Simonsen S, et al. (2010)** Dietary vitamin K2 supplement improves bone status after lung and heart transplantation, *Transplantation* 89:458-464. PMID: 20177349

57. **Iwamoto J, Sato Y, Takeda T, Matsumoto H (2011)** Bone quality and vitamin K2 in type 2 diabetes: review of preclinical and clinical studies, *Nutrition Reviews* 69:162-167. PMID: 21348880
58. **Shiraki M, Shiraki Y, Aoki C, Miura M (2000)** Vitamin K2 (menatetrenone) effectively prevents fractures and sustains lumbar bone mineral density in osteoporosis, *Journal of Bone and Mineral Research* 15:515-521. PMID: 10750566
59. **Ozuru R, Sugimoto T, Yamaguchi T, Chihara K (2002)** Time-dependent effects of vitamin K2 (menatetrenone) on bone metabolism in postmenopausal women, *Endocrine Journal* 49:363-370. PMID: 12201222
60. **Saito M (2009)** [Effect of vitamin K on bone material properties]. [Article in Japanese], *Clinical Calcium* 19:1797-1804. PMID: 19949271
61. **Tsuchie H, Miyakoshi N, Hongo M, et al. (2012)** Amelioration of pregnancy-associated osteoporosis after treatment with vitamin K2: a report of four patients, *Upsala Journal of Medical Sciences* 117:336-341. PMID: 22746299
62. **Koitaya N, Ezaki J, Nishimuta M, et al. (2009)** Effect of low dose vitamin K2 (MK-4) supplementation on bio-indices in postmenopausal Japanese women, *Journal of Nutritional Science and Vitaminology* 55:15-21. PMID: 19352059
63. **Amizuka N, Li M, Kobayashi M, et al. (2008)** Vitamin K2, a gamma-carboxylating factor of GLA-proteins, normalizes the bone crystal nucleation impaired by Mg-insufficiency, *Histology and Histopathology* 23:1353-1366. PMID: 18785118
64. **Kidd P (2010)** Vitamins D and K as pleiotropic nutrients: clinical importance to the skeletal and cardiovascular systems and preliminary evidence for synergy, *Alternative Medicine Review* 15:199-222. PMID: 21155624
65. **Iwamoto J, Sato Y, Takeda T, Matsumoto H (2012)** Strategy for prevention of hip fractures in patients with Parkinson's disease, *World Journal of Orthopedics* 3:137-141. PMID: 23173109
66. **Saito E, Wachi H, Sato F, et al. (2007)** Treatment with vitamin K(2) combined with bisphosphonates synergistically inhibits calcification in cultured smooth muscle cells, *Journal of Atherosclerosis and Thrombosis* 14:317-314. PMID: 18174662
67. **Matsumoto Y, Mikuni-Takagaki Y, Kozai Y, et al. (2009)** Prior treatment with vitamin K(2) significantly improves the efficacy of risedronate, *Osteoporosis International* 20:1863-1872. PMID: 19280272
68. **Kanellakis S, Moschonis G, Tenta R, et al. (2012)** Changes in parameters of bone metabolism in postmenopausal women following a 12-month intervention period using dairy products enriched with calcium, vitamin D, and phylloquinone (vitamin K(1)) or menaquinone-7 (vitamin K(2)): the Postmenopausal Health Study II, *Calcified Tissue International* 90:251-262. PMID: 22392526
69. **Yaegashi Y, Onoda T, Tanno K, et al. (2008)** Association of hip fracture incidence and intake of calcium, magnesium, vitamin D, and vitamin K, *European Journal of Epidemiology* 23:219-225. PMID: 18214692

70. **Masterjohn C (2007)** Vitamin D toxicity redefined: vitamin K and the molecular mechanism, *Medical Hypotheses* 68:1026-1034. PMID: 17145139
71. **Pucaj K, Rasmussen H, Moller M, Preston T (2011)** Safety and toxicological evaluation of a synthetic vitamin K2, menaquinone-7, *Toxicology Mechanisms and Methods* 21:520-532. PMID: 21781006
72. **Shimada H, Himeno K, Michimoto T, et al. (1990)** [Prevention of vitamin K deficiency in the early neonatal period--prophylactic oral administration of VK to the mother]. [Article in Japanese], *Nihon Sanka Fujinka, Gakkai Zasshi* 42:705-710. PMID: 2212808
73. **Tsuchie H, Miyakoshi N, Hongo M, et al. (2012)** Amelioration of pregnancy-associated osteoporosis after treatment with vitamin K2: a report of four patients, *Upsala Journal of Medical Sciences* 117:336-341. PMID: 22746299
74. **Stevenson M, Lloyd-Jones M, Papaioannou D (2009)** Vitamin K to prevent fractures in older women: systemic review and economic evaluation, *Health Technology Assessment* 13:1-134. PMID: 19818211

CHAPTER 8 CITATIONS

1. **Trivedi D, Doll R, Khaw K (2003)** Effect of four monthly oral vitamin D3 (cholecalciferol) supplementation on fractures and mortality in men and women living in the community: randomised double blind controlled trial, *BMJ* 326:469. PMID: 12609940
2. **Bischoff-Ferrari H, Willett W, Orav E, et al. (2012)** A pooled analysis of vitamin D dose requirements for fracture prevention, *The New England Journal of Medicine* 367:40-49. PMID: 22762317
3. **Rizzoli R, Boonen S, Brandi M, et al. (2013)** Vitamin D supplementation in elderly or postmenopausal women: a 2013 update of the 2008 recommendations from the European Society for Clinical and Economic Aspects of Osteoporosis and Osteoarthritis (ESCEO), *Current Medical Research and Opinion* Feb 7 [Epub ahead of print]. PMID: 23320612
4. **Burgi A, Gorham E, Garland C, et al. (2011)** High serum 25-hydroxyvitamin D is associated with a low incidence of stress fractures, *Journal of Bone and Mineral Research* 26:2371-2377. PMID: 21698667
5. **Narula R, Tauseef M, Ahmad I, et al. (2013)** Vitamin D deficiency among postmenopausal women with osteoporosis. *Journal of Clinical and Diagnostic Research* 7:336-338. PMID: 23543783
6. **James J, Massey P, Hollister A, Greber E (2013)** Prevalence of hypovitaminosis D among children with upper extremity fractures, *Journal of Pediatric Orthopedics* 33:159-162. PMID: 23389570
7. **Johnson A, Smith JJ, Smith JM, Sanzone A (2013)** Vitamin D insufficiency in patients with acute hip fractures of all ages and both sexes in a sunny climate, *Journal of Orthopaedic Trauma* Mar 19. [Epub ahead of print]. PMID: 23515125
8. **Mehrotra R, Ranjan A, Lath R, and Ratnam R (2012)** Postmenopausal osteoporosis: our experience, *Indian Journal of Endocrinology and Metabolism* 16:S421-S422. PMID: 23565450
9. **Maierhofer W, Gray R, Cheung H, Lemann J Jr (1983)** Bone resorption stimulated by elevated serum 1,25-(OH)2-vitamin D concentrations in healthy men, *Kidney International* 24:555-560. PMID: 6689038
10. **Allen S, Shah J (1992)** Calcinosis and metastatic calcification due to vitamin D intoxication. A case report and review, *Hormone Research* 37:68-77. PMID: 1398478
11. **Masterjohn C (2007)** Vitamin D toxicity redefined: vitamin K and the molecular mechanism, *Medical Hypotheses* 68:1026-1034. PMID: 17145139
12. **Adams J, Lee G (1997)** Gains in bone mineral density with resolution of vitamin D intoxication, *Annals of Internal Medicine* 127:203-206. PMID: 9245225
13. **Lips P (2001)** Vitamin D deficiency and secondary hyperparathyroidism in the elderly: consequences for bone loss and fractures and therapeutic implications, *Endocrine Reviews* 22:477-501. PMID: 11493580

14. **von Hurst P, Stonehouse W, Kruger M, Coad J (2010)** Vitamin D supplementation suppresses age-induced bone turnover in older women who are vitamin D deficient, *The Journal of Steroid Biochemistry and Molecular Biology* 121:293-296. PMID: 20304051
15. **Adams J, Kantorovich V, Wu C, et al. (1999)** Resolution of vitamin D insufficiency in osteopenic patients results in rapid recovery of bone mineral density, *The Journal of Clinical Endocrinology & Metabolism* 84:2729-2730. PMID: 10443668
16. **Pekkinen M, ViljakainenvH, Saarnio E, et al. (2012)** Vitamin D is a major determinant of bone mineral density at school age, *PLoS One* 7:e40090. PMID: 22768331
17. **Kurabayashi M (2012)** [Is calcium supplement useful in aged persons? Calcium supplement doesn't reduce the fracture and vascular risk in aged persons]. [Article in Japanese], *Clinical Calcium* 22:736-739. PMID: 22549199
18. **Wacker M, Holick M (2013)** Vitamin D – effects on skeletal and extraskeletal health and the need for supplementation, *Nutrients* 5:111-148. PMID: 23306192
19. **Carlberg C, Molnar F (2012)** Current status of vitamin D signaling and its therapeutic applications, *Current Topics in Medicinal Chemistry* 12:528-547. PMID: 22242854
20. **Sakthiswary R, Raymond A (2013)** The clinical significance of vitamin D in systemic lupus erythematosus: a systematic review, *PLoS One* 8:e55275. PMID: 23383135
21. **Jones G (2012)** Metabolism and biomarkers of vitamin D, *Scandinavian Journal of Clinical and Laboratory Investigation. Supplementum* 243:7-13. PMID: 22536757
22. **Blomberg M (2012)** Vitamin D metabolism, sex hormones, and male reproductive function, *Reproduction* (Cambridge, England) 144:135-152. PMID: 22635305
23. **Ceglia L Harris S (2013)** Vitamin D and its role in skeletal muscle, *Calcified Tissue International* 92:151-162. PMID: 22968766
24. **Girgis C, Clifton-Bligh R, Hamrick M, et al. (2013)** The roles of vitamin D in skeletal muscle: form, function, and metabolism, *Endocrine Reviews* 34:33-83. PMID: 23169676
25. **Munger K, Levin L, Hollis B, et al. (2006)** Serum 25-hydroxyvitamin D levels and risk of multiple sclerosis, *The Journal of the American Medical Association* 296:2832-2838. PMID: 17179460
26. **Carlberg C, Campbell M (2013)** Vitamin D receptor signaling mechanisms: integrated actions of a well-defined transcription factor, *Steroids* 78:127-136. PMID: 23178257
27. **Holick M (2013)** Vitamin D, sunlight and cancer connection, *Anti-Cancer Agents in Medicinal Chemistry* 13:70-82. PMID: 23094923
28. **Nemazannikova N, Antonas K, Dass C (2013)** Role of vitamin D metabolism in cutaneous tumour formation and progression, *The Journal of Pharmacy and Pharmacology* 65:2-10. PMID: 23215682
29. **Korn S, Hubner M, Jung M, et al. (2013)** Severe and uncontrolled adult asthma is associated with vitamin D insufficiency and deficiency, *Respiratory Research* 14:25. [Epub ahead of print]. PMID: 23432854

30. **Erten S, Kucuksahin O, Sahin A, et al. (2013)** Decreased plasma vitamin D levels in patients with undifferentiated spondyloarthritis and ankylosing spondylitis. *Internal Medicine* (Tokyo, Japan) 52:339-344. PMID: 23370741
31. **Bearden A, Abad C, Gangnon R, et al. (2013)** Cross-sectional study of vitamin D levels, immunologic and virologic outcomes in HIV-infected adults, *The Journal of Clinical Epidemiology and Metabolism* Mar 1. [Epub ahead of print]. PMID: 23457406
32. **Scragg R, Jackson R, Holdaway I, et al. (1990)** Myocardial infarction is inversely associated with plasma 25-hydroxyvitamin D3 levels: a community-based study, *International Journal of Epidemiology* 19:599-563. PMID: 2262248
33. **Yang L, Ma J, Zhang X, et al. (2012)** Protective role of the vitamin D receptor, *Cellular Immunology* 279:160-166. PMID: 23246677
34. **Arnson Y, Itzhaky D, Mosseri M, et al. (2013)** Vitamin D inflammatory cytokines and coronary events: a comprehensive review, *Clinical Reviews in Allergy & Immunology* Jan 12. [Epub ahead of print]. PMID: 23314982
35. **Grant W, Boucher B (2011)** Requirements for vitamin D across the life span, *Biological Research for Nursing* 13:120-133. PMID: 21242196
36. **Semba R, Houston D, Bandinelli S, et al. (2010)** Relationship of 25-hydroxyvitamin D with all-cause and cardiovascular disease mortality in older community-dwelling adults, *European Journal of Clinical Nutrition* 64:203-209. PMID: 19953106
37. **Ginde A, Scragg R, Schwartz R, Camargo C Jr (2009)** Prospective study of serum 25-hydroxyvitamin D level, cardiovascular disease mortality, and all-cause mortality in older U.S. adults, *Journal of the American Geriatrics Society* 57:1595-1603. PMID: 19549021
38. **Giovannucci E, Liu Y, Hollis B, Rimm E (2008)** 25-hydroxyvitamin D and risk of myocardial infarction in men: a prospective study, *Archives of Internal Medicine* 168:1174-1180. PMID: 18541825
39. **Melamed M, Michos E, Post W, Astor B (2008)** 25-hydroxyl vitamin D levels and the risk of mortality in the general population, *Archives of Internal Medicine* 168:1629-1637. PMID: 18695076
40. **Hutchinson M, Grimnes G, Joakimsen R, et al. (2010)** Low serum 25-hydroxyvitamin D levels are associated with increased all-cause mortality risk in a general population: the Tromso study, *European Journal of Endocrinology* 162:935-942. PMID: 20185562
41. **Saliba W, Barnett O, Rennert H, Rennert G (2012)** The risk of all-cause mortality is inversely related to serum 25(OH)D levels, *The Journal of Clinical Endocrinology and Metabolism* 97:2792-2798. PMID: 22648653
42. **Schierbeck L, Rejnmark L, Tofteng C, et al. (2012)** Vitamin D deficiency in postmenopausal, healthy women predicts increased cardiovascular events: a 16-year follow-up study, *European Journal of Endocrinology* 167:553-560. PMID: 22875588
43. **Thomas G, o Hartaigh B, Bosch J, et al. (2012)** Vitamin D levels predict all-cause and cardiovascular disease mortality in subjects with the metabolic syndrome: the Ludwigshafen Risk and Cardiovascular Health (LURIC) Study, *Diabetes Care* 35:1158-1164. PMID: 22399697

45. **Schottker B, Haug U, Schomburg L, et al. (2013)** Strong associations of 25-hydroxyvitamin D concentrations with all-cause, cardiovascular, cancer, and respiratory disease mortality in a large cohort study, *The American Journal of Clinical Nutrition* 97:782-793. PMID: 23446902
46. **Raisz L, Trummel C, Holick M, DeLuca H (1972)** 1,25-dihydroxycholecalciferol: a potent stimulator of bone resorption in tissue culture, *Science* 175:768-769. PMID: 4333399
47. **Boris A, Hurley J, Trmal T (1979)** In vivo studies in chicks and rats of bone calcium mobilization by 1 alpha,25-dihydroxycholecalciferol (calcitriol) and its congeners, *The Journal of Nutrition* 109:1772-1778. PMID: 226665
48. **Maierhofer W, Gray R, Cheung H, Lemann J Jr. (1983)** Bone resorption stimulated by elevated serum 1,25-(OH)2-vitamin D concentrations in healthy men, *Kidney International* 24:555-560. PMID: 6689038
49. **Adams J, Kantorovich V, Wu C, et al. (1999)** Resolution of vitamin D insufficiency in osteopenic patients results in rapid recovery of bone mineral density, *The Journal of Clinical Endocrinology & Metabolism* 84:2729-2730. PMID: 10443668
50. **Adams J, Lee G (1997)** Gains in bone mineral density with resolution of vitamin D intoxication, *Annals of Internal Medicine* 127:203-206. PMID: 9245225
51. **Allen S, Shah J (1992)** Calcinosis and metastatic calcification due to vitamin D intoxication. A case report and review, *Hormone Research* 37:68-77. PMID: 1398478
52. **Adams J (1989)** Vitamin D metabolite-mediated hypercalcemia, *Endocrinology and Metabolism Clinics of North America* 18:765-778. PMID: 2673772
53. **Shetty K, Ajiouni K, Rosenfeld P, Hagen T (1975)** Protracted vitamin D intoxication, *Archives of Internal Medicine* 135:986-988. PMID: 1080406

References

CHAPTER 9 CITATIONS

1. **Kruger M, Horrobin D (1997)** Calcium metabolism, osteoporosis and essential fatty acids: a review, *Progress in Lipid Research* 36:131-151. PMID: 9624425
2. **No authors listed (2000)** Fish oil. Monograph, *Alternative Medicine Review* 5:576-580. PMID: 11134981
3. **von Schacky C, Angerer P, Kothny W, et al. (1999)** The effect of dietary omega-3 fatty acids on coronary atherosclerosis. A randomized, double-blind, placebo-controlled trial, *Annals of Internal Medicine* 130:554-562. PMID: 10189324
4. **Richardson A, Puri B (2002)** A randomized double-blind, placebo-controlled study of the effects of supplementation with highly unsaturated fatty acids on ADHD-related symptoms in children with specific learning difficulties, *Progress in Neuro-Psychopharmacology & Biological Psychiatry* 26:233-239. PMID: 11817499
5. **Morris M, Evans D, Bienias J, et al. (2003)** Consumption of fish and n-3 fatty acids and risk of incident Alzheimer disease, *Archives of Neurology* 60:940-946. PMID: 12873849
6. **Covington M (2004)** Omega-3 fatty acids, *American Family Physician* 70:133-140. PMID: 15259529
7. **Wu M, Harvey K, Ruzmetov N, et al. (2005)** Omega-3 polyunsaturated fatty acids attenuate breast cancer growth through activation of a neutral sphingomyelinase-mediated pathway, *International Journal of Cancer* 117:340-348. PMID: 15900589
8. **Iso H, Kobayashi M, Ishihara J, et al. (2006)** Intake of fish and n3 fatty acids and risk of coronary heart disease among Japanese: the Japan Public Health Center-Based (JPHC) Study Cohort I, *Circulation* 113:195-202. PMID: 16401768
9. **Hoffman D, Boettcher J, Diersen-Schade D (2009)** Toward optimizing vision and cognition in term infants by dietary docosahexaenoic acid and arachidonic acid supplementation: a review of randomized controlled trials, *Prostaglandins, Leukotrienes, and Essential Fatty Acids* 81:151-158. PMID: 19505812
10. **Yurko-Mauro K (2010)** Cognitive and cardiovascular benefits of docosahexaenoic acid in aging and cognitive decline, *Current Alzheimer Research* 7:190-196. PMID: 20088810
11. **Guttler N, Zheleva K, Parahuleva M, et al. (2012)** Omega-3 fatty acids and vitamin D in cardiology, *Cardiology Research and Practice* 2012:729670. PMID: 23346457
12. **Weitz D, Weintraub H, Fisher E, Schwartzbard A (2010)** Fish oil for the treatment of cardiovascular disease, *Cardiology in Review* 18:258-263. PMID: 20699674
13. **Maskrey B, Megson I, Rossi A, Whitfield P (2013)** Emerging importance of omega-3 fatty acids in the innate immune response: molecular mechanisms and lipidomic strategies for their analysis, *Molecular Nutrition & Food Research* Feb 18. [Epub ahead of print]. PMID: 23417926

14. **Casado-Diaz A, Santiago-Mora R, Dorado G, Quesada-Gomez J (2013)** The omega-6 arachidonic fatty acid, but not the omega-3 fatty acids, inhibits osteoblastogenesis and induces adipogenesis of human mesenchymal stem cells: potential implication in osteoporosis, Osteoporosis International 24:1647-1661. PMID: 23104199
15. **Nikolakopoulou Z, Shaikh M, Dehlawi H, et al. (2013)** The induction of apoptosis in pre-malignant keratinocytes by omega-3 polyunsaturated fatty acids docosahexaenoic acid (DHA) and eicosapentaenoic acid (EPA) in inhibited by albumin, *Toxicology Letters* 218:150-158. PMID: 23391486
16. **Fahrmann J, Hardman W (2013)** Omega 3 fatty acids increase the chemo-sensitivity of B-CLL-derived cell lines EHEB and MEC-2 and of B-PLL-derived cell line JVM-2 to anti-cancer drugs doxorubicin, vincristine and fludarabine, *Lipids in Health and Disease* 12:36. PMID: 23497075
17. **Calder P (2013)** n-3 fatty acids, inflammation and immunity: new mechanisms to explain old actions, *The Proceedings of the Nutrition Society* May 14. [Epub ahead of print]. PMID: 23668691
18. **Flock M, Rogers C, Prabhu K, Kris-Etherton P (2013)** Immunometabolic role of long-chain omega-3 fatty acids in obesity-induced inflammation, *Diabetes/Metabolism Research and Reviews* Apr 16. [Epub ahead of print]. PMID: 23592441
19. **Pages N, Maurois P, Delplanque B, et al. (2011)** Brain protection by rapeseed oil in magnesium-deficient mice, *Prostaglandins, Leukotrienes, and Essential Fatty Acids* 85:53-60. PMID: 21664114
20. **Ye S, Tan L, Ma J, et al. (2010)** Polyunsaturated docosahexaenoic acid suppresses oxidative stress induced endothelial cell calcium influx by altering lipid composition in membrane caveolar rafts, *Prostaglandins, Leukotrienes, and Essential Fatty Acids* 83:37-43. PMID: 20206488
21. **Kruger M, Schollum L (2005)** Is docosahexaenoic acid more effective than eicosapentaenoic acid for increasing calcium bioavailability? *Prostaglandins, Leukotrienes, and Essential Fatty Acids* 73:327-334. PMID: 16154334
22. **Bonnet N, Ferrari S (2011)** Effects of long-term supplementation with omega-3 fatty acids on longitudinal changes in bone mass and microstructure in mice. *The Journal of Nutritional Biochemistry* 22:665-672. PMID: 21036590
23. **Tarlton J, Wilkins L, Toscano M, et al. (2013)** Reduced bone breakage and increased bone strength in free range laying hens fed omega-3 polyunsaturated fatty acid supplemented diets, *Bone* 52:578-586. PMID: 23142806
24. **No authors listed (2009)** Docosahexaenoic acid (DHA). Monograph, *Alternative Medicine Review* 14:391-399. PMID: 20030466
25. **Kruger M, Horrobin D (1997)** Calcium metabolism, osteoporosis and essential fatty acids: a review. *Progress in Lipid Research* 36:131-151. PMID: 9624425
26. **Schlemmer C, Coetzer H, Claassen N, et al. (1998)** Ectopic calcification of rat aortas and kidneys is reduced with n-3 fatty acid supplementation, *Prostaglandins, Leukotrienes, and Essential Fatty Acids* 59:221-227. PMID: 9844996

27. **Burgess N, Reynolds T, Williams N, et al. (1995)** Evaluation of four animal models of intrarenal calcium deposition and assessment of the influence of dietary supplementation with essential fatty acids on calcification, *Urological Research* 23:239-242. PMID: 8533210
28. **Maggio M, Artoni A, Lauretani F, et al. (2009)** The impact of omega-3 fatty acids on osteoporosis, *Current Pharmaceutical Design* 15:4157-4164. PMID: 20041817
29. **Siener R, Jansen B, Watzer B, Hesse A (2011)** Effect of n-3 fatty acid supplementation on urinary risk factors for calcium oxalate stone formation, *The Journal of Urology* 185:719-724. PMID: 21168878
30. **Buck A, Davies R, Harrison T (1991)** The protective role of eicosapentaenoic acid [EPA] in the pathogenesis of nephrolithiasis, *The Journal of Urology* 146:188-194. PMID: 2056589
31. **Ortiz-Alvarado O, Miyaoka R, Kriedberg C, et al. (2012)** Omega-3 fatty acids eicosapentaenoic acid and docosahexaenoic acid in the management of hypercalciuric stone formers, *Urology* 79:282-286. PMID: 22000931
32. **Albertazzi P, Coupland K (2002)** Polyunsaturated fatty acids. Is there a role in postmenopausal osteoporosis prevention? *Maturitas* 42:13-22. PMID: 12020975
33. **Orchard T, Pan X, Cheek F, et al. (2012)** A systematic review of omega-3 fatty acids and osteoporosis, *The British Journal of Nutrition* 107:S253-S260. PMID: 22591899
34. **Farina E, Kiel D, Roubenoff R, et al. (2012)** Plasma phosphatidylcholine concentrations of polyunsaturated fatty acids are differentially associated with hip bone mineral density and hip fracture in older adults: the Framingham Osteoporosis Study, *Journal of Bone and Mineral Research* 27:1222-1230. PMID: 22392875
35. **Kruger M, Coetzer H, de Winter R, et al. (1998)** Calcium, gamma-linolenic acid and eicosapentaenoic acid supplementation in senile osteoporosis, *Aging* (Milan, Italy) 10:385-394. PMID: 9932142
36. **Moon H, Kim T, Byun D, Park Y (2012)** Positive correlation between erythrocyte levels of n-3 polyunsaturated fatty acids and bone mass in postmenopausal Korean women with osteoporosis, *Annals of Nutrition & Metabolism* 60:146-153. PMID: 22507833
37. **Jarvinen R, Tuppurainen M, Erkkila A, et al. (2012)** Associations of dietary polyunsaturated fatty acids with bone mineral density in elderly women. *European Journal of Clinical Nutrition* 66:496-503. PMID: 22113249
38. **Lappe J, Kunz I, Bendik I, et al. (2013)** Effect of a combination of genistein, polyunsaturated fatty acids and vitamins D3 and K1 on bone mineral density in postmenopausal women: a randomized, placebo-controlled, double-blind pilot study, *European Journal of Nutrition* 52:203-215. PMID: 22302614
39. **Delgado-Lista J, Perez-Martinez P, Lopez-Miranda J, Perez-Jimenez F (2012)** Long chain omega-3 fatty acids and cardiovascular disease: a systematic review, *The British Journal of Nutrition* 107:S201-S213. PMID: 22591894
40. **Poole C, Halcox J, Jenkins-Jones S, et al. (2013)** Omega-3 fatty acids and mortality outcome in patients with and without type 2 diabetes after myocardial infarction: a respective, matched-cohort study, *Clinical Therapeutics* 35:40-51. PMID: 23246017

41. **Wang M, Thomas G, Ho S, et al. (2011)** Fish consumption and mortality in Hong Kong Chinese--the LIMOR study, *Annals of Epidemiology* 21:164-169. PMID: 21109449
42. **Einvik G, Klemsdal T, Sandvik L, Hjerkinn E (2010)** A randomized clinical trial on n-3 polyunsaturated fatty acids supplementation and all-cause mortality in elderly men at high cardiovascular risk, *European Journal of Cardiovascular Prevention and Rehabilitation* 17:588-592. PMID: 20389249
43. **Hamazaki K, Terashima Y, Itomura M, et al. (2011)** Docosahexaenoic acid is an independent predictor of all-cause mortality in hemodialysis patients, *American Journal of Nephrology* 33:105-110. PMID: 21196723
44. **Pottala J, Garg S, Cohen B, et al. (2010)** Blood eisosapentaenoic and docosahexaenoic acids predict all-cause mortality in patients with stable coronary artery disease: the Heart and Soul study, *Circulation. Cardiovascular Quality and Outcomes* 3:406-412. PMID: 20551373
45. **Abhyankar B (2002)** Further reduction in mortality following myocardial infarction, *Hospital Medicine* 63:610-614. PMID: 12422496
46. **Patterson R, Flatt S, Newman V, et al. (2011)** Marine fatty acid intake is associated with breast cancer prognosis, *The Journal of Nutrition* 141:201-206. PMID: 21178081
47. **Wendel M, Heller A (2009)** Anticancer actions of omega-3 fatty acids – current state and future perspectives, *Anti-Cancer Agents in Medicinal Chemistry* 9:457-470. PMID: 19442044
48. **Burns C, Halabi S, Clamon G, et al. (1999)** Phase I clinical study of fish oil fatty acid capsules for patients with cancer cachexia: cancer and leukemia group B study 9473, *Clinical Cancer Research* 5:3942-3947. PMID: 10632323
49. **Villani A, Crotty M, Cleland L, et al. (2013)** Fish oil administration in older adults: is there potential for adverse events? A systematic review of the literature, *BMC Geriatrics* 13:41. PMID: 23634646

References

CHAPTER 10 CITATIONS

1. **Osako M, Nakagami H, Koibuchi N, et al. (2010)** Estrogen inhibits vascular calcification via vascular RANKL system: common mechanism of osteoporosis and vascular calcification, *Circulation Research* 107:466-475. PMID: 20595654
2. **Choi B, Vilahur G, Cardoso L, et al. (2008)** Ovariectomy increases vascular calcification via the OPG/RANKL cytokine signalling pathway, *European Journal of Clinical Investigation* 38:211-217. PMID: 18279396
3. **Manson J, Allison M, Rossouw J, et al. (2007)** Estrogen therapy and coronary-artery calcification, *The New England Journal of Medicine* 356:2591-2602. PMID: 17582069
4. **Weinberg N, Young A, Hunter C, et al. (2012)** Physical activity, hormone replacement therapy, and the presence of coronary calcium in midlife women, *Women & Health* 52:423-436. PMID: 22747181
5. **Jeon G, Kim S, Yun S, et al. (2010)** Association between serum estradiol level and coronary artery calcification in postmenopausal women, *Menopause* 17:902-907. PMID: 20512078
6. **Carlsen C, Soerensen T, Eriksen E (2000)** Prevalence of low serum estradiol levels in male osteoporosis, *Osteoporosis International* 11:697-701. PMID: 11095173
7. **Cervellati C, Bonaccorsi G, Cremonini E, et al. (2013)** Bone mass density selectively correlates with serum markers of oxidative damage in post-menopausal women, *Clinical Chemistry and Laboratory Medicine* 51:333-338. PMID: 23089610
8. **Bjarnason N, Alexandersen P, Christiansen C (2002)** Number of years since menopause: spontaneous bone loss is dependent but response to hormone replacement therapy is independent, *Bone* 30:637-642. PMID: 11934658
9. **Hui S, Perkins A, Zhou L, et al. (2002)** Bone loss at the femoral neck in premenopausal white women: effects of weight change and sex-hormone levels, *The Journal of Clinical Endocrinology and Metabolism* 87:1539-1543. PMID: 11932278
10. **Heshmati H, Khosla S, Robins S, et al. (2002)** Role of low levels of endogenous estrogen in regulation of bone resorption in late postmenopausal women, *Journal of Bone and Mineral Research* 17:172-178. PMID: 11771665
11. **Das U (2002)** Nitric oxide as the mediator of the antiosteoporotic actions of estrogen, statins, and essential fatty acids, *Experimental Biology and Medicine* 227:88-93. PMID: 11815671
12. **Barbour K, Boudreau R, Danielson M, et al. (2012)** Inflammatory markers and the risk of hip fracture: the Women's Health Initiative, *Journal of Bone and Mineral Research* 27:1167-1176. PMID: 22392817
13. **de Villiers T, Stevenson J (2012)** The WHI: the effect of hormone replacement therapy on fracture prevention, *Climacteric* 15:263-266. PMID: 22612613

14. **Karim R, Dell R, Greene D, et al.** **(2011)** Hip fracture in postmenopausal women after cessation of hormone therapy: results from a prospective study in a large health management organization, *Menopause* 18:1172-1177. PMID: 21775911
15. **Gambacciani M (2012)** HRT misuse and the osteoporosis epidemic, *Climacteric* 15:10-11. PMID: 22132704
16. **Oliver R, Yu Y, Yee G, et al.** **(2013)** Poor histological healing of a femoral fracture following 12 months of oestrogen deficiency in rats, *Osteoporosis International* Apr 6. [Epub ahead of print]. PMID: 23563933
17. **No authors listed (1996)** Effects of hormone therapy on bone mineral density: results from the postmenopausal estrogen/progestin interventions (PEPI) trial. The Writing Group for the PEPI, *The Journal of the American Medical Association* 276:1389-1396. PMID: 8892713
18. **Lisabeth L, Bushnell C (2012)** Stroke risk in women: the role of menopause and hormone therapy, *Lancet Neurology* 11:82-91. PMID: 22172623
19. **Mansur A, Silva T, Takada J, et al.** **(2012)** Long-term prospective study of the influence of estrone levels on events in postmenopausal women with or at high risk for coronary artery disease, *The Scientific World Journal* 2012:363595. PMID: 22701354
20. **Korljan B, Bagatin J, Kokic S, et al.** **(2010)** The impact of hormone replacement therapy on metabolic syndrome components in perimenopausal women, *Medical Hypotheses* 74:162-163. PMID: 19665311
21. **Alemany M (2012)** Do the interactions between glucocorticoids and sex hormones regulate the development of the metabolic syndrome? Frontiers in Endocrinology 3:27. PMID: 22649414
22. **Mauvais-Jarvis F, Clegg D, Hevener A (2013)** The role of estrogens in control of energy balance and glucose homeostasis, *Endocrine Reviews* 34:309-338. PMID: 23460719
23. **Kilic S, Yilmaz N, Erdogan G, et al.** **(2010)** Effect of non-oral estrogen on risk markers for metabolic syndrome in early surgically menopausal women, *Climacteric* 13:55-62. PMID: 19591007
24. **Finan B, Yang B, Ottaway N, et al.** **(2012)** Targeted estrogen delivery reverses the metabolic syndrome, *Nature Medicine* 18:1847-1856. PMID: 23142820
25. **Xu J, Xiang Q, Lin G, et al.** **(2012)** Estrogen improved metabolic syndrome through down-regulation of VEGF and HIF-1α to inhibit hypoxia of periaortic and intra-abdominal fat in ovariectomized female rats, *Molecular Biology Reports* 39:8177-8185. PMID: 22570111
26. **Wild R, Wu C, Curb J, et al.** **(2013)** Coronary heart disease events in the Women's Health Initiative hormone trials: effect modification by metabolic syndrome: a nested case-control study within the Women's Health Initiative randomized clinical trials, *Menopause* 20:254-260. PMID: 23435021
27. **Alexandersen P, Tanko L, Bagger Y, et al.** **(2006)** The long-term impact of 2-3 years of hormone replacement therapy on cardiovascular mortality and atherosclerosis in healthy women, *Climacteric* 9:108-118. PMID: 16698657

28. **Schairer C, Adami H, Hoover R, Persson I (1997)** Cause-specific mortality in women receiving hormone replacement therapy, *Epidemiology* 8:59-65. PMID: 9116097
29. **Rossouw J, Anderson G, Prentice R, et al. (2002)** Risks and benefits of estrogen plus progestin in healthy postmenopausal women: principal results from the Women's Health Initiative randomized controlled trial, *The Journal of the American Medical Association* 288:321-333. PMID: 12117397
30. **Yang X, Reckelhoff J (2011)** Estrogen, hormonal replacement therapy and cardiovascular disease, *Current Opinion in Nephrology and Hypertension* 20:133-138. PMID: 21178615
31. **Burg M, Fraser K, Gui S, et al. (2006)** Treatment of menopausal symptoms in family medicine settings following the Women's Health Initiative findings, *Journal of the American Board of Family Medicine* 19:122-131. PMID: 16513900
32. **Seelig M, Altura BM, Altura BT (2004)** Benefits and risks of sex hormone replacement in postmenopausal women, Journal of the *American College of Nutrition* 23:482S-496S. PMID: 15466949
33. **Henderson V, Lobo R (2012)** Hormone therapy and the risk of stroke: perspectives 10 years after the Women's Health Initiative trials, *Climacteric* 15:229-234. PMID: 22612608
34. **Sanada M, Higashi Y, Nakagawa K, et al. (2003)** A comparison of low-dose and standard-dose oral estrogen on forearm endothelial function in early postmenopausal women, *The Journal of Clinical Endocrinology and Metabolism* 88:1303-1309. PMID: 12629123
35. **Ziller M, Herwig J, Ziller V, et al. (2012)** Effects of a low-dose oral estrogen only treatment on bone mineral density and quantitative ultrasonometry in postmenopausal women, *Gynecological Endocrinology* 28:1002-1005. PMID: 22835159
36. **Moskowitz D (2006)** A comprehensive review of the safety and efficacy of bioidentical hormones for the management of menopause and related health risks, *Alternative Medicine Review* 11:208-223. PMID: 17217322
37. **Holtorf K (2009)** The bioidentical hormone debate: are bioidentical hormones (estradiol, estriol, and progesterone) safer or more efficacious than commonly used synthetic versions in hormone replacement therapy? *Postgraduate Medicine* 121:73-85. PMID: 19179815
38. **Stevenson J (2011)** Prevention of osteoporosis: one step forward, two steps back, *Menopause International* 17:137-141. PMID: 22120943
39. **Santen R, Song Y, Yue W, et al. (2013)** Effects of menopausal hormonal therapy on occult breast tumors, *The Journal of Steroid Biochemistry and Molecular Biology* Jun 6. [Epub ahead of print]. PMID: 23748149
40. **Stevenson J (2009)** Type and route of estrogen administration, *Climacteric* 12:86-90. PMID: 19811249
41. **Pattison N, Uptin T, Knox B, France J (1989)** Transdermal oestrogen for postmenopausal women: a double blind crossover comparative study with ethinyl oestradiol, *The Australian & New Zealand Journal of Obstetrics and Gynaecology* 29:62-65. PMID: 2562605

42. **Selby, P., H. McGarrigle, and M. Peacock (1989)** Comparison of the effects of oral and transdermal oestradiol administration on oestrogen metabolism, protein synthesis, gonadotrophin release, bone turnover and climacteric symptoms in postmenopausal women. *Clinical Endocrinology* 30:241-249. PMID: 2512035
43. **Nahoul, K., L. Dehennin, M. Jondet, and M. Roger (1993)** Profiles of plasma estrogens, progesterone and their metabolites after oral or vaginal administration of estradiol or progesterone. *Maturitas* 16:185-202. PMID: 8515718
44. **Gadomska, H., E. Barcz, A. Cyganek, et al. (2002)** Efficacy and tolerability of low-dose transdermal estrogen (Oesclim) in the treatment of menopausal symptoms. *Current Medical Research and Opinion* 18:97-102. PMID: 12017217
45. **Vrablik, M., T. Fait, J. Kovar, et al. (2008)** Oral but not transdermal estrogen replacement therapy changes the composition of plasma lipoproteins. *Metabolism* 57:1088-1092. PMID: 18640386
46. **Shifren, J., N. Rifai, S. Desindes, et al. (2008)** A comparison of the short-term effects of oral conjugated equine estrogens versus transdermal estradiol on C-reactive protein, other serum markers of inflammation, and other hepatic proteins in naturally menopausal women. *The Journal of Clinical Endocrinology and Metabolism* 93:1702-1710. PMID: 18303079
47. **Karim, R., F. Stanczyk, H. Hodis, et al. (2010)** Associations between markers of inflammation and physiological and pharmacological levels of circulating sex hormones in postmenopausal women. *Menopause* 17:785-790. PMID: 20632462
48. **Nabham, Z., L. Dimeglio, R. Qi, et al. (2009)** Conjugated oral versus transdermal estrogen replacement in girls with Turner syndrome: a pilot comparative study. *The Journal of Clinical Endocrinology and Metabolism* 94:2009-2014. PMID: 19318455
49. **Cetinkaya, M., A. Kokcu, F. Yanik, et al. (2002)** Comparison of the effects of transdermal estrogen, oral estrogen, and oral estrogen-progestogen therapy on bone mineral density in postmenopausal women. *Journal of Bone and Mineral Metabolism* 20:44-48. PMID: 11810416
50. **Huang, A., B. Ettinger, E. Vittinghoff, et al. (2007)** Endogenous estrogen levels and the effects of ultra-low-dose transdermal estradiol therapy on bone turnover and BMD in postmenopausal women. *Journal of Bone and Mineral Research* 22:1791-1797. PMID: 17620054
51. **Richman, S., V. Edusa, A. Fadiel, and F. Naftolin (2006)** Low-dose estrogen therapy for prevention of osteoporosis: working our way back to monotherapy. *Menopause* 13:148-155. PMID: 16607111
52. **Valenzuela, P. and J. Simon (2012)** Nanoparticle delivery for transdermal HRT. *Nanomedicine* 8:S83-S89. PMID: 22640909
53. **Ni, X., T. Xia, Y. Zhao, et al. (2012)** Postmenopausal hormone therapy is associated with in situ breast cancer risk. Asian Pacific *Journal of Cancer Prevention* 13:3917-3925. PMID: 23098493
54. **Eriksen, E. (2012)** Hormone replacement therapy or SERMS in the long term treatment of osteoporosis. *Minerva Ginecologica* 64:207-221. PMID: 22635016

55. **Olie V, Canonico M, Scarabin P (2010)** Risk of venous thrombosis with oral versus transdermal estrogen therapy among postmenopausal women, *Current Opinion in Hematology* 17:457-463. PMID: 20601871
56. **Renoux C, Dell'Aniello S, Suissa S (2010)** Hormone replacement therapy and the risk of venous thromboembolism: a population-based study, *Journal of Thrombosis and Haemostasis* 8:979-986. PMID: 20230416
57. **Fait T, Vrablik M (2012)** Coronary heart disease and hormone replacement therapy – from primary and secondary prevention to the window of opportunity, *Neuro Endocrinology Letters* 33:17-21. PMID: 23183504
58. **Reslan O, Khalil R (2012)** Vascular effects of estrogenic menopausal hormone therapy, *Reviews on Recent Clinical Trials* 7:47-70. PMID: 21864249
59. **Lopez-Grueso R, Gambini J, Mohamed K, et al. (2013)** Early, but not late-onset estrogen replacement therapy prevents oxidative stress and metabolic alterations caused by ovariectomy, *Antioxidants & Redox Signaling* Jun 2. [Epub ahead of print]. PMID: 23725100
60. **Gambacciani M, Pepe A (2009)** Vasomotor symptoms and cardiovascular risk, *Climacteric* 12:32-35. PMID: 19811238
61. **Thurston R, Kuller L, Edmundowicz D, Matthews K (2010)** History of hot flashes and aortic calcification among postmenopausal women, *Menopause* 17:256-261. PMID: 20042895
62. **Yasui T, Uemura H, Takikawa M, Irahara M (2003)** Hormone replacement therapy in postmenopausal women, *The Journal of Medical Investigation* 50:136-145. PMID: 13678382
63. **Mueck A (2012)** Postmenopausal hormone replacement therapy and cardiovascular disease: the value of transdermal estradiol and micronized progesterone, *Climacteric* 15:11-17. PMID: 22432811
64. **Theodoraki A, Bouloux P (2009)** Testosterone therapy in men, *Menopause International* 15:87-92. PMID: 19465676
65. **Moskovic D, Araujo A, Lipshultz L, Khera M (2013)** The 20-year public health impact and direct cost of testosterone deficiency in U.S. men, *The Journal of Sexual Medicine* 10:562-569. PMID: 23035926
66. **Traish A, Miner M, Morgentaler A, Zitzmann M (2011)** Testosterone deficiency, *The American Journal of Medicine* 124:578-587. PMID: 21683825
67. **Ogbera O, Sonny C, Olufemi F, Wale A (2011)** Hypogonadism and subnormal total testosterone levels in men with type 2 diabetes mellitus, *Journal of the College of Physicians and Surgeons – Pakistan* 21:517-521. PMID: 21914405
68. **Torremade-Barreda J, Rodriguez-Tolra J, Roman-Romera I, et al. (2013)** Testosterone-deficiency as a risk factor for hip fracture in elderly men, *Actas Urologicas Españolas* 37:142-146. PMID: 23246104
69. **Gullberg B, Johnell O, Kanis J (1997)** World-wide projections for hip fracture, *Osteoporosis International* 7:407-413. PMID: 9425497
70. **Herrera A, Lobo-Escolar A, Mateo J, et al. (2012)** Male osteoporosis: a review. *World Journal of Orthopedics* 3:223-234. PMID: 23362466

71. **Campion J, Maricic M (2003)** Osteoporosis in men, *American Family Physician* 67:1521-1526. PMID: 12722852
72. **Rao S, Budhwar N, Ashfaque A (2010)** Osteoporosis in men. *American Family Physician* 82:503-508. PMID: 20822086
73. **Tuck S, Francis R (2009)** Testosterone, bone and osteoporosis, *Frontiers of Hormone Research* 37:123-132. PMID: 19011293
74. **van den Beld A, de Jong F, Grobbee D, et al. (2000)** Measures of bioavailable serum testosterone and estradiol and their relationships with muscle strength, bone density, and body composition in elderly men, *The Journal of Clinical Endocrinology and Metabolism* 85:3276-3282. PMID: 10999822
75. **Paller C, Shiels M, Rohrmann S, et al. (2009)** Relationship of sex steroid hormones with bone mineral density (BMD) in a nationally representative sample of men, *Clinical Endocrinology* 70:26-34. PMID: 18485120
76. **Woo J, Kwok T, Leung J, et al. (2012)** Sex steroids and bone health in older Chinese men, *Osteoporosis International* 23:1553-1562. PMID: 21318439
77. **Wang Y, Zhan J, Huang W, et al. (2013)** Effects of low-dose testosterone undecanoate treatment on bone mineral density and bone turnover markers in elderly male osteoporosis with low serum testosterone, *International Journal of Endocrinology* 2013:570413. PMID: 23533404
78. **Aversa A, Bruzziches R, Francomano D, et al. (2012)** Effects of long-acting testosterone undecanoate on bone mineral density in middle-aged men with late-onset hypogonadism and metabolic syndrome: results from a 36 months controlled study, *The Aging Male* 15:96-102. PMID: 22439807
79. **Deb P, Gupta S, Godbole M (2012)** Effects of short-term testosterone replacement on areal bone mineral density and bone turnover in young hypogonadal males, *Indian Journal of Endocrinology and Metabolism* 16:947-951. PMID: 23226640
80. **Chin K, Ima-Nirwana S (2012)** Sex steroids and bone health status in men, *International Journal of Endocrinology* 2012:208719. PMID: 23150727
81. **Akishita M, Fukai S, Hashimoto M, et al. (2010)** Association of low testosterone with metabolic syndrome and its components in middle-aged Japanese men, *Hypertension Research* 33:587-591. PMID: 20339372
82. **Jones T (2010)** Testosterone deficiency: a risk factor for cardiovascular disease? *Trends in Endocrinology and Metabolism* 21:496-503. PMID: 20381374
83. **Muraleedharan V, Jones T (2010)** Testosterone and the metabolic syndrome, *Therapeutic Advances in Endocrinology and Metabolism* 1:207-223. PMID: 23148165
84. **Malkin C, Pugh P, Morris P, et al. (2010)** Low serum testosterone and increased mortality in men with coronary heart disease, *Heart* 96:1821-1825. PMID: 20959649

85. **Ponikowska B, Jankowska E, Maj J, et al. (2010)** Gonadal and adrenal androgen deficiencies as independent predictors of increased cardiovascular mortality in men with type II diabetes mellitus and stable coronary artery disease, *International Journal of Cardiology* 143:343-348. PMID: 19395096
86. **Cattabiani C, Basaria S, Ceda G, et al. (2012)** Relationship between testosterone deficiency and cardiovascular risk and mortality in adult men, *Journal of Endocrinological Investigation* 35:104-120. PMID: 22082684
87. **Hackett G (2012)** Testosterone and the heart, *International Journal of Clinical Practice* 66:648-655. PMID: 22698417
88. **Khaw K, Dowsett M, Folkerd E, et al. (2007)** Endogenous testosterone and mortality due to all causes, cardiovascular disease, and cancer in men: European prospective investigation into cancer in Norfolk (EPIC-Norfolk) Prospective Population Study, *Circulation* 116:2694-2701. PMID: 18040028
89. **Laughlin G, Barrett-Connor E, Bergstrom J (2008)** Low serum testosterone and mortality in older men, *The Journal of Clinical Endocrinology* 93:68-75. PMID: 17911176
90. **Tivesten A, Vandenput L, Labrie F, et al. (2009)** Low serum testosterone and estradiol predict mortality in elderly men, *The Journal of Clinical Endocrinology and Metabolism* 94:2482-2488. PMID: 19401373
91. **Vikan T, Schirmer H, Njolstad I, Svartberg J (2009)** Endogenous sex hormones and the prospective association with cardiovascular disease and mortality in men: the Tronso Study, *European Journal of Endocrinology* 161:435-442. PMID: 19542243
92. **Fukai S, Akishita M, Yamada S, et al. (2011)** Plasma sex hormone levels and mortality in disabled older men and women, *Geriatrics & Gerontology International* 11:196-203. PMID: 21143567
93. **Grossman M, Hoermann R, Gani L, et al. (2012)** Low testosterone levels as an independent predictor of mortality in men with chronic liver disease, *Clinical Endocrinology* 77:323-328. PMID: 22280063
94. **Corona G, Monami M, Boddi V, et al. (2010)** Low testosterone is associated with an increased risk of MACE lethality in subjects with erectile dysfunction, *The Journal of Sexual Medicine* 7:1557-1564. PMID: 20102478
95. **Vlachopoulos C, Loakeimidis N, Terentes-Printzios D, et al. (2013)** Plasma total testosterone and incident cardiovascular events in hypertensive patients, *American Journal of Hypertension* 26:373-381. PMID: 23382488
96. **Lerchbaum E, Pilz S, Boehm B, et al. (2012)** Combination of low free testosterone and low vitamin D predicts mortality in older men referred for coronary angiography, *Clinical Endocrinology* 77:475-483. PMID: 22356136
97. **Saad F (2012)** Androgen therapy in men with testosterone deficiency: can testosterone reduce the risk of cardiovascular disease? *Diabetes/Metabolism Research and Reviews* 28:52-59. PMID: 23280867
98. **Keating N, O'Malley A, Smith M (2006)** Diabetes and cardiovascular disease during androgen deprivation therapy for prostate cancer, *Journal of Clinical Oncology* 24:4448-4456. PMID: 16983113

99. **Levine G, D'Amico A, Berger P, et al.** (2010) Androgen-deprivation therapy in prostate cancer and cardiovascular risk: a science advisory from the American Heart Association, American Cancer Society, and American Urological Association: endorsed by the American Society for Radiation Oncology, *Circulation* 121:833-840. PMID: 20124128
100. **Jones T (2011)** Cardiovascular risk during androgen deprivation therapy for prostate cancer, *BMJ* 342:d3105. PMID: 21610041
101. **Hall J, Jones R, Jones T, et al.** (2006) Selective inhibition of L-type Ca2+ channels in A7r5 cells by physiological levels of testosterone, *Endocrinology* 147:2675-2680. PMID: 16527846
102. **Scragg J, Dallas M, Peers C (2007)** Molecular requirements for L-type Ca2+ channel blockade by testosterone, *Cell Calcium* 42:11-15. PMID: 17173968
103. **Oloyo A, Sofola O, Nair R, et al.** (2011) Testosterone relaxes abdominal aorta in mal Sprague-Dawley rats by opening potassium (K(+)) channel and blockage of calcium (Ca(2+)) channel, *Pathophysiology* 18:247-253. PMID: 21439799
104. **Kelly D, Jones T (2013)** Testosterone: a vascular hormone in health and disease, *The Journal of Endocrinology* 217:R47-R71. PMID: 23549841
105. **Gillman M, Ross-Degnan D, McLaughlin T, et al.** (1999) Effects of long-acting versus short-acting calcium channel blockers among older survivors of acute myocardial infarction, *Journal of the American Geriatrics Society* 47:512-517. PMID: 10323641
106. **Gibson R, Hansen J, Messerli F, et al.** (2000) Long-term effects of diltiazem and verapamil on mortality and cardiac events in a non-Q-wave acute myocardial infarction without pulmonary congestion: post hoc subset analysis of the multicenter diltiazem postinfarction trial and the second Danish verapamil infarction trial studies, *The American Journal of Cardiology* 86:275-279. PMID: 10922432
107. **Lubsen J, Wagener G, Kirwan B, et al.** (2005) Effect of long-acting nifedipine on mortality and cardiovascular morbidity in patients with symptomatic stable angina and hypertension: the ACTION trial, *Journal of Hypertension* 23:641-648. PMID: 15716708
108. **Costanzo P, Perrone-Filardi P, Petretta M, et al.** (2009) Calcium channel blockers and cardiovascular outcomes: a meta-analysis of 175,634 patients, *Journal of Hypertension* 27:1136-1151. PMID: 19451836
109. **Park B, Shim J, Lee Y, et al.** (2012) Inverse relationship between bioavailable testosterone and subclinical coronary artery calcification in non-obese Korean men, *Asian Journal of Andrology* 14:612-615. PMID: 22522505
110. **Holyoak J, Crawford E, Meacham R (2008)** Testosterone and the prostate: implications for the treatment of hypogonadal men, *Current Urology Reports* 9:500-505. PMID: 18947516
111. **Coward R, Simhan J, Carson C, 3rd (2009)** Prostate-specific antigen changes and prostate cancer in hypogonadal men treated with testosterone replacement therapy, *BJU International* 103:1179-1183. PMID: 19154450
112. **Raynaud J (2009)** Testosterone deficiency syndrome: treatment and cancer risk, *The Journal of Steroid Biochemistry and Molecular Biology* 114:96-105. PMID: 19429438

113. **Mearini L, Zucchi A, Nunzi E, et al. (2013)** Low serum testosterone levels are predictive of prostate cancer, *World Journal of Urology* 31:247-252. PMID: 22068548
114. **Holmang S, Marin P, Lindstedt G, Hedelin H (1993)** Effect of long-term oral testosterone undecanoate treatment on prostate volume and serum prostate-specific antigen concentration in eugonadal middle-aged men, *The Prostate* 23:99-106. PMID: 7690956
115. **Wang Y, Zhan J, Huang W, et al. (2013)** Effects of low-dose testosterone undecanoate treatment on bone mineral density and bone turnover markers in elderly male osteoporosis with low serum testosterone, *International Journal of Endocrinology* 2013:570413. PMID: 23533404
116. **Pearl J, Berhanu D, Francois N, et al. (2013)** Testosterone supplementation does not worsen lower urinary tract symptoms, *The Journal of Urology* Jun 10. [Epub ahead of print]. PMID: 23764078
117. **Vignozzi L, Morelli A, Sarchielli E, et al. (2012)** Testosterone protects from metabolic syndrome-associated prostate inflammation: an experimental study in rabbit, *The Journal of Endocrinology* 212:71-84. PMID: 22010203
118. **Basaria S, Coviello A, Travison T, et al. (2010)** Adverse events associated with testosterone administration, *The New England Journal of Medicine* 363:109-122. PMID: 20592293
119. **Zitzmann M, Mattern A, Hanisch J, et al. (2013)** IPASS: a study on the tolerability and effectiveness of injectable testosterone undecanoate for the treatment of male hypogonadism in a worldwide sample of 1,438 men, *The Journal of Sexual Medicine* 10:579-588. PMID: 22812645
120. **Theodoraki A, Bouloux P (2009)** Testosterone therapy in men, *Menopause International* 15:87-92. PMID: 19465676
121. **Morales A, Bella A, Chun S, et al. (2010)** A practical guide to diagnosis, management and treatment of testosterone deficiency for Canadian physicians, *Canadian Urological Association Journal* 4:269-275. PMID: 20694106
122. **Snyder P, Peachey H, Hannoush P, et al. (1999)** Effect of testosterone treatment on bone mineral density in men over 65 years of age, *The Journal of Clinical Endocrinology and Metabolism* 84:1966-1972. PMID: 10372695
123. **Boelaert K, Franklyn J (2005)** Thyroid hormone in health and disease, *Journal of Endocrinology* 187:1-15. PMID: 16214936
124. **Williams G (2009)** Actions of thyroid hormones in bone, *Endokrynologia Polska* 60:380-388. PMID: 19885809
125. **Vestergaard P, Mosekilde L (2002)** Fractures in patients with hyperthyroidism and hypothyroidism: a nationwide follow-up study in 16,249 patients, *Thyroid* 12:411-419. PMID: 12097203
126. **Wojcicka A, Bassett J, Williams G (2013)** Mechanisms of action of thyroid hormones in the skeleton, *Biochimica et Biophysica Acta* 1830:3979-3986. PMID: 22634735
127. **Dhanwal D (2011)** Thyroid disorders and bone mineral metabolism, *Indian Journal of Endocrinology and Metabolism* 15:S107-S112. PMID: 21966645

128. **Nicholls J, Brassill M, Williams G, Bassett J (2012)** The skeletal consequences of thyrotoxicosis, *The Journal of Endocrinology* 213:209-221. PMID: 22454529

129. **Reddy P, Harinarayan C, Sachan A, et al. (2012)** Bone disease in thyrotoxicosis, *The Indian Journal of Medical Research* 135:277-286. PMID: 22561612

130. **Gonzalez-Rodriguez L, Felici-Giovanini M, Haddock L (2013)** Thyroid dysfunction in an adult female population: a population-based study of Latin American Vertebral Osteoporosis Study (LAVOS)--Puerto Rico site, *Puerto Rico Health Sciences Journal* 32:57-62. PMID: 23781620

131. **Tuchendler D, Bolanowski M (2013)** Assessment of bone metabolism in premenopausal females with hyperthyroidism and hypothyroidism, *Endokrynologia Polska* 64:40-44. PMID: 23450446

132. **Krolner B, Jorgensen J, Nielsen S (1983)** Spinal bone mineral content in myxoedema and thyrotoxicosis, Effects of thyroid hormone(s) and antithyroid treatment. *Clinical Endocrinology* 18:439-446. PMID: 6603290

133. **Tarraga Lopez P, Lopez C, de Mora F, et al. (2011)** Osteoporosis in patients with subclinical hypothyroidism treated with thyroid hormone, *Clinical Cases in Mineral and Bone Metabolism* 8:44-48. PMID: 22461829

134. **Murphy E, Gluer C, Reid D, et al. (2010)** Thyroid function within the upper normal range is associated with reduced bone mineral density and an increased risk of nonvertebral fractures in healthy euthyroid postmenopausal women, *The Journal of Clinical Endocrinology and Metabolism* 95:3173-3181. PMID: 20410228

135. **Mazziotti G, Porcelli T, Patelli I, et al. (2010)** Serum TSH levels and risk of vertebral fractures in euthyroid postmenopausal women with low bone mineral density, *Bone* 46:747-751. PMID: 19892039

136. **Murphy E, Gluer C, Reid D, et al. (2010)** Thyroid function within the upper normal range is associated with reduced bone mineral density and an increased risk of nonvertebral fractures in healthy euthyroid postmenopausal women, *The Journal of Clinical Endocrinology and Metabolism* 95:3173-3181. PMID: 20410228

137. **Flynn R, Bonellie S, Jung R, et al. (2010)** Serum thyroid-stimulating hormone concentration and morbidity from cardiovascular disease and fractures in patients on long-term thyroxine therapy, *The Journal of Clinical Endocrinology and Metabolism* 95:186-193. PMID: 19906785

138. **Zaidi M, Davies T, Zallone A, et al. (2009)** Thyroid-stimulating hormone, thyroid hormones, and bone loss, *Current Osteoporosis Reports* 7:47-52. PMID: 19631028

139. **Ma R, Morshed R, Latif R, et al. (2011)** The influence of thyroid-stimulating hormone and thyroid-stimulating hormone receptor antibodies on osteoclastogenesis, *Thyroid* 21:897-906. PMID: 21745106.

140. **Baliram R, Sun L, Li J, et al. (2012)** Hyperthyroid-associated osteoporosis is exacerbated by the loss of TSH signaling, *The Journal of Clinical Investigation* 122:3737-3741. PMID: 22996689

141. **Sun L, Zhu L, Lu P, et al. (2013)** Genetic confirmation for a central role for TNFα in the direct action of thyroid stimulating hormone on the skeleton, *Proceedings of the National Academy of Sciences of the United States of America May 28*. [Epub ahead of print]. PMID: 23716650

142. **Zofkova I (2013)** [Drug induced osteoporosis]. [Article in Czech], *Vnitrni Lekarstvi* 59:59-63. PMID: 23565522

143. **Tseng F, Lin W, Lin C, et al. (2012)** Subclinical hypothyroidism is associated with increased risk for all-cause and cardiovascular mortality in adults, *Journal of the American College of Cardiology* 60:730-737. PMID: 22726629

144. **Ceresini G, Ceda G, Lauretani F, et al. (2013)** Thyroid status and 6-year mortality in elderly people living in a mildly iodine-deficient area: the aging in the Chianti Area Study, *Journal of the American Geriatrics Society* 61:868-874. PMID: 23647402

145. **McQuade C, Skugor M, Brennan D, et al. (2011)** Hypothyroidism and moderate subclinical hypothyroidism are associated with increased all-cause mortality independent of coronary heart disease risk factors: a PreCIS database study, *Thyroid* 21:837-843. PMID: 21745107

146. **Tseng F, Lin W, Lin C, et al. (2012)** Subclinical hypothyroidism is associated with increased risk for all-cause and cardiovascular mortality in adults, *Journal of the American College of Cardiology* 60:730-737. PMID: 22726629

147. **Haentjens P, Van Meerhaeghe A, Poppe K, Velkeniers B (2008)** Subclinical thyroid dysfunction and mortality: an estimate of relative and absolute excess all-cause mortality based on time-to-event data from cohort studies, *European Journal of Endocrinology* 159:329-341. PMID: 18511471

148. **Sgarbi J, Matsumura L, Kasamatsu T, et al. (2010)** Subclinical thyroid dysfunctions are independent risk factors for mortality in a 7.5-year follow-up: the Japanese-Brazilian thyroid study, *European Journal of Endocrinology* 162:569-577. PMID: 19966035

149. **McQuade C, Skugor M, Brennan D, et al. (2011)** Hypothyroidism and moderate subclinical hypothyroidism are associated with increased all-cause mortality independent of coronary heart disease risk factors: a PreCIS database study, *Thyroid* 21:837-843. PMID: 21745107

150. **Tseng F, Lin W, Lin C, et al. (2012)** Subclinical hypothyroidism is associated with increased risk for all-cause and cardiovascular mortality in adults, *Journal of the American College of Cardiology* 60:730-737. PMID: 22726629

151. **Razvi S, Weaver J, Vanderpump M, Pearce S (2010)** The incidence of ischemic heart disease and mortality in people with subclinical hypothyroidism: reanalysis of the Whickham Survey cohort, *The Journal of Clinical Endocrinology and Metabolism* 95:1734-1740. PMID: 20150579

152. **Rhee C, Alexander E, Bhan I, Brunelli S (2013)** Hypothyroidism and mortality among dialysis patients. *Clinical Journal of the American Society of Nephrology* 8:593-601. PMID: 23258793

153. **Yang J, Han S, Song S, et al. (2012)** Serum T3 level can predict cardiovascular events and all-cause mortality rates in CKD patients with proteinuria, *Renal Failure* 34:364-372. PMID: 22260378
154. **Pereg D, Tirosh A, Elis A, et al. (2012)** Mortality and coronary heart disease in euthyroid patients, *The American Journal of Medicine* 125:e7-e12. PMID: 22608790
155. **Westerink J, van der Graaf Y, Faber D, et al. (2012)** Relation between thyroid-stimulating hormone and the occurrence of cardiovascular events and mortality in patients with manifest vascular diseases, *European Journal of Preventive Cardiology* 19:864-873. PMID: 21724680
156. **Clarke N, Kabadi U (2004)** Optimizing treatment of hypothyroidism, *Treatments in Endocrinology* 3:217-221. PMID: 16026104

References

CHAPTER 11 CITATIONS

1. **Christakos S, Dhawan P, Porta A, et al. (2011)** Vitamin D and intestinal calcium absorption, *Molecular and Cellular Endocrinology* 347:25-29. PMID: 21664413
2. **Hoenderop J, Nilius B, Bindels R (2005)** Calcium absorption across epithelia, *Physiological Reviews* 85:373-422. PMID: 15618484
3. **Lisse T, Chun R, Rieger S, et al. (2013)** Vitamin D activation of functionally distinct regulatory miRNAs in primary human osteoblasts, *Journal of Bone and Mineral Research* Jan 29 [Epub ahead of print]. PMID: 23362149
4. **Yamamoto Y, Yoshizawa T, Fukuda T, et al. (2013)** Vitamin D receptor in osteoblasts is a negative regulator of bone mass control, *Endocrinology* 154:1008-1020. PMID: 23389957
5. **Cheng M, Gupta V (2012)** Teriparatide--indications beyond osteoporosis, *Indian Journal of Endocrinology and Metabolism* 16:343-348. PMID: 22629497
6. **Vescini F, Grimaldi F (2012)** PTH 1-84: bone rebuilding as a target for the therapy of severe osteoporosis, *Clinical Cases in Mineral and Bone Metabolism* 9:31-36. PMID: 22783333
7. **Kozai M, Yamamoto H, Ishiguro M, et al. (2013)** Thyroid hormones decrease plasma 1α,25-dihydroxyvitamin D levels through transcriptional repression of the renal 25-hydroxyvitamin D3 1α-hydroxylase gene (CYP27B1), *Endocrinology* 154:609-622. PMID: 23307792
8. **Rejnmark L, Vestergaard P, Brot C, Mosekilde L (2011)** Increased fracture risk in normocalcemic postmenopausal women with high parathyroid hormone levels: a 16-year study, *Calcified Tissue International* 88:238-245. PMID: 21181400
9. **Foster G, Baghdiantz A, Kumar M, et al. (1964)** Thyroid origin of calcitonin, *Nature* 202:1303-1305. PMID: 14210962
10. **Friedman J, Raisz L (1965)** Thyrocalcitonin: inhibitor of bone resorption in tissue culture, *Science* 150:1465-1467. PMID: 5892553
11. **Hamdy R, Daley D (2012)** Oral calcitonin, *International Journal of Women's Health* 4:471-479. PMID: 23071417
12. **Singer F (1977)** Human calcitonin treatment of Paget's disease of bone, *Clinical Orthopaedics and Related Research* 127:86-93. PMID: 912995
13. **Civitelli R, Gonnelli S, Zacchei F, et al. (1988)** Bone turnover in postmenopausal osteoporosis. Effect of calcitonin treatment, *The Journal of Clinical Investigation* 82:1268-1274. PMID: 3262626
14. **Mittleman R, Chausmer A, Bellavia J, Wallach S (1967)** Thyrocalcitonin activity in hypercalcemia produced by calcium salts, parathyroid hormone and vitamin D, *Endocrinology* 81:599-604. PMID: 4291806
15. **Wagner G, Guiraudon C, Milliken C, Copp D (1995)** Immunological and biological evidence for a stanniocalcin-like hormone in human kidney, *Proceedings of the National Academy of Sciences of the United States of America* 92:1871-1875. PMID: 7892193

16. **Ookata K, Tojo A, Onozato M, et al.** (2001) Distribution of stanniocalcin 1 in rat kidney and its regulation by vitamin D3, *Experimental Nephrology* 9:428-435. PMID: 11702003
17. **Honda S, Kashiwagi M, Ookata K, et al.** (1999) Regulation by 1alpha,25-dihydroxyvitamin D(3) of expression of stanniocalcin messages in the rat kidney and ovary, *FEBS Letters* 459:119-122. PMID: 10508929
18. **Hung N, Yamamoto H, Takei Y, et al.** (2012) Up-regulation of stanniocalcin 1 expression by 1,25-dihydroxy vitamin D(3) and parathyroid hormone in renal proximal tubular cells, *Journal of Clinical Biochemistry and Nutrition* 50:227-233. PMID: 22573926
19. **Nordin B, Horsman A, Marshall D, et al.** (1979) Calcium requirement and calcium therapy, *Clinical Orthopaedics and Related Research* 140:216-239. PMID: 477077
20. **Nordin B, Need A, Morris H, et al.** (1991) Evidence for a renal calcium leak in postmenopausal women, *The Journal of Clinical Endocrinology and Metabolism* 72:401-407. PMID: 1991810
21. **Papavasiliou K, Kenanidis E, Potoupnis M, et al.** (2009) Incidence of secondary hyperparathyroidism among postmenopausal women with end-stage knee osteoarthritis, *Journal of Orthopaedic Surgery* (Hong Kong) 17:310-312. PMID: 20065370
22. **Jamal S, Miller P (2013)** Secondary and tertiary hyperparathyroidism, *Journal of Clinical Densitometry* 16:64-68. PMID: 23267748
23. **Vincent A, Riggs B, Atkinson E, et al.** (2003) Effect of estrogen replacement therapy on parathyroid hormone secretion in elderly postmenopausal women, *Menopause* 10:165-171. PMID: 12627043
24. **Kelly, D. and T. Jones (2013)** Testosterone: a vascular hormone in health and disease, *The Journal of Endocrinology* Apr 2. [Epub ahead of print]. PMID: 23549841
25. **Son B, Akishita M, Iijima K, et al.** (2010) Androgen receptor-dependent transactivation of growth arrest-specific gene 6 mediates inhibitory effects of testosterone on vascular calcification, *The Journal of Biological Chemistry* 285:7537-7544. PMID: 20048160
26. **Park B, Shim J, Lee Y, et al.** (2012) Inverse relationship between bioavailable testosterone and subclinical coronary artery calcification in non-obese Korean men, *Asian Journal of Andrology* 14:612-615. PMID: 22522505
27. **Kumar V, Prasad R (2002)** Molecular basis of renal handling of calcium in response to thyroid hormone status of rat, *Biochimica et Biophysica Acta* 1586:331-343. PMID: 11997084
28. **Kumar V, Prasad R (2003)** Thyroid hormones stimulate calcium transport systems in rat intestine, *Biochimica et Biophysica Acta* 1639:185-194. PMID: 14636950
29. **Kozai M, Yamamoto H, Ishiguro M, et al.** (2013) Thyroid hormones decrease plasma 1α,25-dihydroxyvitamin D levels through transcriptional repression of the renal 25-hydroxyvitamin D3 1α-hydroxylase gene (CYP27B1), *Endocrinology* 154:609-622. PMID: 23307792

30. **Moeller L, Haselhorst N, Dumitrescu A, et al. (2011)** Stanniocalcin 1 induction by thyroid hormone depends on thyroid hormone receptor β and phosphatidylinositol 3-kinase activation, *Experimental and Clinical Endocrinology & Diabetes* 119:81-85. PMID: 20827662
31. **Wofl C, Englert S, Moghaddam A, et al. (2013)** Time course of 25(OH)D3 vitamin D3 as well as PTH (parathyroid hormone) during fracture healing of patients with normal and low bone mineral density (BMD), *BMC Musculoskeletal Disorders* 14:6. PMID: 23286544

CHAPTER 12 CITATIONS

1. **Hite AH, et al. (2010)** In the face of contradictory evidence: report of the Dietary Guidelines for Americans Committee, *Nutrition* Oct;26(10):915-24. PMID: 20888548
2. **Seeley S (1991)** Is calcium excess in Western diet a major cause of arterial disease? *International Journal of Cardiology* Nov;33(2):191-8, PMID: 1743778

References

CHAPTER 14 CITATIONS

1. **Siqueira J, Rocas I (2009)** Diversity of endodontic microbiota revisited, *Journal of Dental Research* 88:969-981. PMID: 19828883
2. **Issels J (2005)** *Cancer: A Second Opinion*, Garden City Park, NY: Square One Publishers, Inc.
3. **Caplan D, Pankow J, Cai J, et al. (2009)** The relationship between self-reported history of endodontic therapy and coronary heart disease in the Atherosclerosis Risk in Communities Study, *Journal of the American Dental Association* 140:1004-1012. PMID: 19654253
4. **Caplan D, Chasen J, Krall E, et al. (2006)** Lesions of endodontic origin and risk of coronary heart disease, *Journal of Dental Research* 85:996-1000. PMID: 17062738
5. **Pasqualini D, Bergandi L, Palumbo L, et al. (2012)** Association among oral health, apical periodontitis, CD14 polymorphisms, and coronary artery disease in middle-aged adults, *Journal of Endodontics* 38:1570-1577. PMID: 23146639
6. **Pessi T, Karhunen V, Karjalainen P, et al. (2013)** Bacterial signatures in thrombus aspirates of patients with myocardial infarction, *Circulation* 127:1219-1228. PMID: 23418311
7. **Willershausen I, Weyer V, Peter M, et al. (2013)** Association between chronic periodontal and apical inflammation and acute myocardial infarction, *Odontology* Apr 21. [Epub ahead of print]. PMID: 23604464
8. **Kulacz R, Levy T (2002)** *The Roots of Disease. Connecting Dentistry and Medicine*, Philadelphia, PA: Xlibris Corporation.
9. **Levy T, Huggins H (1996)** Routine dental extractions routinely produce cavitations, *Journal of Advancement in Medicine* 9:235-249.
10. **Bouquot J, Roberts A, Person P, Christian J (1992)** Neuralgia-inducing cavitational osteonecrosis (NICO). Osteomyelitis in 224 jawbone samples from patients with facial neuralgia, *Oral Surgery, Oral Medicine, and Oral Pathology* 73:307-319. PMID: 1545963
11. **Elter J, Champagne C, Offenbacher S, Beck J (2004)** Relationship of periodontal disease and tooth loss to prevalence of coronary heart disease, *Journal of Periodontology* 75:782-790. PMID: 15295942
12. **Holmlund A, Holm G, Lind L (2010)** Number of teeth as a predictor of cardiovascular mortality in a cohort of 7,674 subjects followed for 12 years, *Journal of Periodontology* 81:870-876. PMID: 20350152
13. **Holmlund A, Hulthe J, Lind L (2007)** Tooth loss is related to the presence of metabolic syndrome and inflammation in elderly subjects: a prospective study of the vasculature in Uppsala seniors (PIVUS), *Oral Health & Preventive Dentistry* 5:125-130. PMID: 17722439
14. **Huggins H, Levy T (1999)** *Uninformed Consent. The Hidden Dangers in Dental Care*, Charlottesville, VA: Hampton Roads Publishing Company, Inc.
15. **Humphrey L, Fu R, Buckley D, et al. (2008)** Periodontal disease and coronary heart disease incidence: a systemic review and meta-analysis, *Journal of General Internal Medicine* 23:2079-2086. PMID: 18807098

16. **Kshirsagar A, Craig R, Moss K, et al. (2009)** Periodontal disease adversely affects the survival of patients with end-stage renal disease, *Kidney International* 75:746-751. PMID: 19165177
17. **Dorn J, Genco R, Grossi S, et al. (2010)** Periodontal disease and recurrent cardiovascular events in survivors of myocardial infarction (MI): the Western New York Acute MI Study, *Journal of Periodontology* 84:502-511. PMID: 20367093
18. **Ameet M, Avneesh H, Babita R, Pramod P (2013)** The relationship between periodontitis and systemic diseases--hype or hope? *Journal of Clinical and Diagnostic Research* 7:758-762. PMID: 23730671
19. **Hanaoka Y, Soejima H, Yasuda O, et al. (2013)** Level of serum antibody against a periodontal pathogen is associated with atherosclerosis and hypertension, *Hypertension Research* May 16. [Epub ahead of print]. PMID: 23676848
20. **Kodovazenitis G, Pitsavos C, Papadimitriou L, et al. (2013)** Association between periodontitis and acute myocardial infarction: a case-control study of a nondiabetic population, *Journal of Periodontal Research* May 29. [Epub ahead of print]. PMID: 23713486
21. **Berent R, Auer J, Schmid P, et al. (2011)** Periodontal and coronary heart disease in patients undergoing coronary angiography, *Metabolism* 60:127-133. PMID: 20096894
22. **Jimenez M, Krall E, Garcia R, et al. (2009)** Periodontitis and incidence of cerebrovascular disease in men, *Annals of Neurology* 66:505-512. PMID: 19847898
23. **Iwai T (2009)** Periodontal bacteremia and various vascular diseases, *Journal of Periodontal Research* 44:689-694. PMID: 19874452

CHAPTER 20 CITATIONS

1 **Seely S (1991)** Is calcium excess in Western diet a major cause of arterial disease? *International Journal of Cardiology* 33:191-198. PMID: 1743778
2 **Ely M, Kenefick R, Cheuvront S, et al. (2013)** The effect of heat acclimation on sweat micro-minerals: artifact of surface contamination, *International Journal of Sport Nutrition and Exercise Metabolism* Mar 26. [Epub ahead of print] PMID: 23535853
3 **Guder H, Karaca S, Cemek M, et al. (2011)** Evaluation of trace elements, calcium, and magnesium levels in the plasma and erythrocytes of patients with essential hyperhidrosis, *International Journal of Dermatology* 50:1071-1074. PMID: 22126867
4 **Barry D, Hansen K, van Pelt R, et al. (2011)** Acute calcium ingestion attenuates exercise-induced disruption of calcium homeostasis, *Medicine and Science in Sports and Exercise* 43:617-623. PMID: 20798655
5 **Omokhodion F, Howard J (1994)** Trace elements in the sweat of acclimatized persons, *Clinica Chimica Acta* 231:23-28. PMID: 7704945
6 **Sears M, Kerr K, Bray R (2012)** Arsenic, cadmium, lead, and mercury in sweat: a systematic review, *Journal of Environmental and Public Health* 2012:184745. PMID: 22505948
7 **Imamura M, Biro S, Kihara T, et al. (2001)** Repeated thermal therapy improves vascular endothelial function in patients with coronary risk factors, *Journal of the American College of Cardiology* 38:10831088. PMID: 11583886
8 **Gutierrez E, Vazquez R (2001)** Heat in the treatment of patients with anorexia nervosa, *Eating and Weight Disorders* 6:49-52. PMID: 11300546
9 **Kihara T, Miyata M, Fukudome T, et al. (2009)** Waon therapy improves the prognosis of patients with chronic heart failure, *Journal of Cardiology* 53:214-218. PMID: 19304125
10 **Ernst E, Pecho E, Wirz P, Saradeth T (1990)** Regular sauna bathing and the incidence of common colds, *Annals of Medicine* 22:225-227. PMID: 2248758
11 **Umehara M, Yamaguchi A, Itakura S, et al. (2008)** Repeated waon therapy improves pulmonary hypertension during exercise in patients with severe chronic obstructive pulmonary disease, *Journal of Cardiology* 51:106-113. PMID: 18522783
12 **Masuda A, Kihara T, Fukudome T, et al. (2005)** The effects of repeated thermal therapy for two patients with chronic fatigue syndrome, *Journal of Psychosomatic Research* 58:383-387. PMID: 15992574
13 **Masuda A, Koga Y, Hattanmaru M, et al. (2005)** The effects of repeated thermal therapy for patients with chronic pain, *Psychotherapy and Psychosomatics* 74:288-294. PMID: 16088266
14 **Auersperger I, Skof B, Leskosek B, et al. (2013)** Exercise-induced changes in iron status and hepcidin response in female runners, *PLoS One* 8:e58090. PMID: 23472137

15 **Garvican L, Saunders P, Cardoso T, et al. (2013)** Intravenous iron supplementation in distance runners with low or suboptimal ferritin, *Medicine and Science in Sports and Exercise* Jul 18. [Epub ahead of print] PMID: 23872938

APPENDIX A CITATIONS

1. **Mason R, Marche P, Hintze T (2003)** Novel vascular biology of third-generation L-type calcium channel antagonists: ancillary actions of amlodipine, *Arteriosclerosis, Thrombosis, and Vascular Biology* 23:2155-2163. PMID: 14512371
2. **Staessen J, Fagard R, Thijs L, et al. (1997)** Randomised double-blind comparison of placebo and active treatment for older patients with isolated systolic hypertension, *The Systolic Hypertension in Europe* (Syst-Eur) Trial Investigators. Lancet 350:757-764. PMID: 9297994
3. **Brown M, Palmer C, Castaigne A, et al. (2000)** Morbidity and mortality in patients randomised to double-blind treatment with a long-acting calcium-channel blocker or diuretic in the International Nifedipine GITS Study: Intervention as a Goal in Hypertension Treatment (INSIGHT), *Lancet* 356:366-372. PMID: 10972368
4. **Hansson L, Hedner T, Lund-Johansen P, et al. (2000)** Randomised trial of effects of calcium antagonists compared with diuretics and beta-blockers on cardiovascular morbidity and mortality in hypertension: the Nordic Diltiazem (NORDIL) study, *Lancet* 356:359-365. PMID: 10972367
5. **Nissen S, Tuzcu E, Libby P, et al. (2004)** Effect of antihypertensive agents on cardiovascular events in patients with coronary disease and normal blood pressure: the CAMELOT study: a randomized controlled trial, *The Journal of the American Medical Association* 292:2217-2225. PMID: 15536108
6. **Truitt C, Brooks D, Dommer P, LoVecchio F (2012)** Outcomes of unintentional beta-blocker or calcium channel blocker overdoses: a retrospective review of poison center data, *Journal of Medical Toxicology* 8:135-139. PMID: 22311669
7. **No Authors Listed (2010)** Morbidity & Mortality; 2012 Chart Book on Cardiovascular, Lung, and Blood Diseases, National Institutes of Health, 2012, p13.
8. **Goldberg J, Guzman J, Estep C, et al. (2012)** Calcium entry induces mitochondrial oxidant stress in vagal neurons at risk in Parkinson's disease, *Nature Neuroscience* 15:1414-1421. PMID: 22941107
9. **Kim J, Kang J, Lee W (2012)** Vitamin C induces apoptosis in human colon cancer cell line, HCT-8 via the modulation of calcium influx in endoplasmic reticulum and the dissociation of Bad from 14-3-3β, *Immune Network* 12:189-195. PMID: 23213312
10. **Smaili S, Hirata H, Ureshino R, et al. (2009)** Calcium and cell death signaling in neurodegeneration and aging, *Anais da Academia Brasileira de Ciencias* 81:467-475. PMID: 19722016
11. **Kolev M, Alov P (1996)** Effect of multiple administration of calcium antagonists on lipid peroxidation in rat liver microsomes, *General Pharmacology* 27:891-893. PMID: 8842695
12. **Mason R, Walter M, Trumbore M, et al. (1999)** Membrane antioxidant effects of the charged dihydropyridine calcium antagonist amlodipine, *Journal of Molecular and Cellular Cardiology* 31:275-281. PMID: 10072734

13. **Godfraind T (2005)** Antioxidant effects and the therapeutic mode of action of calcium channel blockers in hypertension and atherosclerosis. Philosophical Transactions of the Royal Society of London. Series B, *Biological Sciences* 360:2259-2272. PMID: 16321796
14. **Naito Y, Shimozawa M, Manabe H, et al.** (2006) Azelnidipine, a new calcium channel blocker, inhibits endothelial inflammatory response by reducing intracellular levels of reactive oxygen species, European *Journal of Pharmacology* 546:11-18. PMID: 16919261
15. **Eagleton M, Bishop P, Bena J, et al.** (2008) Calcium channel blockers and angiotensin-converting enzyme inhibitors may be associated with altered atherosclerotic plaque size and morphology, *Vascular* 16:171-178. PMID: 18674467
16. **Brovkovych V, Kalinowski L, Muller-Peddinghaus R, Malinski T (2001)** Synergistic antihypertensive effects of nifedipine on endothelium: concurrent release of NO and scavenging of superoxide, *Hypertension* 37:34-39. PMID: 11208753
17. **Berkels R, Breitenbach T, Bartels H, et al. (2005)** Different antioxidative potencies of dihydropyridine calcium channel modulators in various models, *Vascular Pharmacology* 42:145-152. PMID: 15820440
18. **Munaron L, Antoniotti S, Fiorio Pla A, Lovisolo D (2004)** Blocking Ca2+ entry: a way to control cell proliferation, *Current Medicinal Chemistry* 11:1533-1543. PMID: 15180562
19. **Roderick H, CookS (2008)** Ca2+ signalling checkpoints in cancer: remodelling Ca2+ for cancer cell proliferation and survival, *Nature Reviews. Cancer* 8:361-375. PMID: 18432251
20. **Santoni G, Santoni M, Nabissi M (2012)** Functional role of T-type calcium channels in tumour growth and progression: prospective in cancer therapy, *British Journal of Pharmacology* 166:1244-1246. PMID: 22352795
21. **Keir S, Friedman H, Reardon D, et al. (2013)** Mibefradil, a novel therapy for glioblastoma multiforme: cell cycle synchronization and interlaced therapy in a murine model, *Journal of Neuro-Oncology* 111:97-102. PMID: 23086436
22. **Taylor J, Zeng X, Pottle J, et al., (2008)** Calcium signaling and T-type calcium channels in cancer cell cycling, *World Journal of Gastroenterology* 14:4984-4991. PMID: 18763278
23. **Poch M, Mehedint D, Green D, et al. (2012)** The association between calcium blocker use and prostate cancer outcome, *The Prostate* Dec 31 [Epub ahead of print]. PMID: 23280547
24. **Monteith G, Davis F, Roberts-Thomson S (2012)** Calcium channels and pumps in cancer: changes and consequences, *The Journal of Biological Chemistry* 287:31666-31673. PMID: 22822055
25. **Chattipakorn N, Kumfu S, Fucharoen S, Chattipakorn S (2011)** Calcium channels and iron uptake into the heart, *World Journal of Cardiology* 3:215-218. PMID: 21860702
26. **Bangalore S, Parkar S, Messerli F (2009)** Long-acting calcium antagonists in patients with coronary artery disease: a meta-analysis, *The American Journal of Medicine* 122:356-365. PMID: 19332231

References

27. **Mason R (2012)** Pleiotropic effects of calcium channel blockers, *Current Hypertension Reports* 14:293-303. PMID: 22610475
28. **Ishii N, Matsumura T, Shimoda S, Araki E (2012)** Anti-atherosclerotic potential of dihydropyridine calcium channel blockers, *Journal of Atherosclerosis and Thrombosis* 19:693-704. PMID: 22653165

APPENDIX B CITATIONS

1. **Levy T (2002)** *Curing the Incurable. Vitamin C, Infectious Diseases, and Toxins.* Henderson, NV: MedFox Publishing
2. **Klenner F (1971)** Observations of the dose and administration of ascorbic acid when employed beyond the range of a vitamin in human pathology, *Journal of Applied Nutrition* 23:61-88.
3. **Ayre S, Perez D, Perez D Jr.** (1986) Insulin potentiation therapy: a new concept in the management of chronic degenerative disease, *Medical Hypotheses* 20:199-210. PMID: 3526099
4. **Qutob S, Dixon S, Wilson J (1998)** Insulin stimulates vitamin C recycling and ascorbate accumulation in osteoblastic cells, *Endocrinology* 139:51-56. PMID: 9421397
5. **Rumsey S, Daruwala R, Al-Hasani H, et al.** (2000) Dehydroascorbic acid transport by GLUT4 in Xenopus oocytes and isolated rat adipocytes, *The Journal of Biological Chemistry* 275:28246-28253. PMID: 10862609
6. **Musselmann K, Kane B, Alexandrou B, Hassell J (2006)** Stimulation of collagen synthesis by insulin and proteoglycan accumulation by ascorbate in bovine keratocytes in vitro, *Investigative Ophthalmology & Visual Science* 47:5260-5266. PMID: 17122111
7. **Klenner F (1971)** Observations of the dose and administration of ascorbic acid when employed beyond the range of a vitamin in human pathology, *Journal of Applied Nutrition* 23:61-88.
8. **Cathcart R (1981)** Vitamin C, titrating to bowel tolerance, anascorbemia, and acute induced scurvy, *Medical Hypotheses* 7:1359-1376. PMID: 7321921
9. **Cathcart R (1985)** Vitamin C: the nontoxic, nonrate-limited, antioxidant free radical scavenger, *Medical Hypotheses* 18:61-77. PMID: 4069036
10. **Kurtz T, Morris R Jr.** (1983) Dietary chloride as a determinant of "sodium-dependent" hypertension, *Science* 222:1139-1141. PMID: 6648527
11. **Kurtz T, Al-Bander H, Morris R Jr.** (1987) "Salt-sensitive" essential hypertension in men. Is the sodium ion alone important? *The New England Journal of Medicine* 317:1043-1048. PMID: 3309653
12. **Pokorski M, Marczak M, Dymecka A, Suchocki P (2003)** Ascorbyl palmitate as a carrier of ascorbate into neural tissues, *Journal of Biomedical Science* 10:193-198. PMID: 12595755
13. **Pokorski M, Gonet B (2004)** Capacity of ascorbyl palmitate to produce the ascorbyl radical in vitro: an electron spin resonance investigation, *Physiological Research* 53:311-316. PMID: 15209539
14. **Pokorski M, Ramadan A, Marczak M (2004)** Ascorbyl palmitate augments hypoxic respiratory response in the cat, *Journal of Biomedical Science* 11:465-471. PMID: 15153781
15. **Ross D, Mendiratta S, Qu Z, et al.** (1999) Ascorbate 6-palmitate protects human erythrocytes from oxidative damage, *Free Radical Biology & Medicine* 26:81-89. PMID: 9890643

16. **Loyd D, Lynch S (2011)** Lipid-soluble vitamin C palmitate and protection of human high-density lipoprotein from hypochlorite-mediated oxidation, *International Journal of Cardiology* 152:256-257. PMID: 21872949
17. **Gosenca M, Bester-Rogac M, Gasperlin M (2013)** Lecithin based lamellar liquid crystals as a physiologically acceptable dermal delivery system for ascorbyl palmitate, *European Journal of Pharmaceutical Sciences* May 3. [Epub ahead of print]. PMID: 23643736
18. **Sawant R, Vaze O, Wang T, et al. (2012)** Palmitoyl ascorbate liposomes and free ascorbic acid: comparison of anticancer therapeutic effects upon parenteral administration, *Pharmaceutical Research* 29:375-383. PMID: 21845505
19. **Levy T (2002)** *Curing the Incurable. Vitamin C, Infectious Diseases, and Toxins.* Henderson, NV: MedFox Publishing
20. **Levy T (2011)** *Primal Panacea.* Henderson, NV: MedFox Publishing
21. **Padayatty S, Sun A, Chen Q, et al. (2010)** Vitamin C: intravenous use by complementary and alternative medicine practitioners and adverse effects, *PLoS One* 5:e11414. PMID: 20628650
22. **Rawat A, Vaidya B, Khatri K, et al. (2007)** Targeted intracellular delivery of therapeutics: an overview, *Die Pharmazie* 62:643-658. PMID: 17944316
23. **Yamada Y, Harashima H (2008)** Mitochondrial drug delivery systems for macromolecule and their therapeutic application to mitochondrial diseases, *Advanced Drug Delivery Reviews* 60:1439-1462. PMID: 18655816
24. **Goldenberg H, Schweinzer E (1994)** Transport of vitamin C in animal and human cells, *Journal of Bioenergetics and Biomembranes* 26:359-367. PMID: 7844110
25. **Liang W, Johnson D, Jarvis S (2001)** Vitamin C transport systems of mammalian cells, *Molecular Membrane Biology* 18:87-95. PMID: 11396616
26. **Welch R, Wang Y, Crossman A Jr. (1995)** Accumulation of vitamin C (ascorbate) and its oxidized metabolite dehydroascorbic acid occurs by separate mechanisms, *The Journal of Biological Chemistry* 270:12584-12592. PMID: 7759506
27. **Ling S, Magosso E, Khan N, et al. (2006)** Enhanced oral bioavailability and intestinal lymphatic transport of a hydrophilic drug using liposomes, *Drug Development and Industrial Pharmacy* 32:335-345. PMID: 16556538
28. **Lubin B, Shohet S, Nathan D (1972)** Changes in fatty acid metabolism after erythrocyte peroxidation: stimulation of a membrane repair process, *The Journal of Clinical Investigation* 51:338-344. PMID: 5009118
29. **Mastellone I, Polichetti E, Gres S, et al., (2000)** Dietary soybean phosphatidylcholines lower lipidemia: mechanisms at the levels of intestine, endothelial cell, and hepato-biliary axis, *The Journal of Nutritional Biochemistry* 11:461-466. PMID: 11091102
30. **Buang Y, Wang Y, Cha J, et al. (2005)** Dietary phosphatidylcholine alleviates fatty liver induced by orotic acid, *Nutrition* 21:867-873. PMID: 15975496

31. **Demirbilek S, Karaman A, Baykarabulut A, et al. (2006)** Polyenylphosphatidylcholine pretreatment ameliorates ischemic acute renal injury in rats, *International Journal of Urology* 13:747-753. PMID: 16834655
32. **Levy T (2002)** *Curing the Incurable. Vitamin C, Infectious Diseases, and Toxins.* Henderson, NV: MedFox Publishing
33. **Klenner F (1971)** Observations of the dose and administration of ascorbic acid when employed beyond the range of a vitamin in human pathology, *Journal of Applied Nutrition* 23:61-88.

References

APPENDIX C CITATIONS

1. **Stone I (1972)** *The Healing Factor. "Vitamin C" Against Disease.* New York, NY: Grosset & Dunlap
2. **Levy T. (2002)** *Curing the Incurable. Vitamin C, Infectious Diseases, and Toxins.* Henderson, NV: MedFox Publishing
3. **Frazao B, Vasconcelos V, Antunes A (2012)** Sea anemone (Cnidaria, Anthozoa, Actiniaria) toxins: an overview, *Marine Drugs* 10:1812-1851. PMID: 23015776
4. **Lekawanvijit S, Kompa A, Wang B, et al. (2012)** Cardiorenal syndrome: the emerging role of protein-bound uremic toxins, *Circulation Research* 111:1470-1483. PMID: 23139286
5. **Pedraza M, Possani L (2013)** Scorpion beta-toxins and voltage-gated sodium channels: interactions and effects, *Frontiers in Bioscience: A Journal and Virtual Library* 18:572-587. PMID: 23276943
6. **Krolik M, Milnerowicz H (2012)** The effect of using estrogens in the light of scientific research, *Advances in Clinical and Experimental Medicine* 21:535-543. PMID: 23240460
7. **Angelini D, Dorsey R, Willis J, et al. (2013)** Chemical warfare agent and biological toxin-induced pulmonary toxicity: could stem cells provide potential therapies? *Inhalation Toxicity* 25:37-62. PMID: 23293972
8. **Smith D, Anderson R (2013)** Toxicity and metabolism of nitroalkanes and substituted nitroalkanes, *Journal of Agricultural and Food Chemistry* 61:763-779. PMID: 23294468
9. **Liu S, Zhang Y, Hoover B, Leppla S (2012)** The receptors that mediate the direct lethality of anthrax toxin, *Toxins* 27:1-8. PMID: 23271637
10. **Reeves C, Charles-Horvath P, Kitajewski J (2013)** Studies in mice reveal a role for anthrax toxin receptors in matrix metalloproteinase function and extracellular matrix homeostasis, *Toxins* 5:315-326. PMID: 23389402
11. **Berthiller F, Crews C, Dall'Asta C, et al. (2013)** Masked mycotoxins: a review, *Molecular Nutrition & Food Research* 57:165-186. PMID: 23047235
12. **Garcia-Prieto C, Riaz Ahmed K, Chen Z, et al. (2013)** Effective killing of leukemia cells by the natural product OSW-1 through disruption of cellular calcium homeostasis, *The Journal of Biological Chemistry* 288:3240-3250. PMID: 23250754
13. **Schwartz E, Qu B, Hoth M (2013)** Calcium, cancer and killing: the role of calcium in killing cancer cells by cytotoxic T lymphocytes and natural killer cells, *Biochimica et Biophysica Acta* 1833:1603-1611. PMID: 23220009
14. **Santos C, Anilkumar N, Zhang M, et al. (2011)** Redox signaling in cardiac myocytes, *Free Radical Biology & Medicine* 50:777-793. PMID: 21236334
15. **Bogeski I, Kappl R, Kummerow C, et al. (2011)** Redox regulation of calcium ion channels: chemical and physiological aspects, *Cell Calcium* 50:407-423. PMID: 21930299

16. **Zhou S, Liu R, Yuan K, et al. (2012)** Proteomics analysis of tumor microenvironment: implications of metabolic and oxidative stresses in tumorigenesis, *Mass Spectrometry Reviews* Nov 19 [Epub ahead of print]. PMID: 23165949
17. **Parri M, Chiarugi P (2013)** Redox molecular machines involved in tumor progression, *Antioxidants & Redox Signaling* Jan 8 [Epub ahead of print]. PMID: 23146119
18. **Shen P, Lin X, Zheng W, et al. (2013)** Oxidative stress in malignant melanoma enhances TNF-α secretion of tumor-associated macrophages that promote cancer cell invasion, *Antioxidants & Redox Signaling* Feb 2 [Epub ahead of print]. PMID: 23373752

Resources

Here's help for finding...

Serum Biocompatibility Testing
This is to help minimize the toxicity of dental materials and products to be used in your dental treatments:
> http://www.shslab.com/

Revision Dentistry
A dentist who will be open to helping you in the removal of dental infections and toxins, and also for a Total Dental Revision:
> www.hugginsappliedhealing.com
> www.iaomt.org
> www.biologicaldent.com
> www.biodentist.com

Physicians
A doctor who might be open to some or all of the treatment options discussed in this book:
> www.acamnet.org
> www.orthomolecular.org
> www.a4m.com
> www.icimed.com
> www.acimconnect.com
> www.grossmanwellness.com

Quality Products and Supplements
Find health products like those discussed in this book:
> www.lef.org
> www.livonlabs.com
> www.altrient-europe.com

www.swansonvitamins.com
www.mcguff.com
torrancecompany.com
hightechhealth.com
www.nationalpoolwholesalers.com/_Saunas_
--CAT_SAUN.html
www.meritpharm.com

Further Information and for Medical Care:
www.doctoryourself.com
www.gordonresearch.com
www.riordanclinic.org
www.vitamincfoundation.org
www.drwhitaker.com
www.peakenergy.com
www.medfoxpub.com
www.oasisofhope.com
www.patrickholford.com
www.naturalhealth365.com
www.garynull.com
www.naturalnews.com

These websites are for general reference only, and any information or treatments that might result from their use cannot be guaranteed to be in complete agreement with the information provided in this book. In fact, consider bringing this book to the attention of any dentist, physician, or other healthcare provider who you decide to see as a patient.

Index

A

Vitamin "A" - *see under "Vitamins" below*

Alzheimer's
channel blocker benefits – 50

Angina
channel blocker benefits – 50

Apoptosis
excess calcium related – 42 (see also "necrosis")

Atherosclerotic Plaque
and calcium channel blockers – 290

B

Biophosphonates
benefit of – 124
caution on side effects of – 125

Bones
as structural support, protection, red cell factory, and mineral bank – 73
absorption/resorption defined – 73
effect of dietary vitamin C on density of – 90
effect of supplemental vitamin C on density of – 90-91
in homeostasis – 73
osteoblasts, defined – 74
osteoclasts, defined – 75
oxidative stress – 76
scurvy of – 73

C

Vitamin "C" - *see under "Vitamins" below*

Calcium
250% death rate for high versus low calcium consumption – 45
absorption enhanced by omega 3's – 141
absorption increased by presence of vitamin D – 130
allopathic medicine's denial of dangers of excess – 27
as a conducting medium – 185
avoidance important for cardiac healing – 252
balance of improved by EFA supplementation – 142
"banked" in bones unless needed – 184
bone-released calcium linked to heart disease, all disease, decreased longevity – 67
calcification lessened by estrogen – 150-151
calcitonin -187
calcium channel blocker effect on testosterone – 167
calcium/coronary disease by country (illustration) – 197
cautions against joint supplementation with vitamin D – 129-130
common denominator in degenerative diseases – 197
connection to cancer – 38
contributory factor in ALS (Lou Gerhig's disease), Parkinson's, and Alzheimer's – 43
critical analysis of calcium dietary recommendations – 194
daily need for easily met – 58
dangers of excess – 27

deposition linked to thyroid cancer – 39
determining effectiveness – 297
dietary need, (table) – 196
dietary need, actual – 195
dietary need, government recommendations (RDA) – 193
dietary sources (table) 199-204
dosing recommendations – 294-295
EFA's inhibit abnormal calcification – 141
effect on heart valves – 44
estrogen – 189
excess calcium detrimental to health, nearly impossible to create deficiency – 183
excess deposited in bones, organs, tissues, or excreted – 184
forms of – 296
heart disease related stats – 36
high content no guarantee of bone strength – 63-64
high presence in plaque deposits – 37
hormones as regulators – 185
level correlates to heart disease and all-cause mortality – 43
level limiting cellular processes – 48
linked to "vascular events" – 36
linked to heart disease – 35
low calcium consumption – 45
milk/dairy warning – 196
necessity as an electrolyte – 287
necrosis – 42
non-bone deposition directly linked to a significantly increased cancer, high blood pressure, stroke, and many other chronic degenerative diseases – 71-72
non-bone functions listed – 185
RDA based on bad science – 194-195
repercussions expected to mimic tobacco's denial – 33
research peer-reviewed scientific data – 34
role in arterial plaque formation – 80
role in atherosclerosis – 289
role in hypertension – 287
role in oxidative stress – 80
role in prostate cancer – 290
role of excess in apoptosis/necrosis – 42
stanniocalcin – 188
strong warning about supplementation – 52
success and negative results of milk marketing hype – 54-55
supplementation increases all-cause mortality – 65
supplementation ineffective without vitamin D – 132
testosterone's role in calcium distribution – 168
thyroid hormone – 190
tied to chronic degenerative diseases – 29
transferred from bones to blood and soft tissues caused by excess vitamin D – 134-135
universal deficiency proclaimed – 34
vitamin C critical to heart and bone management – 82
vitamin C for all degenerative diseases – 293
vitamin D critical to absorption – 58
vitamin D, parathyroid hormone – 186
vitamin D/calcium caution – 196

Cancer
about antioxidants – 268
avoid dairy/vitamin D in combination – 282
balancing hormones – 267
be selective about foods – 283
benefits of sweating for calcium removal – 283-285
breast cancer/calcium connections – 40
calcification related – 71, 289
calcium-related metastatic spread – 41
calcium/metastatic spread

Index

connection? – 40
connection to calcium – 38
dangers related to HRT (hormone replacement therapy) – 153
dietary guidelines – 265-266
disease commonalities – 280
eliminating toxins – 266
estrogen therapy and – 163
far infrared sauna therapy – 267
general disease tests – 278-279
K2 effective on leukemia – 119
K2 effective on some forms of liver cancer – 118-119
list of treatment goals – 263
measuring progress – 275
minimizing new toxin exposure – 264
more antioxidants – 270-271
need to limit diary – 281
of colon, pancreas, prostrate, and breast slowed by omega 3's – 146
oxidative stress related – 89
possible calcium/prostate connection – 39
prescription meds – 272-273
related to excess calcium – 35
resolving infections – 266
root canal connection – 216
root canals high risk – 264-265
small cell carcinoma and calcium – 39
specific cancer tests – 277-278
supplement dosing (table) – 269
testosterone therapy and – 166
thyroid/calcium deposition related – 39
treatment protocol – 263-273
Unified Theory of Disease,
summary/overview – 329-348
vitamin C compatibility with other therapies – 309-310
vitamin C dosing recommendations – 294-295
vitamin C effectiveness determination – 297
vitamin C for all degenerative diseases – 293
vitamin C form selection

considerations – 303-309
vitamin C frequency and duration guidelines – 302-303
vitamin C lowers all cause mortality – 97- 98
vitamin C route and speed of administration – 298-301
vitamin C safety – 310-311
vitamin C, forms of – 296
vitamin C: in depth discussion of forms, pluses, minuses, whys, and wherefores – 313-319
vitamin K3 with vitamin C effective – 115

Channel Blockers

anti-atherosclerotic effect – 49
antioxidant properties of – 290
beneficial in limiting toxin-induced (formaldehyde, methyl mercury, arsenic, glucose, etc.) cellular calcium uptake – 43
beneficial when used in conjunction with vitamin C therapy – 100
effects on atherosclerotic plaque – 290
efficacy in treatment of stroke, heart attack, angina, and heart failure – 49
fibrous plaque – 290
free radical suppression – 290
iron absorption – 291
limit cellular calcium uptake 42
list for hypertension treatment – 291
medical issues that benefit from: preterm labor, coronary artery spasm, angina pectoris, pulmonary arterial hypertension, Raynaud's phenomenon, acute head trauma, epilepsy, chemotherapy induced peripheral neuropathy, Alzheimer's, Parkinson's – 50
positive effect on misc. diseases – 288
programmed cell death – 290
prostate cancer – 290
safety of – 288-290

study indicates significant
  decrease in all cause
  mortality – 51
summary of benefits – 51
testosterone's natural channel
  blocking ability – 167
Cholesterol
deposition enhanced by calcium
  supplementation – 36
Collagen
K2 efficacy in collagen
  formation – 123
vitamin C necessary for
  production of – 87-88
Coronary Artery Disease
aortic calcification increases
  mortality – 117
bone-released calcium linked to
  heart disease, all disease,
  decreased longevity – 67
calcium, iron, copper avoidance
  extremely important – 252
channel blocker benefits – 50
estrogen therapy may contribute
  to – 154
higher estrogen/lower calcium
  scores – 151
increases focal scurvy, non-bone
  calcium deposition – 80
predicted by high calcium
  score regardless of other
  factors – 44
Unified Theory of Disease,
  summary/overview – 329-348
vitamin C compatibility with other
  therapies – 309-310
vitamin C dosing
  recommendations – 294-295
vitamin C effectiveness
  determination – 297
vitamin C for all degenerative
  diseases – 293
vitamin C form selection
  considerations – 303-309
vitamin C frequency and duration
  guidelines – 302-303
vitamin C lowers mortality – 97
vitamin C route and speed of
  administration – 298-301
vitamin C safety – 310-311
vitamin C, forms of – 296

vitamin C: in depth discussion of
  forms, pluses, minuses, whys,
  and wherefores – 313-319
C-Reactive Protein
as a fracture predictor in elderly
  women – 90
as an inflammation marker – 90
oxidative stress related – 89-90
Cross-Linking
connection to vitamin C – 123
necessity of – 88

D

Vitamin "D" - *see under
"Vitamins" below*

Dental Related Issues
amalgam fillings,
  cavitations – 253
biocompatibility testing – 231
"dead teeth" and cancer – 216
dental cavitations
  addressed – 223
dental toxicity/rheumatoid
  arthritis/infected tonsils – 243
diseases – 293
futility of laser sterilization – 219
futility of root canal laser
  "sterilization" – 219
"how" and "why" of
  toxicity – 217-218
implant dangers – 227-228
importance of periodontal
  ligament removal – 223-224
largely ignored by dental
  profession – 221
periodontal disease
  hazards – 231
root canal/coronary artery
  disease – 253
root canal/heart
  disease connection
  established – 220-221
root canals as "toxin
  pumps" – 220
root canals/"death
  sentence" – 214
statistical scope of problem – 222
study validates root canal
  toxicity – 220

Index

toxic reconstruction
materials – 230
toxicity – 213
toxicity and consequences of
jawbone cavitations – 224-226
toxicity of amalgam ("silver")
fillings – 229-230
Unified Theory of Disease,
summary/overview – 329-348
vitamin C compatibility with other
therapies – 309-310
vitamin C dosing
recommendations – 294-295
vitamin C effectiveness
determination – 297
vitamin C form selection
considerations – 303-309
vitamin C frequency and duration
guidelines – 302-303
vitamin C route and speed of
administration – 298-301
vitamin C safety – 310-311
vitamin C, forms of – 296
vitamin C, in depth discussion of
forms, pluses, minuses, whys,
and wherefores – 313-319

Diabetes

diabetic deficiencies,
osteoporosis
connection – 164-165
testosterone deficiency
contributes to impaired
glucose metabolism – 164

E

EFA's - see "Omega 3 fatty acids"
below

Epilepsy: channel blocker
benefits – 50
Estrogen: see under "Hormones"
below

F

Fracture Risk
substantially lowered
with vitamin C
supplementation – 91

Fractures
Framingham Osteoporosis Study
and vitamin C – 77-78

healing enhanced by
vitamin C – 92
osteoporotic bone loss – 77-78
vitamin C deficiency – 78
vitamin E – 78

H

Heart Attack
aortic calcification increases
mortality – 117
channel blocker benefits – 50
EFA supplementation lowers
mortality from – 144
EFA's inhibit abnormal
calcification – 141
estrogen therapy should
lessen – 163
oral estrogen therapy with
metabolic syndrome may
increase risk – 154
oxidative stress related – 89
relationship to metabolic
syndrome – 166

Heart Disease
amalgam fillings,
cavitations – 253
anti-angina drugs with
vitamin C – 100
antioxidant dosing
methodology – 260
antioxidant recommendations
(illustrated) – 259
antioxidant support minimizes
complications – 161
avoid dairy/vitamin D in
combination – 282
be selective about foods – 283
benefits of sweating for calcium
removal – 283-285
bone-released calcium linked to
heart disease, all disease,
decreased longevity – 67
calcification reduced by
EFA's – 141-142
calcium channel blockers'
efficacy in treatment of stroke,
heart attack, angina, and
heart failure – 49

calcium level correlates to heart disease and all-cause mortality – 43
calcium related stats – 36
calcium, iron, copper avoidance extremely important – 252
cardiovascular considerations in pre- and postmenopausal women – 161
coronary artery calcium (CAC) score – 275
dietary recommendations – 254
disease commonalities – 280
EFA supplementation lowers mortality – 144
effects of metabolic syndrome on – 166
eliminate old infections – 254-255
eliminating toxins (iron) – 255-256
estrogen reduces coronary calcification – 150-151
evaluate and correct hormone levels – 256-258
explanation of coronary arteries as repository for released calcium – 80-82
general disease tests – 278-279
importance of monitoring during hormone replacement therapy (HRT) – 153
linked to excess calcium – 35
measuring progress – 275
misc. antioxidant therapies – 258
misc. cancer tests – 276-277
misc. heart-related tests – 276
monitoring protocols – 161-162
need to limit diary – 281
prescription drug dosing recommendations – 260-261
root canal worst offender – 253
statin drug warnings – 261
testing protocols – 162
tonsils – 255
Unified Theory of Disease, summary/overview – 329-348
vitamin C compatibility with other therapies – 309-310
vitamin C dosing recommendations – 294-295
vitamin C effectiveness determination – 297
vitamin C for all degenerative diseases – 293
vitamin C form selection considerations – 303-309
vitamin C frequency and duration guidelines – 302-303
vitamin C lowers all cause mortality rate – 97-98
vitamin C route and speed of administration – 298-301
vitamin C safety – 310-311
vitamin C, forms of – 296
vitamin C: in depth discussion of forms, pluses, minuses, whys, and wherefores – 313-319

Hemodialysis
patients' benefit from vitamin C – 98

Hypercalcemia
related to milk/alkali treatment of peptic ulcers and resultant renal failure – 46

Hormones

Estrogen
administration options – 158
age-related timing considerations – 161
and osteoporotic bone loss – 77
as calcium regulator – 189
beneficial even after menopause – 151
combination cautions (venous thromboembolism)- 158
correct deficiencies – 245
deficiency in osteoporotic men more common than testosterone deficiency – 151
deficiency may contribute to metabolic syndrome, abdominal obesity, increased triglycerides, low HDL lipoproteins, high blood pressure, elevated fasting blood sugar – 154
deficiency raises all-cause mortality – 154
duration of therapy – 160
efficacy comparison – 158

Index

estrogen deficiency equates to increased cytokine production – 152
estrogen summary and recommendations – 163
formulations – 158
higher levels in post-menopausal women equals lower coronary artery calcification – 150-151
HRT equals reduction in all-cause mortality – 154
importance of proper dosing levels – 151-152
in conjunction with progesterone – 153
list of critical supplementation considerations – 156
loss equates to onset of osteoporosis – 151
monitoring requirements – 153
necessity of aggressive anti-oxidant therapy during HRT – 155
oral administration/coronary events – 154
oral/non-oral comparisons – 158-159
osteoporosis connection – 150
poor results attributable to hormone combinations and/or calcium supplementation – 156
postmenopausal transdermal effectiveness – 160
real dangers of HRT – 153
recommendations – 157
role in inhibiting calcification – 150
transdermal considerations – 159
transdermal preferred for osteoporosis-prone estrogen-deficient girls – 159
types – 157-158
vitamin C's compensation for – 77-78
Women's Health Initiative study – 155

Parathyroid Hormone
increases calcium concentration in blood, raises all-cause mortality – 45

Progestin
used in conjunction with estrogen – 155

Progesterone
used in conjunction with estrogen – 153

Testosterone
additional dosing and side effect data – 171-172
affects many organs/areas/functions – 164
as calcium regulator – 190
calcium channel blocker effect – 167
cautions, adverse events and adjustments – 171-172
connection between androgen lowering therapy and cardiovascular risk – 167
deficiency in osteoporotic men less influential than estrogen deficiency – 151
deficiency increases all-cause mortality – 166
dosing considerations – 170
general treatment protocols – 169
male bone mass T related – 165
multiple health issues related to T deficiency – 164
percentage of men deficient in T – 164
possible results – 170-171
possible side effects of T therapy – 168
role in calcium deposition – 168
summary and protocols, osteoporosis recommendations, vitamin supplementation – 173
T related to cardiovascular/coronary/metabolic syndrome issues – 166
T supplementation recommendations – 165
T supplementation stats – 170

Thyroid
as calcium regulator – 290
critical nature of thyroid function, lab testing – 177

critical to bone health – 174
either excess or deficient levels raise mortality – 174
high or low levels can affect bone density and strength without indications of osteoporosis – 175
regulates metabolism – 174

TSH (thyroid stimulating hormone)
balancing bone and cardiovascular issues – 177
bone protecting effect – 176
level affects fracture rates and cardiovascular issues – 175-176
side effects and dosing – 178
summary of thyroid function on osteoporosis, nutritional supplement recommendations – 179-180
T3, T4, dosing recommendations, need to recognize individuality of patients – 179
TSH effect on morbidity rates – 178

Hypertension (high blood pressure)
calcium related – 71
channel blocker benefits for pulmonary arterial – 50
estrogen related – 156
treatment with calcium channel blockers – 50-71, 250-291
vitamin C for all degenerative diseases – 293
vitamin C in conjunction with hypertensive drugs – 100

K

Vitamin "K" - *see under "Vitamins" below*

Kidney
calcification reduced by EFA's – 141-142
kidney failure vitamin C caution – 98
stones reduced by vitamin C – 99

M

Metabolic Syndrome
connection of metabolic syndrome to cardiac/coronary issues – 166
estrogen therapy may benefit – 154
estrogen therapy may increase coronary events during oral estrogen therapy -154
increased risk of heart disease and/or diabetes mellitus – 154

N

Necrosis
excess calcium related – 42 (see also "apoptosis")

O

Omega 3 fatty acids (EFA's)
beneficial to hemodialysis and coronary artery disease patients – 145
body-wide benefits listed – 140
decrease urinary calcium oxalate excretion – 142
dosing considerations – 147
EFA safety – 146
EPA and DHA decrease bone loss, promote bone mass – 143
high EFA's equal lower breast cancer death rates – 146
high omega 3's equal lower mortality rate – 145
inhibit calcium uptake – 139
inhibit inflammation by reduction of cytokine activity – 142
lowers all cause mortality rate – 143-144
reduce cancers of colon, pancreas, prostate, and breast – 146
summary – 147

Osteocalcin
function in bone mineralization – 121

Osteoporosis
addressing dental toxicities – 241

Index

aggravated by excess vitamin D causing calcium transfer from bones to blood – 134
antioxidant deficiency equates to osteoporosis – 151
antioxidant recommendations – 245-246
avoid dairy/vitamin D in combination – 282
avoid dairy/vitamin D in combination – 282
be selective about foods – 283
benefits of sweating for calcium removal – 283-285
bone density improved by omega 3's – 141
bone-released calcium linked to heart disease, all disease, decreased longevity – 67
calcium without vitamin D will not alleviate – 60-61
caution advised – 249
defined – 34, 71
density and fracture incidence affected by thyroid – 175
dietary advice – 243
dietary cautions – 240-241
discontinuance of HRT increases fracture risk – 152
drug protocols and table – 248
effects of estrogen decline on – 151
estrogen decline equates to increased cytokine production – 152
fracture related statistics, costs – 85
futility of calcium supplementation for – 85
guidelines for bone protection/ restoration – 239
high calcium content no guarantee of bone strength – 63-64
higher mortality linked to excess calcium than to fractures – 65
hormone replacement therapy (HRT) beneficial in fracture prevention – 152
importance of vitamin C and other anti-oxidant supplementation – 101-102
lack of calcium in bones generally unrelated to levels in body – 56
linked to stroke, intracerebral hemorrhage, occlusions, atherosclerosis, arterial calcification – 66
male bone mass/ testosterone levels – 165
may also caused by vitamin D deficiency – 134-135
minimal suggestions for improved dental health – 242
need to limit diary – 281
nutritional recommendations – 179-180
osteoblast activity increased by EFA's – 142
other than bones, calcium deficiency nearly impossible to achieve – 183
oxidative stress – 76, 101
positive effects of osteoporosis treatment on other issues – 144
strong warning against calcium supplementation for – 52
supplement table and recommendations – 247
testosterone deficiency linked to 50% of male hip fractures, mortality rate double women – 165
testosterone related – 164-165
, summary/overview – 329-348
vitamin C compatibility with other therapies – 309-310
vitamin C critical to calcium management of heart and bones – 82
vitamin C deficiency related – 92
vitamin C dosing recommendations – 294-295
vitamin C effectiveness determination – 297
vitamin C for all degenerative diseases – 293
vitamin C form selection considerations – 303-309

vitamin C frequency and duration guidelines – 302-303
vitamin C lowers all cause mortality rate – 97-98
vitamin C lowers mortality – 97
vitamin C route and speed of administration – 298-301
vitamin C safety – 310-311
vitamin C, forms of – 296
vitamin C: in depth discussion of forms, pluses, minuses, whys, and wherefores – 313-319
vitamin D toxicity caution – 180
vitamin D, toxins, hormonal issues critical to resolution of – 58-59

Oxidative Stress (OS)
and cancer – 41
connection to all diseases – 51
constipation equated to root canal for OS – 210
dental considerations – 212
dietary recommendations – 211-212
electron donation/OS neutralization – 209
elevates C-reactive protein – 89-90
explained – 42
importance of all anti-oxidants (AO) – 102
importance of OS/AO balance – 208
misc. disease related – 89
oral/digestive tract sources of OS – 209
OS/bowel function – 210
relationship to all diseases – 207-208
relationship to degenerative diseases/cancer – 39
Unified Theory of Disease, summary/overview – 329-348
vitamin C compatibility with other therapies – 309-310
vitamin C deficiency related – 89, 101
vitamin C dosing recommendations – 294-295

vitamin C effectiveness determination – 297
vitamin C for all degenerative diseases – 293
vitamin C form selection considerations – 303-309
vitamin C frequency and duration guidelines – 302-303
vitamin C lowers all cause mortality rate – 97-98
vitamin C lowers mortality – 97
vitamin C route and speed of administration – 298-301
vitamin C safety – 310-311
vitamin C, forms of – 296
vitamin C: in depth discussion of forms, pluses, minuses, whys, and wherefores – 313-319

P

Parkinson's
channel blocker benefits – 50, 288, 289
K, D, biophosphonates efficacy in preventing hip fractures – 124

R

Raynaud's Phenomenon
channel blocker benefits – 50
RDA
"Food pyramid" not science-based – 194-195
Root Canals - see "Dental issues" above
Rheumatoid Arthritis
possible dental connections – 243

S

Scurvy
and vitamin C – 74
of bones – 74

Stroke
HRT (hormone replacement therapy) related – 153
lower bone density linked to stroke, intracerebral hemorrhages, occlusions,

Index

atherosclerosis, arterial calcification – 66
non-bone deposition related – 72

Synergism
complementary effects of K, D, magnesium, biophosphonates, etc. – 123-124
K, D synergism – 125

T

Testosterone - see under "Hormones" above

Thyroid
calcium deposition linked to malignancy – 39

Tonsils
adversely affected by dental issues – 244

Toxins
means of elimination – 244
Unified Theory of Disease, summary/overview – 329-348
vitamin C compatibility with other therapies – 309-310
vitamin C dosing instructions – 294-295
vitamin C effectiveness determination – 297
vitamin C for all degenerative disease – 293
vitamin C forms – 296
vitamin C forms and selection considerations – 303-309
vitamin C frequency and duration guidelines (IMPORTANT) – 302-303
vitamin C protocols administration – 312-313
vitamin C route and speed of administration – 298-301
vitamin C safety – 310-311
vitamin C: in depth discussion of forms, pluses, minuses, whys, and wherefores – 313-319

V

Vitamin A
efficacy in preventing D toxicity – 126

Vitamin C
ability to dissolve dangerous calcium deposits – 93
and bone scurvy – 75-76
and post-menopausal bone loss – 77-78
benefits hemodialysis patients – 98
benefits of multiple sources of – 100
compatibility with other therapies – 309-310
critical to calcium management in heart and bones – 82
deficiencies implicated in most if not all chronic degenerative diseases – 293
deficiency and calcium excretion – 93
deficiency related to arterial lesions – 80
deficiency related to poor quality bone formation – 94
determining effectiveness – 297
dosing – 294-295
enhances healing of fractures – 92
falsely linked to the formation of calcium oxalate kidney stones, resists formation of calcium oxalate stones – 9, 95
for all degenerative diseases – 293
forms of – 296
IMPORTANT: frequency and duration guidelines – 302-303
in arterial calcium deposition – 77
in bone calcium deposition – 77
in collagen synthesis – 76
in cross linking – 77
in depth discussion of C forms, pluses, minuses, whys, and wherefores – 313-319
inhibits stone formation – 97
kidney stone formation inhibited by – 99
lowers all-cause mortality – 97-98
may be effective channel blocker – 93
multiple forms and selection

considerations – 303-309
necessary for all aspects of bone physiology – 86-87
necessity in cross-linking – 88
no known toxicity level – 99
Other Must Read Considerations! – 319-328
oxidative stress – 76
protocols of administration – 312 - 313
role in collagen quality/quantity – 87-88
role in fracture prevention – 78
route and speed of C administration – 298-301
safety – 310-311
summary of benefits – 101
toxicity stats – 98
Unified Theory of Disease, summary/overview – 329-348

Vitamin D

as calcium regulator – 186
calcium supplementation useless without – 132
caution when used in thyroid therapies – 180
contributor to calcification of kidneys, renal failure – 46
D directly affects about 200 genes, indirectly affects about 2000 – 68
D, K synergism – 125
D, K, biophosphonate therapy – 124
D's role in calcium absorption and overdosing – 69
dangers of joint D/calcium supplementation – 129-130
deficiency contributes to osteoporosis – 135
either excess or deficiency contribute to calcium transfer from bones to elsewhere in the body – 135-136
essential to calcium absorption/utilization – 58
excess D always results in calcium assimilation – 134
excess long-lasting in soft tissues – 136
excess results in calcium transfer from bones to blood – 134
importance for health – 133
importance in fracture prevention – 130-131
important to monitor – 136-137
list of positively affected health issues – 133
lowers all-cause mortality – 133-134
necessity of supplementation even in tropic regions – 70
recommended blood levels and dosing – 137
role in gene expression – 133
summary of benefits – 137-138
toxicity cautions – 126

Vitamin K

antidote to warfarin – 115
considerations and summary – 127
dosing recommendations – 125
explanation of various forms of K – 114
for osteoporosis – 113
high K2 = less coronary artery calcification – 117
in blood coagulation – 115
K, D, synergism – 125
K1 efficacy in increasing bone density – 121
K1/K2 efficacy in bone deposition/fracture prevention – 122
K2 critical to bone health – 125
K2 effective on at least some forms of liver cancer – 118-119
K2 efficacy for diabetic bone issues – 123
K2 in bone formation/repair – 119
K2 inversely related to all cause mortality – 118
known inhibitor of calcification outside of bones – 115-116
lack of proven toxicity, list of proven benefits – 128
MK7 as parathyroid blocker – 121
no established toxicity at any dose – 114
safety stats – 126

Index

suitability of various forms of K – 120
synergistic effect of K, D, bisphosphonates, on bone size and strength – 124
useful for D toxicity amelioration – 126
warfarin calcification reversed with K – 116
warfarin calcification without K – 116

Warfarin

causes arterial calcification – 116
calcification reversed with vitamin K – 116

Other Books by Thomas E. Levy, MD, JD
From MedFox Publishing

PRIMAL PANACEA
Overwhelming documentation proves that in high enough doses this substance prevents and cures
- *Cancer*
- *Heart Disease*
- *Infectious & Degenerative Diseases*

and can neutralize and even reverse damage from virtually all toxins, venoms, and radiation!

Just hours before his scheduled removal from life support, and upon advice from the author, Allan Smith was brought back from the dead with massive doses of the "Primal Panacea." A news segment by *60 Minutes* in New Zealand documented Allan's full recovery in graphic detail and revealed his "one-in-a-billion-miracle" to the world. Since that time the FDA has ordered the supplier to stop selling this natural, perfectly safe substance. Why?

Is the FDA protecting us from "bad" medicine or protecting Big Pharma's interests and mega-profits? The answer will become obvious as this well-documented book proves that high-dose treatment with vitamin C is one of the most important medical discoveries of all time. Documented evidence also shows that powerful men have purposely ignored and tried to discredit the facts about high-dose vitamin C. They have lied, bribed, and even sacrificed innocent lives to keep this incredible substance hidden from those who would be helped by Nature's "Primal Panacea."

CURING THE INCURABLE: *Vitamin C, Infectious Diseases, and Toxins*

Don't just accept a casual, unenlightened assessment of what vitamin C can and cannot do. Read the truth for yourself...

Vitamin C has been able to cure or contribute to the cure of many common infectious diseases, such as hepatitis and polio. *Curing the Incurable* presents the documented evidence that vitamin C is the treatment of choice for many potentially fatal diseases and toxins.

"Dr. Levy's book presents clear evidence that vitamin C cures disease. It contains over 1,200 scientific references, presented chapter by

chapter. It does not mince words. It is disease specific. It is dose specific. It is practical. It is readable. It is excellent."
Review in *Journal of Orthomolecular Medicine*

"With the current book, Thomas E. Levy, MD, JD, joins Albert Szent-Gyorgyi, MD, PhD, Linus Pauling, PhD, and Frederick R. Klenner, MD, among others, on the list of vitamin C's heroic researchers."
International Council for Health Freedom

"Levy's book is unmatched in the medical literature. The Vitamin C Foundation credits Levy with "doing an almost impossible feat of reading, analyzing, and clearly explaining the meaning of the massive science behind vitamin C."
Owen Fonorow
in the *Townsend Letter*

STOP AMERICA'S #1 KILLER
PROOF that the Origin of ALL Coronary Heart Disease is a Clearly Reversible Arterial Scurvy

In the next 24 hours, over 2,500 Americans will die from Coronary Heart Disease (CHD). The financial impact of CHD during that same 24 hours will approach $5,500,000. Based on government health statistics, over 25 million Americans are currently diagnosed with CHD and during the next 12 months over 600,000 of us will die from this disease.

Beyond the age of 50, your chances of suffering from CHD are greater than the chance of getting heads in a simple coin toss. That means most of us are heading down a dark, threatening road. It's time to take a safe detour!

This book also offers a protocol for preventing and reversing the arterial blockages that cause heart attacks.

All three of these ground-breaking books are available at www.MedFoxPub.com

Information on more books authored or co-authored by Dr. Levy, along with how to purchase them, is available on his website at
http://peakenergy.com/books.php